Clinical Implications of Laboratory Tests

Clinical Implications of Laboratory Tests

4th Edition
with 111 illustrations

Sarko M. Tilkian, M.D.

Director of Medical Education, Northridge Hospital Medical Center; Staff Physician, Northridge Hospital Foundation, Northridge, California, and Tarzana Medical Center, Tarzana, California

Mary Boudreau Conover, R.N., B.S.

Instructor and Education Consultant, West Hills Hospital, Canoga Park, California, Instructor of ECG Workshops, Santa Terisita Hospital, Duarte, California

Ara G. Tilkian, M.D., F.A.C.C.

Assistant Clinical Professor of Medicine, University of California, Los Angeles; Co-Director of Cardiology, Holy Cross Hospital, Mission Hills, California.

The C. V. Mosby Company
ST. LOUIS • WASHINGTON, D.C. • TORONTO 1987

Lovingly dedicated to
our parents
Garabed and Nevart Tilkian
Essel and Eleanor Boudreau

Preface

This fourth edition has been completely rewritten with the special needs of the nurse in mind. Experts have been consulted and have contributed to most of the chapters on specialized tests (pulmonary, renal, gastrointestinal, hematological, endocrine, neurological, and rheumatological diseases and sleep disorders). New tests have been included if they are clinically applicable or on the brink of entering clinical practice. Under each test the reader will find an explanation of the test, its value and limitations, interfering factors, and nursing action. Throughout the book there are highlighted sections reminding the nurse of a particularly important nursing action.

The routine screening blood tests in Chapter 1 have been listed alphabetically for easy access. In the other chapters the tests are listed in order of clinical importance or grouped with a certain organ, since this is the easiest way to remember them and learn their clinical application. An alphabetical list of all tests, with their page number, is provided in the front of the book so that individual tests can be found rapidly.

In Section II the discussions of anatomy, physiology, and pathophysiology of the organ systems have been retained in response to reader input. Diagnostic laboratory tests for each disease are briefly mentioned in the order of choice; the tests themselves are then detailed. We have expanded the chapter on the rapidly moving field of infectious diseases and have added a new chapter on perinatal diagnostic tests.

We are grateful to the physicians and nurses who reviewed our manuscript and especially for the contributions and reviews of Drs. Mugurdich Balabanian (Nephrology), Karl Blau, (Gastroenterology), Harry W. Rein (Neurology), Michael M. Stevenson (Sleep Disorders), Paul Sussman (Rheumatology), Ellen I. Tamagna (Endocrinology), and Jeffrey Aaronson (Pulmonary Medicine). We also appreciate the suggestions and contributions from Joan Grant, R.N., M.S.N., Norma Pinnell, R.N., M.S., and the cheerful assistance of librarians Lucille Moss, Cati Kreie, and Angela D'Amico.

Sarko M. Tilkian
Mary Conover
Ara G. Tilkian

Table of Contents

Alphabetized List of Tests

UNIT 1
Routine Multisystem Screening Tests

REFERENCE RANGES

Normal ranges have been listed with each test and in the appendix because of reader demand for such a list, not because it is of any practical value. These values should not be applied to the laboratory tests performed in your own hospital unless they have been compared and do in fact agree; to do otherwise will cause erroneous diagnoses. Except for a few tests (electrolytes, BUN, and others), normal values vary with methods and local population factors. Each laboratory should provide for its clinicians normal ranges relative to the techniques used in that particular laboratory and to the geographical location served.

SI UNITS

The Système International d'Unités (SI units), proposed in 1967, is based on the metric system and designed to create uniformity and aid in the interpreting of clinical chemistry assays. These recommendations were revised in 1974, finalized in 1979, and should be implemented by 1987, the conversion having been mandated by the House of Delegates of the American Medical Association in December of 1984.

NURSING ACTION FOR THE SMAC OR SMA12

Although the individual blood chemistry tests differ as to fasting requirements and whether or not anticoagulants are used, they are usually done as a unit on the fasting patient, using one venous puncture and filling a series of three or four color-coded tubes.

For most of the blood chemistry tests either serum or plasma may be used, except for enzymes or electrophoresis when serum must be used. *Serum* is the liquid part of clotted blood; *plasma* is the liquid part of anticoagulated blood.

1. Explain to the patient that a single venous blood sample will be taken, permitting multiple biochemical determinations and providing information about a broad area of body function.
2. Instruct the patient to fast, except for water, 8 to 12 hours before the test. Tests that are influenced directly by food intake are serum phosphorus, cholesterol, glucose, triglycerides, potassium, and serum urea.
3. Instruct the patient regarding diet before the test. The patient should avoid alcohol and foods high in cholesterol such as eggs, organ meats, shellfish, bacon, butter, fatty meat, and coconut.
4. If liver dysfunction is suspected, be especially vigilant regarding the venipuncture site because the patient may have a prolonged clotting time.
5. List any intramuscular injection in the last 8 hours, since these will affect creatine kinase (CK) and lactic dehydrogenase (LDH) levels.
6. Withhold medications as ordered until the blood is collected.
7. Do not leave the tourniquet on more than 1 minute. If possible, remove the venous blood without a tourniquet. If a tourniquet is needed, release it 1 to 2 minutes before the blood is drawn. Prolonged application of the tourniquet produces an increase in blood cell concentration by causing a shift of plasma into the interstitial fluid. Blood pH, electrolytes, and lactate levels are particularly sensitive to the pressure of the tourniquet.
8. Hemolysis may invalidate test results; guard against it by avoiding air bubbles and unnecessary shaking. Release of hemoglobin and cholesterol contained in the red blood cells can produce inaccurate test results.
9. Protect the sample from bright light and refrigerate it. Bright light has a deteriorating effect on bilirubin, and room temperature causes creatinine, an unstable compound, to decompose.

10. Withdraw the blood into color-coded collection tubes:
    First draw: red-top tube without additive
    Second draw: red-top tube with additive
    Third draw: lavender-top tube
    Fourth draw: green-top tube
11. Label all tubes and deliver them to the laboratory immediately so that the serum can be removed within the hour; notify the laboratory that the specimen has arrived. Allowing the specimen to stand for a prolonged time has the same effect as does leaving the tourniquet on too long.
12. Drugs that may cause decreased or increased values are listed under the individual tests.

COLOR-CODED TUBE TOPS

The color-coded rubber stoppers indicate the presence or absence of additives, commonly preservatives and anticoagulants, in the tube. A *preservative* prevents changes in the specimen. An *anticoagulant* inhibits clot formation or coagulation (examples are citrates, EDTA, oxalates).

Red-top tube without additives

Use: Blood bank, chemistry, and serology

Precaution: Do not mix, invert, or agitate the blood.

Red-top tube with additives

Use: Serology, immunology, chemistry

Precaution: Do not use for blood bank; invert gently 5 times.

Lavender-top tube

Use: Hematology, immunohematology/blood bank, chemistry when plasma is needed

Precaution: Mix thoroughly but gently (tube contains sodium EDTA, which is not as soluble as liquid potassium EDTA).

Green-top tube

Use: pH, blood gases, electrolytes, hormones, amino acids, chromosome karyotype, drug level, G6PD, lupus erythematosus

Precaution: The additives are heparin salts; therefore do not use for differential smears. If testing for lupus erythematosus use a green-top tube with glass beads (contains less heparin).

Blue-top tube

Use: Coagulation studies, plasma hemoglobin

Precaution: Fill tube to maximal level for coagulation studies. Collect without a tourniquet to prevent tissue fluid contamination. Use a second tube for coagulation studies.

Gray-top tube

Use: Glucose determinations

Precaution: Contains various additives to preserve the glucose concentration

GENERAL COMMENTS REGARDING ELECTROLYTE PANEL

The serum electrolyte panel traditionally has included tests for sodium (Na^+), potassium (K^+), and chloride (Cl^-) levels and carbon dioxide (CO_2) content. Recently, however, there has been increased awareness that electrolyte disorders often involve abnormalities in the levels of magnesium (Mg^{++}) and, to a lesser degree, phosphorus (PO_4) and calcium (Ca^{++}). It is likely that in the near future a *complete* electrolyte panel will include all seven.

The levels of electrolytes in the blood result from the fine regulation of ionic charges and the osmotic balance of the extracellular fluid. This regulation is accomplished through the marvelous adaptation of the kidneys, the lungs, and the endocrine system to varying and multidirectional forces. The kidneys and the lungs are involved in acid-base balance, while osmotic balance is finely governed by the endocrine system, with the hypothalamus, the posterior pituitary gland, and the kidneys being intricately interrelated.

It is apparent, then, that the determination of the serum level of a single electrolyte is insufficient for an overall evaluation of a patient's metabolic state. When one wishes to determine the serum level of any electrolyte, the whole series should be ordered. This approach will have a profound bearing on the correct interpretation and evaluation of the patient's electrolyte status.

The following example is given to emphasize the importance of a complete electrolyte analysis. A serum potassium level of 4.5 mEq/L means one thing if the CO_2 content is 35 mEq/L and something altogether different if the CO_2 content is 10 mEq/L. In the first case, the patient probably has a metabolic alkalosis. This would cause the potassium to migrate into the cells and be excreted in the urine. A serum potassium level of 4.5 mEq/L does not then reflect a true potassium homeostasis, since when the alkalosis is corrected the potassium will return to its extracellular position, with a possible decrease in total body potassium.

In the second case (CO_2 content of 10 mEq/L), the patient probably has a metabolic acidosis. This would cause the potassium to leave the cells. A serum potassium level of 4.5 mEq/L would then reflect a much lower potassium level when acidosis is corrected, since the available potassium will migrate back into the cells when the acidosis is corrected.

In addition to electrolyte level determination, it is extremely important that the blood urea nitrogen (BUN) and creatinine levels be determined as well. These serve two purposes. First, serum electrolyte values have one implication in the presence of an elevated BUN level with the associated metabolic acidosis, but when the BUN level is normal the implication changes. In addition, the BUN level is a relatively good indication of a patient's overall water metabolism and hydration status, which has a pronounced effect on the levels of the various electrolytes. Second, if therapy must be instituted, particularly potassium replacement, it is essential to know kidney function. It is preferable that a creatinine clearance test be ordered. However, if this is not available, at least one BUN determination should be ordered so that the patient's condition may be managed safely.

It is preferable to measure the arterial pH, Po_2, and Pco_2 directly, because the pH affects and is affected by the serum electrolyte levels. This is particularly true in complex metabolic and/or respiratory acid-base problems, in which it is extremely difficult to evaluate the patient's electrolyte levels without knowing the arterial blood gas levels and pH.

Serum electrolyte levels may vary from moment to moment; therefore they are only rough indicators of the total body content of the ions. For example, in the condition known as dilutional hyponatremia the serum sodium level is below normal, but the total body sodium content is increased.

There is no direct way of measuring intracellular levels of electrolytes. It is known, however, that an electrocardiogram reflects the ratio of intracellular electrolytes to extracellular electrolytes. Initial information about a patient's overall electrolyte and acid-base state, therefore, may be drawn from this source.

By keeping in mind the above principles and problems, one can evaluate electrolyte levels much more rationally and obtain a more significant insight into a patient's overall metabolic state. At the present time electrolyte level determinations are usually performed in critical care units and in hospital environments. However, the value of these determinations is being appreciated more and more in the daily office practice of physicians, particularly in view of the large number of medications that alter electrolyte levels and body water metabolism.

ANION GAP

The anion gap is the number of unmeasurable anions in the serum. Since serum has a neutral pH, the numbers of cations and anions are equal. The measurable electrolytes contributing to this anion-cation electroneutrality are sodium, chloride, and bicarbonate. Potassium, being an intracellular ion, contributes minimally and is not considered. The totals of measurable anions plus cations are not equal, the sum of the cations always being normally greater than the sum of the anions—thus the *anion gap*. The difference is accounted for by the unmeasured anions (sulfates and phosphates). These unmeasured anions (anion gap) are calculated by subtracting the sum of plasma bicarbonate and chloride from plasma sodium concentration; the normal value is 8 to 16 mmol/L. This measurement may help in the differential diagnosis of normal anion gap acidosis versus wide anion gap acidosis, in which case the cause is not chloride but another anion (for example, in lactic acidosis, diabetic ketoacidosis).

1

Routine blood chemistry

ACID PHOSPHATASE (ACP) (SERUM)

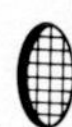

Adult reference range

Conventional:	*SI units:*
Male: Total: 0.13-0.63 sigma U/ml	36-175 nmol · sec^{-1}/L
Female: Total: 0.01-0.56 sigma U/ml	2.8-156 nmol · sec^{-1}/L
Prostatic: 0-0.5 Fishman-Lerner U/dl	

Infant and adolescent reference range

Up to 104 U/L

PHYSIOLOGY

Acid phosphatase is an enzyme of a group of related phosphate transfer enzymes. In the healthy individual, serum levels are from formed elements in blood, histiocytes, and epithelioid tissue. It is found in the prostate gland in high concentration and is similar to the enzyme alkaline phosphatase, differing in physiology according to the pH.

VALUE OF THE TEST

Detection of prostatic carcinoma
Monitoring the response to treatment

NURSING ACTION

1. Unless the test is part of the SMAC or SMA12, instruct the patient that he or she may eat and drink before the collection of the specimen.
2. Explain to the patient that this test helps to evaluate prostatic function.
3. Collect 5 to 10 ml of venous blood in a red-top tube and transport to the laboratory immediately. Handle the specimen gently to prevent hemolysis. The specimen should be examined within 1 hour if it is not refrigerated. With refrigeration acid phosphatase remains stable for up to 1 week.
4. Make a complete list of all drugs being taken by the patient on the laboratory slip.
5. Do not collect the specimen if the patient has received clofibrate in the past 24 hours, or has had a transurethral resection, prostatic massage, or extensive palpation of the prostate in the past 24 hours.

INTERFERING FACTORS

Hemolysis of the specimen or exposure to air and room temperature for more than an hour

Drugs causing decreased levels: fluorides, oxalates, phosphates, and alcohol

CLINICAL IMPLICATIONS

Elevated in about 5% to 10% of patients with prostate adenocarcinoma without metastases, in 20% to 25% of patients with metastases to nearby tissue, and in 75% to 80% of patients with bone metastases

May be elevated in:
- Prostatic infarct (temporary elevation)
- Benign prostatic hypertrophy (5% to 10%)
- Nonprostatic metastatic carcinoma to bone
- Paget's disease
- Primary hyperparathyroidism
- Gaucher's disease
- Thrombocytosis
- Disorders of platelet destruction

ALANINE AMINOTRANSFERASE (ALT) (SERUM) (FORMERLY SERUM GLUTAMIC PYRUVIC TRANSAMINASE [SGPT])

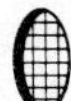

Adult reference range

1-21 U/L (SI units: 17-350 nmol · sec^{-1}/L)

PHYSIOLOGY

Alanine aminotransferase (ALT) is an enzyme found in high concentrations in the liver, with moderate concentrations in kidney tissue and small quantities in myocardium and skeletal muscle.

Serum ALT levels are 30 to 50 times normal values in toxic hepatitis and 20 times normal in infectious mononucleosis. In myocardial infarction there are no, or only minor, elevations.

VALUE OF THE TEST

To confirm liver origin of an elevated AST

The AST/ALT ratio is occasionally used in the differential diagnosis of liver disease.

NURSING ACTION

1. Unless the test is part of the SMAC or SMA12, instruct the patient that he or she may eat and drink before collection of the specimen.

2. Explain to the patient that this test helps to evaluate liver and bone function.
3. Collect 5 to 10 ml of venous blood in a red-top tube and transport to the laboratory immediately. Handle the specimen gently to prevent hemolysis.
4. List drugs being taken by the patient on the laboratory slip.

INTERFERING FACTORS

Hemolysis

Drugs causing decreased levels: carbenicillin, clindamycin, erythromycin, gentamicin, lincomycin, mithramycin, spectinomycin, tetracycline, meperdine (Demerol), morphine, codeine, methyldopa, granethidine, digitalis indomethacin (Indocin), salicylates, rifampin, flurazepam (Dalmane), propranolol (Inderal), oral contraceptives.

CLINICAL IMPLICATIONS

Elevated along with AST:

In viral hepatitis
In infectious mononucleosis
In drug-induced acute liver cell injury

Elevated to a lesser degree and frequency than AST:

In acute alcoholic liver disease
In active cirrhosis
In liver passive congestion
In long-standing extrahepatic bile duct obstruction
In metastatic tumor to the liver

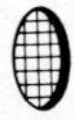

ALKALINE PHOSPHATASE (ALP) (SERUM)

Adult reference range

13-39 U/liter (SI units: 217-650 nmol · sec^{-1}/L)

Infant and adolescent reference range

Up to 104 FU/L (SI units: up to 1.26 μmol · sec^{-1}/L)

PHYSIOLOGY

Alkaline phosphatase is an enzyme from a group of several related isoenzymes that is thought to be involved in the calcification process during bone formation, in the transport of metabolites across cell membranes, and in the transport of lipid. It is normally elevated in infants, during the adolescent skeletal growth period, and during pregnancy. Alkaline phosphatase isoenzymes are relatively specific for bone, liver, placenta, and intestine.

VALUE OF THE TEST

Reflects hepatobiliary disease
An index of bone involvement in nonneoplastic calcium disorders

NURSING ACTION

1. Instruct the patient to fast 8 to 12 hours before the test. Food can increase alkaline phosphatase levels up to 25%.
2. Explain to the patient that this test helps to evaluate liver and bone function.
3. Collect 5 to 10 ml of venous blood in a red-top tube and transport to the laboratory immediately. Handle the specimen gently to prevent hemolysis.
4. With the physician's approval, there is a 24-hour hold on medications that would increase alkaline phosphatase levels.
5. Do not collect the specimen if the patient has received hepatotoxic drugs within the past 12 hours.
6. List drugs being taken by the patient on the laboratory slip.

INTERFERING FACTORS

Intravenous albumin may elevate serum ALP 5 to 10 times normal.
From the third trimester of pregnancy to 4 weeks postpartum serum ALP may be elevated up to 3 times the upper limit of normal.
Drugs causing increased levels: intravenous albumin, allopurinol, colchicine, erythromycin, indomethacin (Indocin), isoniazid (INH), lincomycin, methyldopa (Aldomet), some oral contraceptives, oxacillin, PAS, penicillin, phenothiazine tranquilizers, procainamide, tolbutamide
Drugs causing decreased levels: propranolol, fluoride, oxalate
BSP dye increases ALP levels.

CLINICAL IMPLICATIONS

Elevation of ALP 3 to 5 times upper limit of reference range

Metastatic carcinoma to the liver (75% to 80% of cases)
Space-occupying lesions of the liver (hepatoma, liver abscess, liver granulomas)

Extrahepatic biliary tract obstruction and primary biliary cirrhosis (100% of cases unless obstruction is intermittent). In such a case the patient initially has a slight bilirubinemia, which gradually increases and is accompanied by the extremely high ALP level.

Elevation less than 3 times upper limit of normal

Cholangiolitic hepatitis
Cirrhosis of the liver with some active hepatitis (elevations may be greater than 3 times normal)
Active liver cell damage in nonjaundiced patients

Extreme elevation with normal liver function tests suggests

Paget's disease. The levels may be 10 to 25 times normal along with other indications of bone pathology.
Hyperparathyroidism
Rickets
Osteomalacia
Osteoblastic metastatic carcinoma to the bone

Low ALP

A low ALP level is usually not of much clinical significance. However, if it persists one should consider some extremely rare entities such as hypophosphatasia, achondroplasia, cretinism, and vitamin C deficiency. The isoenzymes of alkaline phosphatase may be evaluated for a definitive diagnosis.

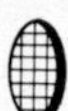

ASPARTATE AMINOTRANSFERASE (AST) (SERUM) (FORMERLY SERUM GLUTAMIC OXALOACETIC TRANSAMINASE [SGOT])

Adult reference range

7-27 U/L (SI units: 117-450 nmol · sec^{-1}/L)

PHYSIOLOGY

AST is an enzyme of the transaminase class found in high concentrations in heart muscle, liver, skeletal muscle, kidneys, and pancreas. Elevated AST levels may be found 8 to 12 hours after injury to the parenchymal cells of these organs, and is frequently found in acute pancreatitis. The serum levels peak in 24 to 36 hours after the injury, falling to normal in 4 to 6 days.

VALUE AND LIMITATIONS OF THE TEST

Used in conjunction with other enzyme analyses to determine the progress and prognosis of patients with myocardial infarction and liver disease

Elevated in many conditions

NURSING ACTION

1. Unless the test is part of the SMAC or SMA12, instruct the patient that he or she may eat and drink before collection of the specimen.
2. Explain to the patient that this test helps to evaluate heart and liver function and that a venous specimen will be taken once a day for 3 days.
3. Collect 5 to 10 ml of venous blood in a red-top tube and transport to the laboratory immediately. Handle the specimen gently to prevent hemolysis. If refrigerated, the enzyme remains stable for 4 days.
4. List drugs being taken by the patient on the laboratory slip.

INTERFERING FACTORS

Intramuscular injections

Hemolysis of the blood specimen

Salicylates may alter test results.

Drugs causing increased levels: ampicillin, carbenicillin, clindamycin, cloxacillin, erythromycin, gentamicin, lincomycin, nafcillin, oxacillin, polycillin, tetracycline, folic acid, pyridoxine, vitamin A codeine, morphine, meperidine (Demerol), methyldopa (Aldomet), guanethidine, mithramycin, digitalis, flurazepam (Dalmane), indomethacin (Indocin), isoniazid (INH), rifampin, oral contraceptives, salicylates, theophylline

CLINICAL IMPLICATIONS

Elevations are seen 8 to 12 hours after the onset of acute myocardial infarction. The elevation usually peaks at 24 to 36 hours, and the level is close to normal by 3 to 7 days. Damage to liver, skeletal muscle, lungs, or kidneys may elevate AST levels, limiting the specificity of the test. There are no myocardial-specific isoenzymes.

Extreme elevation

Acute stage of severe fulminating hepatitis
Severe liver necrosis
Skeletal muscle damage
Acute myocardial infarction (level determined by size of infarction and by time between onset of infarct and drawing of blood sample)

Minor elevation

Chronic hypokalemia (CPK levels elevated too)
Morphine and meperidine may cause temporary elevations
Warfarin or large doses of salicylates (occasionally)
Congestive heart failure
Tachyarrhythmias in the presence of shock
Pericarditis
Pulmonary infarction
Dissecting aneurysm
Cirrhosis
Cholangiolitic jaundice
Metastic liver disease
Skeletal muscle disease
Posttraumatic states
Generalized infections (such as infectious mononucleosis)

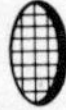

BILIRUBIN (SERUM)

Adult reference range

Total: 0.1-1.2 mg/dl (SI units: 1.7-20.5 μmol/L)
Conjugated (direct): Up to 0.3 mg/dl (SI units: Up to 5.1 μmol/L)
Unconjugated (indirect): 0.1-1.0 mg/dl (SI units: 1.7-17.1 μmol/L)

Pediatric reference range

Newborn total: 1-12 mg/dl (SI units: 17.1-205.0 μmol/L)

PHYSIOLOGY

Bilirubin, the major pigment of bile, is formed by the reticuloendothelial system from the breakdown of hemoglobin. The parenchymal cells of the liver withdraw the bilirubin from the blood, where it was circulating bound to serum albumin. In the liver the bilirubin is conjugated with two glucuronide molecules and excreted in the bile.

The total bilirubin does not distinguish between the bilirubin before and after it has passed through the liver cells, a distinction that permits a means of differentiating among the etiologies of jaundice. Since the posthepatic, conjugated (direct-reacting) form of bilirubin requires only one reagent, it can be measured more easily than the prehepatic, unconjugated (indirect-reacting) form. The SMAC measures only the total and the direct forms of bilirubin. The indirect form can be derived from the difference between these two.

Serum bilirubin concentrations rise when the liver is unable to conjugate and excrete it. When bilirubin concentrations are above 2 mg/dl jaundice can be noted. The three major causes of jaundice are hemolysis (hemolytic jaundice), liver cell damage (hepatic jaundice), and biliary tract obstruction (obstructive jaundice). The type of bilirubin elevation in the serum determines the type of jaundice. In all cases of jaundice the total bilirubin is elevated, but the differential diagnosis is made because:

1. In hemolytic jaundice the unconjugated (indirect) bilirubin is elevated. Severe hemolysis releases into the plasma more unconjugated bilirubin than the liver can excrete. Conjugated bilirubin is normal or only slightly elevated.
2. In hepatic jaundice both conjugated (direct) and unconjugated (indirect) are elevated. Liver cell damage causes both types of bilirubin to rise.
3. In obstructive jaundice the conjugated (direct) bilirubin is elevated. This obstruction to the flow of bile may be extrahepatic or intrahepatic.

VALUE OF THE TEST

Diagnosing liver disease
Detecting hemolytic anemia
Evaluating degrees of jaundice

NURSING ACTION

1. Instruct the patient to fast, except for water, for 4 hours before collection of the specimen.

2. Explain to the patient that this test helps to evaluate liver and red blood cell function.
3. Collect 5 to 10 ml of venous blood in a red-top tube and transport to the laboratory immediately. Handle the specimen gently to prevent hemolysis and protect the specimen from bright light, sunlight, or high-intensity artificial light, lest bilirubin be broken down.
4. With the physician's approval, there is a 24-hour hold on medications that would increase serum bilirubin.
5. Make a complete list of drugs being taken by the patient on the laboratory slip.

INTERFERING FACTORS

Yellow foods. Foods or drugs that give orange or yellow color to the serum (such as yams and carrots) should be avoided because they may produce a false high bilirubin level.

Radiopaque contrast media for x-ray studies will interfere with the color reaction of the test for a maximum of 24 hours.

Drugs causing increased levels: acetazolamide (Diamox), allopurinol, amphotericin B, antiTB-PAS, barbiturate, clindamycin, codeine, dextran, diazepam (Valium), erythromycin, ethacrynic acid (Edecrin), flurazepam (Dalmane), gentamicin, indomethacin (Indocin), isoniazid (INH), lincomycin, meperidine (Demerol), methotrexate, methyldopa (Aldomet), mithramycin, morphine, oral contraceptives, oxacillin, papaverine, procainamide (Pronestyl), sulfonamides, steroids, tetracyclines, tolbutamide (Orinase), vitamins A, C, and K.

Drugs causing decreased levels: barbiturates, salicylates, penicillin, caffeine.

CLINICAL IMPLICATIONS
Elevated total bilirubin

An elevated total bilirubin could be due to an elevation of the indirect- or the direct-reacting bilirubin. Massive hemolysis is suggested if there is a marked elevation in total bilirubin along with a significant drop in hemoglobin and significant reticulocytosis. In such a case the elevation would be that of the unconjugated (indirect) type.

Elevated unconjugated (indirect) bilirubin

Hemolysis caused by congenital hemolytic anemia, drug-induced causes, autoimmune disease, and transfusion reactions.

Absorption of hemoglobin from extravascular hematomas or pulmonary infarction.

Other conditions with obscure connections to jaundice are cholecystitis, cardiac disease, acute or chronic infection, gastrointestinal tract disease (mostly ulcerative or inflammatory), and cancer.

Elevated conjugated (direct) bilirubin

Common bile duct obstruction caused by a stone or pancreatic carcinoma. Only the conjugated bilirubin level rises in obstructive jaundice.

Elevation of both types of bilirubin

Active (decompensated) cirrhosis

Acute viral hepatitis

Other etiologies are alcohol or drug-induced liver injury, chronic hepatitis, liver passive congestion, primary or metastatic liver tumor, and infectious mononucleosis.

NURSING ALERT

Maintain good isolation technique because the patient may have hepatitis.

CALCIUM (CA)

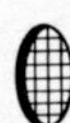

Adult reference range

Total: 8.5-10.5 mg/dl (SI units 2.1-2.6 mmol/L)

Ionized: 4-4.8 mg/dl (SI units 1.0-1.2 mmol/L)
2.0-2.4 mEq/L
30-58% of total (SI units: 0.30-0.58 of total)

Pediatric reference range

Newborn: 3.7-7.0 mEq/L
7.4-14.0 mg/dl

Infant: 5.0-6.0 mEq/L
10-12 mg/dl
Child: 4.5-5.8 mEq/L
9-11.5 mg/dl

PHYSIOLOGY

About 99% of the calcium in the body is in the bones and teeth where it gives structural strength in the form of calcium salts. Of the total plasma calcium, 50% is ionized and physiologically active, while the rest is either nondiffusible protein-bound calcium or diffusible complexed calcium. The ionized calcium is required for blood coagulation (factor IV) and is important to muscle contraction. Calcium also acts as an intracellular second messenger for hormones.

Parathyroid hormone, calcitonin, and vitamin D control the concentration of ionized calcium in the extracellular fluid by a negative feedback mechanism. Parathyroid hormone (PTH) raises the plasma-ionized calcium concentration by increasing the rate of reabsorption of calcium from the renal tubules so that calcium is saved and phosphorus is lost, and by acting directly on osteoclasts to release bone salts into the extracellular fluid, thus affecting both calcium and phosphorus levels in the plasma. Parathyroid hormone also increases the rate of absorption of calcium from the intestines.

Vitamin D increases the efficiency of intestinal calcium absorption, and calcitonin is a potent hypocalcemic hormone that causes a decrease in the resorption of calcium from bone by decreasing osteoclast activity and preventing their formation.

VALUE OF THE TEST

Detection of bone disease
Detection of parathyroid disorders
Detection of nonspecific hypercalcemic states

NURSING ACTION

1. Unless the test is part of the SMAC or SMA12, instruct the patient that he or she may eat and drink before collection of the specimen.
2. Explain to the patient that this test measures blood calcium levels.
3. Collect 5 to 10 ml of venous blood in a red-top tube and transport

to the laboratory immediately. Handle the specimen gently to prevent hemolysis.

4. List drugs being taken by the patient on the laboratory slip.

INTERFERING FACTORS

Radiopaque material. These substances interfere with the color reaction of the test. If the patient has received an injection of radiopaque contrast media, delay the test until 24 hours have elapsed since that injection.

Milk products. Consumption of large quantities of milk products in the last several weeks before the test (milk-alkali syndrome).

Drugs causing increased levels: alkaline antacids, estrogen preparations, calcium salts, vitamin D.

Drugs causing decreased levels: cortisone preparations, gentamicin, methicillin, antacids (magnesium, excessive laxative use), heparin, insulin, mithramycin, acetazolamide (Diamox), phenytoin (Dilantin).

CLINICAL IMPLICATIONS

Reference range serum calcium combined with:

1. *Normal biochemical screening panel* rules out any significant disease entity involving calcium metabolism.
2. *Abnormal serum phosphorus* may indicate a significant disease entity involving calcium metabolism (see Table 1-1).
3. *Elevated blood urea nitrogen (BUN)* suggests either
   a. Secondary hyperparathyroidism, in which case uremia and acidosis have initially lowered the serum calcium level, which in turn stimulates the parathyroid resulting in a normal calcium level, or
   b. Primary hyperparathyroidism, which initially elevates the serum calcium level. The development of secondary kidney disease and uremia then lower the elevated calcium level to normal by phosphate retention.
4. *Marked decrease in serum albumin* should be considered abnormal hypercalcemia. Since about 50% of the total serum calcium is protein bound, the blood level of calcium should be depressed in the presence of hypoproteinemia. Free calcium ions are not measured directly; therefore the concentra-

Table 1-1 Laboratory findings in certain conditions affecting serum calcium and phosphorus*

	Serum Ca	Serum Phos	ALP	Acidosis	Urine Ca
Primary hyperparathyroidism	H	N/L†	N/H†		H
Ectopic PTH syndrome	H	L	H		H
Hypervitaminosis D	H	N/L	N/H		H
Sarcoidosis	N/H	N	H		N/H
Secondary hyperparathyroidism	L/N	H	H	+	H
Renal acidosis	L/N	N/L	H	+	H
Sprue	L/N	N/L	H		L
Osteomalacia	L/N	L/N	H		L
Paget's disease	N	N	H		N/H
Metastatic neoplasm to bone‡	N/H	N	N/H		N/H
Hypoparathyroidism	L	H	N		L
Osteoporosis	N	N	N		N/H
Hyperparathyroidism	N/H	N/H	N/H		N/H

From Ravel, R.: Clinical laboratory medicine, Chicago, 1984, Year Book Medical Publisher, Inc., p. 304.
*Findings vary with individuals.
†ALP is high and serum phosphorus low in textbook cases of primary hyperparathyroidism.
‡Depends on primary tumor and type of bone lesion produced. Metastatic carcinoma to bone is one of the most common etiologies of hypercalcemia, perhaps the most common.

tion of serum proteins is an important factor in estimating the level of ionized calcium in the blood. This level is not affected by serum protein if it is determined ionically.

Hypercalcemia

- Neoplasia (noncutaneous)
  - Bone primary: myeloma and acute leukemia
  - Bone metastatic: breast, lung, kidney
  - Neoplasm secretion of PTH
- Primary hyperparathyroidism (associated with hypophosphatemia)
- Sarcoidosis (associated with hypergammaglobulinemia)
- Thiazide diuretics
- Tertiary (renal) hyperparathyroidism
- Idiopathic
- Artificial (related to laboratory error, dehydration, serum protein elevation)

Less common causes

Severe thyrotoxicosis
Bone fractures, especially during bed rest
Milk-alkali syndrome
Acromegaly
Addison's disease
Hypervitaminosis D
Diuretic phase of acute renal tubular necrosis
Lithium therapy
Idiopathic hypercalcemia of infancy

> **NURSING ALERT**
>
> Serum calcium levels of less than 6 mg/dl or more than 14 mg/dl should be immediately reported to the physician.

Hypocalcemia

Primary hypoparathyroidism (PTH deficiency; decreased PTH levels)
Pseudohypoparathyroidism (renal or skeletal nonresponse to PTH with increased PTH levels)
Malabsorption (serum carotene to screen for fat-soluble vitamin absorption)
Renal failure (BUN and phosphorus levels elevated, pH decreased)
Respiratory or metabolic alkalosis
Magnesium deficiency (exclude with serum magnesium assay)
Vitamin D deficiency
Tumor
Acute pancreatitis
Drugs (anticonvulsants, phosphate infusion, mithramycin, gentamicin, large doses of magnesium sulfate); excluded with patient history
Artifactual (hemodilution, hypoalbuminemia)

CARBON DIOXIDE CONTENT

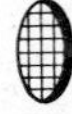

Reference range

Whole blood (venous): 22-26 mM/L (SI units: 22-26 mmol/L)

Venous plasma or serum: 24-30 mM/L (SI units: 24-30 mmol/L)

PHYSIOLOGY

Total carbon dioxide (CO_2) content determination measures the combined concentrations of bicarbonate (HCO_3), carbamino CO_2, carbonic acid, and dissolved CO_2 in blood.

Cellular respiration produces CO_2, which is released into the bloodstream where it diffuses into the red blood cells (RBCs) to be hydrated to carbonic acid (H_2CO_3). Carbonic acid in turn dissociates into hydrogen ions (H^+) and bicarbonate ions (HCO_3^-). Only about 5% of the CO_2 remains in solution, the remainder being carried in the blood as bicarbonate and then to the lungs to be removed. A small fraction is carried by the plasma as dissolved CO_2, carbonic acid (H_2CO_3), bicarbonate (HCO_3), or carbamino compounds (CO_2 coupled with hemoglobin). This bicarbonate/carbonic acid system is one of the buffers that binds hydrogen ions without causing changes in pH. Other buffers are hemoglobin, plasma proteins, and phosphates.

The hydrogen ion concentration of blood is expressed as pH (power of hydrogen or *puissance hydrogen* from the French). If hydrogen ion concentration were to be expressed in hydrogen moles/L it would be awkward to communicate since it is so much less than 1. Thus the simplified negative logarithm pH was developed in which a tenfold change in hydrogen ion concentration translated into a change of 1.0 pH unit. The normal range for blood is between 7.36 and 7.44. When this is decreased acidosis exists, and when increased there is alkalosis. These conditions can be either metabolic or respiratory.

VALUE OF THE TEST

The usual laboratory test done in conjunction with arterial pH for the detection of acid-base abnormalities.

A more accurate result than CO_2 content is that of CO_2 combining power, since the specimen is drawn and processed anaerobically.

NURSING ACTION

1. Unless the test is part of the SMAC or SMA12, instruct the patient that he or she may eat and drink before collection of the specimen.
2. Explain to the patient that this test helps to evaluate the pH of the blood.

3. If electrolytes are also being done, collect 10 to 15 ml of venous blood in a red-top tube. If only CO_2 levels are to be measured, collect 7 to 10 ml of venous blood in a green-top tube. Withdraw the blood anaerobically in a vacuum tube, filling the tube completely to prevent loss of CO_2 into the vacuum. If a tourniquet is needed, the fist should be kept closed without straining.
4. List drugs being taken by the patient on the laboratory slip.

INTERFERING FACTORS

Drugs causing increased levels: excessive ACTH, cortisone, mercurial or chlorothiazide diuretics, excessive ingestion of alkalis or licorice

Drugs causing decreased levels: salicylates, methicillin, dimercaprol, ammonium chloride, acetazolamide.

CLINICAL IMPLICATIONS

Elevated CO_2 content

Metabolic alkalosis. In the absence of chronic obstructive lung disease, elevated CO_2 content indicates *serum alkalosis and intracellular acidosis,* which are most frequently associated with hypokalemia and hypochloremia. Metabolic alkalosis can be divided into two groups, chloride responsive and chloride nonresponsive.

Chloride-responsive metabolic alkalosis constitutes 90% of all hypochloremic alkalosis, is usually caused by vomiting, diarrhea, or diuretics, and can be corrected with potassium chloride administration.

Chloride-nonresponsive metabolic alkalosis occurs with Cushing's syndrome (particularly resulting from the ectopic ACTH production syndrome), primary aldosteronism, Bartter's syndrome, and licorice ingestion.

Differential diagnosis. The two groups of metabolic alkalosis can be differentiated by a 24-hour urine chloride measurement, which will be less than 10 mEq/L in chloride-responsive alkalosis. Calculation of the anion gap (see beginning of chapter) may help in the differential diagnosis of metabolic acidosis.

Low CO_2 content

Metabolic acidosis. A low CO_2 content occurs in conditions associated with metabolic acidosis and renal tubular acidosis, unless the arterial blood pH is elevated (alkalosis), and then a low CO_2 content indicates respiratory alkalosis as seen in hyperventilation syndrome.

Metabolic acidosis (uremic, diabetic, lactic, renal tubular) may be divided into two types: (a) with normal anion gap and (b) with increased anion gap.

Metabolic acidosis with *normal anion gap* may be due to:

Diarrhea (because of loss of bicarbonate)
Chronic interstitial nephritis
Mild renal failure
Renal tubular acidosis with hyperchloremia
Urethrosigmoidostomy
Therapeutic ammonium chloride
Acetazolamide

Metabolic acidosis with *increased anion gap* is usually caused by:

Diabetic ketoacidosis
Lactic acidosis
Azotemic renal failure
Ingestion of toxins such as salicylates, ethylene glycol, paraldehyde, or methyl alcohol

NURSING ALERT

Serum CO_2 levels of less than 10 mEq/L or more than 40 mEq/L should be immediately reported to the physician.

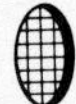

CHLORIDE (Cl) (SERUM)

Adult reference range

100-106 meq/L (SI units: 100-106 mmol/L)

Pediatric reference range

Newborn: 94-112 mEq/L
Infant: 95-110 mEq/L
Child: 98-108 mEq/L

PHYSIOLOGY

Chloride is the most abundant extracellular anion. It exerts important influence on acid-base balance, osmotic pressure, and the regulation of water distribution, as does its cation counterpart, sodium.

VALUE OF THE TEST

Serum chloride levels may be ordered as part of the electrolyte panel.

NURSING ACTION

1. Unless the test is part of the SMAC or SMA12, instruct the patient that he or she may eat and drink before collection of the specimen.
2. Explain to the patient that this test measures blood chloride levels.
3. Collect 5 to 10 ml of venous blood in a red-top or green-top tube and transport to the laboratory immediately. Handle the specimen gently to prevent hemolysis.
4. List drugs being taken by the patient on the laboratory slip.

INTERFERING FACTORS

Drugs causing increased levels: acetazolamide, ammonium chloride, boric acid, cortisone preparations, ion exchange resins, triamterene, chlorothiazide, phenylbutazone, guanethidine

Drugs causing decreased levels: mercurial, thiazide, and loop diuretics, bicarbonates, aldosterone, prednisolone, corticotropin

CLINICAL IMPLICATIONS

Hyperchloremia

Primary hyperparathyroidism
Renal tubular acidosis
Decreased CO_2 content
Hypokalemia

Hypochloremia

Most often, hypochloremia is associated with hypokalemia and alkalosis; this condition has been termed *hypokalemic-chloremic alkalosis*. In such a situation the electrolyte analysis reflects low potassium and chloride levels and elevated CO_2 content. Most of the conditions associated with hypokalemia and alkalosis are also associated with hypochloremia.

Hypochloremia may also be associated with a normal serum potassium level if the patient's potassium deficiency is being corrected with potassium preparations that do not contain chloride, or if the patient is receiving potassium-saving diuretics. These facts bring into focus two points of clinical importance: (1) potassium replacement therapy should be accompanied by a 1:1 ratio of potassium to chloride, and (2) when potassium-saving diuretics are used one should watch very closely for the possible development of hypochloremia and hypochloremic alkalosis.

The development of hypochloremic alkalosis may occur when chronic respiratory acidosis is very rapidly corrected, precipitating significant chloride attrition from the kidneys.

NURSING ALERT

1. Potassium replacement therapy should be accompanied by a 1:1 ratio of potassium to chloride.
2. When potassium-saving diuretics are being used, be alert to the possible development of hypochloremia and hypochloremic alkalosis.

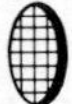

CHOLESTEROL, TOTAL

Adult reference range

120-220 mg/dl (varies with diet and age, and from country to country) (SI units: 3.10-5.69 mmol/L)

Pediatric reference range

Infant: 70-175 mg/dl
Child: 120-240 mg/dl

PHYSIOLOGY

Total serum cholesterol is all of the cholesterol found in the various lipoproteins. It is an essential cellular constituent found in all body tissues, especially in animal fats. It circulates largely in low-density lipoproteins (LDL), which transport the cholesterol from the liver to peripheral cells, which have LDL receptors that permit the cell to ingest cholesterol and protein. High-density lipoproteins (HDL) carry cholesterol from the periphery back to the liver. It has been demonstrated that reduction of plasma LDL is associated with a reduction in myocardial infarction and death, and HDL concentration is inversely related to cardiovascular disease.

VALUE OF THE TEST

Assists in the evaluation of the tendency to atherosclerosis

NURSING ACTION

1. Instruct the patient that, except for water, he or she must fast overnight and abstain from alcohol for 24 hours before collection of the specimen. Direct the patient to remain recumbent in the morning until the specimen is drawn. The patient must remain recumbent because serial specimens should be drawn after the patient has been in the same body position for several hours. The patient must fast because the same specimen may be used for triglyceride assay.
2. Explain to the patient that this test measures blood cholesterol levels.
3. Collect 5 to 10 ml of venous blood in a red-top tube and transport to the laboratory immediately.
4. Make a complete list of drugs being taken by the patient on the laboratory slip.

INTERFERING FACTORS

Radiopaque material. These substances interfere with the color reaction of the test. If the patient has received an injection of radiopaque contrast media, delay the test until 24 hours have elapsed since that injection.

Drugs causing increased levels: aspirin, corticosteroids, oral contraceptives, epinephrine, norepinephrine, bromides, phenothiazines, trifluoperazine (Stelazine), vitamins A and D, sulfonamides, phenytoin (Dilantin).

CLINICAL IMPLICATIONS
Hypercholesterolemia

If the cholesterol level is increased, the cholesterol and triglyceride levels should be determined again following a 12- to 14-hour fast. If these levels are also elevated the secondary causes of hyperlipidemia should be evaluated (hepatic disease, renal failure, hypothyroidism, diabetes mellitus, obesity, alcohol use, and medications).

Significant hypocholesterolemia (<150 mg/dl)

Diet
Malnutrition
Extensive liver disease. In this clinical situation it is advisable to fractionate the cholesterol to the esterified form, since esterification is affected by liver damage much more than is the total cholesterol level.
Hyperthyroidism
Severe sepsis
Anemia (megaloblastic and hypochromic)
Serum α- and β-lipoprotein deficiency
Certain enzyme deficiencies associated with cholesterol metabolism

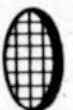

CREATININE (CR) (SERUM)

Adult reference range

0.6-1.5 mg/dl (SI units: 53-133 μmol/L)
Female: 0.2-0.7 mg/dl (SI units: 15.3-53.4 μmol/L)

Pediatric reference range

Infant to 6 years: 0.3-0.6 mg/dl (SI units: 27-34 μM/L)
Older child: 0.4-1.2 mg/dl (SI units: 36-106 μM/L)

PHYSIOLOGY

Creatinine is derived from muscle metabolism, and as such serum creatinine levels are dependent on body muscle mass. Creatinine is excreted in the urine by glomerular filtration and some tubular secretion with a small amount being reabsorbed by the tubules. Blood levels tend to be higher in the afternoon than in the morning. Determination of serum creatinine level is a test of renal function; it reflects the balance between the production of creatinine and its filtration by the renal glomerulus.

VALUE OF THE TEST

A screening test for evaluating renal function, the serum creatinine level has the same clinical value as does the blood urea nitrogen (BUN) but rises later and thus may suggest a chronic condition.

NURSING ACTION

1. Instruct the patient not to eat or drink for 8 hours before collection of the specimen.
2. Explain to the patient that this test assesses kidney function.
3. Collect 5 to 10 ml of venous blood in a red-top tube and transport to the laboratory immediately. Handle the specimen gently to prevent hemolysis.
4. Make a complete list of drugs being taken by the patient on the laboratory slip.

INTERFERING FACTORS

Pregnancy, eclampsia (decreased levels)

Drugs causing decreased levels: amphotericin B, cephalosporin (Ancef, Keflin), gentamicin, kanamycin, methicillin, ascorbic acid, barbiturates, lithium carbonate, mithramycin, methyldopa (Aldomet), glucose, protein, ketone bodies, phenolsulfonphthalein (PSP), bromsulphalein (BSP) tests, triamterene (Dyrenium)

CLINICAL IMPLICATIONS

The serum creatinine concentration is elevated in all diseases of the kidney in which 50% or more of the nephrons are destroyed. Nonrenal causes are few, making the creatinine test fairly specific for renal failure.

People with large muscle mass or patients with acromegaly may have values slightly above the normal range and still have normal kidney function.

GLUCOSE (BLOOD)

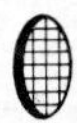

Adult reference range

Serum and plasma: 70-110 mg/dl (SI units: 3.85-6.05 mmol/L)

Whole blood: 60-100 mg/dl (SI units: 3.30-5.50 mmol/L)

Pediatric reference range

Newborn: 30-80 mg/dl
Child: 60-100 mg/dl

PHYSIOLOGY

Most carbohydrates in the diet are digested to form glucose and fructose and are taken by the portal vein to the liver, where fructose is converted to glucose. The utilization of glucose by the body cells is intimately related to the blood level of insulin, the hormone secreted from the islets of Langerhans in the pancreas.

VALUE OF THE TEST

Helps to detect diabetes mellitus but a normal value does not rule out diabetes
Helps to evaluate the clinical status of patients with diabetes mellitus

NURSING ACTION

1. Instruct the patient not to eat or drink for 12 hours before collection of the specimen.
2. Explain to the patient that this test measures blood sugar levels.
3. Collect 5 to 10 ml of venous blood in a gray-top tube (contains fluoride to diminish glycolysis). Insulin may be given as ordered after the blood sample is taken.
4. List drugs being taken by the patient on the laboratory slip.

INTERFERING FACTORS

Drugs causing increased levels: ACTH, cortisone preparations, thiazide and loop diuretics, anesthesia drugs, levodopa
Insulin excess (decreased levels)
Trauma (elevated blood sugar)

CLINICAL IMPLICATIONS

Normal blood glucose

Although a normal value rules out any significant diabetic problem, it does not rule out diabetes as such. Patients who have latent diabetes or prediabetes have normal fasting blood sugar levels even though they are, by definition, diabetic. A patient has latent diabetes or prediabetes if both parents are known to be diabetic, if an identical twin is a known diabetic, or if the patient has diabetic vascular changes.

Hyperglycemia

Hyperglycemia is usually equated with diabetes. In most cases any elevation in blood glucose level does indicate diabetes, whether the elevation is transitory or permanent. However, in always equating hyperglycemia with diabetes, one runs the risk of forgetting other diseases that may be associated with hyperglycemia. For example, hyperglycemia is present in Cushing's disease and in patients being treated with steroids. It is uncertain whether the hyperglycemia in the latter situation represents latent diabetes manifested as a clinical diabetes because of the excessive levels of steroids, or whether this kind of elevated blood glucose concentration represents a pathophysiological entity that is altogether different from the well-known, inherited form of diabetes—diabetes mellitus. The uncertainty is compounded by the fact that one of the tests employed in the diagnosis of latent diabetes is the steroid stimulation test.

It is probably best simply to define diabetes mellitus as the hereditary disease associated with fasting hyperglycemia and found in the majority of hyperglycemic patients. However, it bears repeating that hyperglycemia may not necessarily mean diabetes. A reasonably diligent search for other possible causes of hyperglycemia may produce the correct diagnosis. A glucose tolerance test is indicated when blood glucose levels are borderline or there is clinical evidence of hereditary diabetes.

Mild hyperglycemia (120-130 mg/dl)

Entities (other than diabetes) associated with mild hyperglycemia are:

Conditions causing elevation of blood catecholamine and steroid levels. The most frequent cause is acute stress (acute infection, myocardial infarction, and the like), which may herald the onset of hereditary diabetes.

Pheochromocytoma, a tumor producing epinephrine (adrenalin) and norepinephrine (noradrenalin).

Cushing's syndrome and Cushing's disease, both of which cause hyperglycemia because of elevated glucocorticoid levels. In Cushing's syndrome, which may be caused by a pituitary adenoma, growth hormones may be involved, which definitely elevate the blood glucose level.

Hyperthyroidism, which is suggested when mild hyperglycemia is associated with hypocholesterolemia. The increase in blood glucose concentration is probably mediated through an increase in catecholamine levels.

Adenoma of the pancreas, producing only glucagon that antagonizes insulin, causing hyperglycemia.

Diuretics, mainly the thiazide diuretics and the loop diuretics, most likely by inducing hypokalemia, which is known to suppress the release of insulin.

Acute or chronic pancreatic insufficiency, the mechanism of which may be the destruction of islet cells.

Moderate hyperglycemia (300-500 mg/dl)

A moderate elevation in blood glucose concentration usually leaves no doubt as to the diagnosis of diabetes mellitus. Depending on the age of the patient and other findings, a moderate hyperglycemia usually becomes a management problem.

Marked hyperglycemia (>500 mg/dl)

When a marked elevation in blood glucose level is encountered, attention should immediately be directed to the CO_2 content. This is extremely important, because if the CO_2 content is low the patient has uncontrolled diabetes associated with ketoacidosis, a potentially dangerous situation.

A second possibility, which is relatively rare, is a marked hyperglycemia without ketoacidosis (reflected by a normal CO_2 content). This entity, also serious, is called nonketotic and nonacidotic hyperglycemia; it is not necessarily associated with diabetes. The patient is usually very ill, with significantly abnormal intermediary carbohydrate metabolism caused by the uncoupling of oxidative phosphorylation. This condition is usually found in elderly patients with advanced vascular disease and anoxemia. There is associated dehydration with hypernatremia.

Hypoglycemia

The finding of a fasting hypoglycemia is quite unusual. However, once it is encountered the following conditions should be considered:

Pancreatic islet cell tumor, which independently secretes insulin without the associated check and balance of a normal metabolism

Large tumors of nonpancreatic origin, particularly large retroperitoneal sarcomas or large hepatomas

Pituitary hypofunction

Adrenocortical hypofunction (Addison's disease). If this is the cause, the patient will also have slight hyperkalemia and hyponatremia and a slightly elevated BUN level.

Acquired extensive liver disease

Other relatively rare conditions associated with hypoglycemia include glycogen storage disease; postnatal hypoglycemia, in infants of diabetic mothers; and alcoholic hypoglycemia, which is usually associated with substantial alcohol ingestion after a period of fasting.

Rarer still is hypoglycemia caused by certain amino acids (leucine hypoglycemia). One should also be aware of patients who are taking oral hypoglycemics or insulin and who may have a fasting hypoglycemia in the morning.

Reactive hypoglycemia

In functional reactive hypoglycemia, a rising blood glucose level stimulates excessive insulin secretion. In this syndrome the insulin continues to act after most of the carbohydrate has been stored or metabolized, and hypoglycemia results. A 5-hour glucose tolerance test usually shows a lowering of the blood glucose level between 3 and 5 hours. Preferably, samples should be drawn every half hour. For the 5-hour glucose tolerance test to be diagnostic, the blood glucose level must drop below 40 mg/dl and the patient must have symptoms of hypoglycemia.

NURSING ALERT

Serum glucose levels of less than 40 mg/dl or more than 400 mg/dl should be immediately reported to the physician.

*LACTIC DEHYDROGENASE (LD; LDH)**

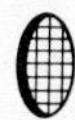

Adult reference range (total LD)

45-90 U/L (SI units: 750-1500 nmol·sec^{-1}/L)

PHYSIOLOGY

LD is an enzyme that is present in nearly all metabolizing cells. However, activity in some tissues may be as much as 500 times that

**LD isoenzymes are discussed in Chapter 4.*

of serum. Damaged cell tissues, therefore, will produce increased levels in the serum.

VALUE OF THE TEST

Total serum LD is not specific; however, there are five LD isoenzymes that may be separated by electrophoresis and are specific for certain tissue (see Chapter 4).

NURSING ACTION

1. Unless the test is part of the SMAC or SMA12, instruct the patient that he or she may eat and drink before collection of the specimen.
2. Explain to the patient that this test helps to evaluate certain activities in tissue. If the patient has had a myocardial infarction, explain that the test will be repeated on the next 2 days.
3. Collect 5 to 10 ml of venous blood in a red-top tube and transport to the laboratory immediately. Handle the specimen gently to prevent hemolysis.
4. List on the laboratory slip narcotics or intramuscular injections received by the patient within the previous 8 hours.

INTERFERING FACTORS

Hemolysis (causes elevated levels).
Narcotics (causes elevated levels).
Intramuscular injections can cause an elevated level.

CLINICAL IMPLICATIONS

An elevated LD when all other parameters are normal should raise the possibility of a hemolyzed blood specimen, and the test should be repeated before any further investigation is undertaken.

Extreme elevation of LD

Myocardial infarction
Hemolytic anemia
Megaloblastic anemia

Persistent slight elevation of LD

Chronic viral hepatitis
Malignancies of skeletal muscles, liver, kidney, brain, blood, and heart

Destruction of pulmonary tissue (pneumonia and pulmonary emboli)
Generalized viral infection involving multiple organs (infectious mononucleosis)
Low-grade hemolytic disorders
Cerebrovascular accidents with brain damage
Renal tissue destruction (renal infarcts, infections, or malignancies)

MAGNESIUM (Mg), SERUM

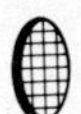

Adult reference range

1.5-2.0 meq/L (SI units: 0.8-1.3 mmol/L)

Pediatric reference range

Newborn: 1.4-2.9 mEq/L
Child: 1.6-2.6 mEq/L

PHYSIOLOGY

Next to potassium, magnesium is the most abundant intracellular cation. It is important in preserving intracellular potassium, a necessary cofactor for ATPase, and participates in the transport of potassium in and sodium out of the cell. Of the total body magnesium 35% is in the cells, 64% is in the bones, and only 1% is in the extracellular fluid.

VALUE OF THE TEST

Detection of early magnesium deficiency
Assessment of severity of existing deficiency
Monitoring of patients receiving prolonged magnesium-free intravenous therapy

NURSING ACTION

1. Unless the test is part of the SMAC or SMA12, instruct the patient that he or she may eat and drink before the collection of the specimen.
2. Explain to the patient that this test measures blood magnesium levels.
3. Collect 5 to 10 ml of venous blood in a red-top tube and transport to the laboratory immediately. Handle the specimen gently to prevent hemolysis.

4. List on the laboratory slip any medications being taken by the patient.

INTERFERING FACTORS

Drugs causing increased levels: Maalox, Mylanta, Aludrox, DiGel, epsom salts, milk of magnesium, magnesium citrate

Drugs causing decreased levels: mercurial and ethacrynic acid diuretics, calcium gluconate, amphotericin B, neomycin, insulin

CLINICAL IMPLICATIONS

Mild hypermagnesemia (2.5-3.0 mEq/L)

Excess intake of magnesium (antacids or cathartics)

Decreased renal function

Severe (symptomatic) hypermagnesemia (>4.0-5.0 mEq/L) (infrequently seen)

Excess intake with poor renal function

Parenteral administration of Mg with poor control

Hypomagnesemia

Loss from the kidney

Diuretics of various types

Diabetic ketoacidosis

Aldosteronism

Congestive heart failure

Hypercalcemia

Drugs (cisplatin, gentamicin, digoxin)

Alcohol

Renal diseases including pyelonephritis, glomerulonephritis, and tubular disorders

Loss from the gastrointestinal tract or because of gastrointestinal diseases

Malabsorption syndromes

Bowel resection

Chronic diarrhea

Intestinal and biliary fistulae

Nasogastric suction

Pancreatitis

Protein-caloric malnutrition

Severe malnutrition (rare)

In association with parenteral alimentation

Endocrine and metabolic causes (infrequent)

Hypoparathyroidism
Hyperthyroidism
Hypothyroidism
Phosphate deficiency

NURSING ALERT

Serum magnesium levels of less than 1 mEq/L or more than 5 mEq/L should be reported to the physician.

Be aware of the guiding values for serum magnesium:
Some degree of magnesium depletion: 1.5-1.8 mEq/L
Definite hypomagnesemia: <:1.5 mEq/L
Life-threatening hypomagnesemia: <1.0 mEq/L

PHOSPHORUS (SERUM)

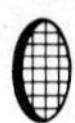

Adult reference range

3.0-4.5 mg/dl (SI units: 1.0-1.5 mmol/L)

Pediatric reference range

4.0-7.0 mg/dl (SI units: 1.29-2.26 mmol/L)

PHYSIOLOGY

Phosphorus is one component of phosphate, and the two are often confused. Of the total body phosphorus, 85% is found in bone and 10% in skeletal muscle. It is found abundantly in all tissues and is involved in almost all metabolic processes.

The phosphorus level is always correlated with the calcium level; the optimal ratio is 1:1, which exists when vitamin D intake is adequate. Calcium and phosphorus determinations are always ordered together because of their close relationships. Parathyroid hormone causes increased rates of absorption of calcium and phosphorus, and causes phosphate to be lost in the urine and calcium to be saved as a result of its effect on renal tubular reabsorption. Phosphorus is ingested with food; the kidney then filters about 90% from the blood and then reabsorbs most of that in the proximal tubules.

Phosphorus is a threshhold substance, and as such its loss in the urine is dependent on both its level in the serum and the level of calcium, since if either element is in excess the other is excreted. Serum phosphorus levels are higher in the afternoon and evening than they are in the morning owing to diet and to shifts across cell membranes.

VALUE OF THE TEST

Important in diagnosing hypoparathyroidism
Important in the evaluation of calcium levels
In the absence of significant glomerular disease (normal BUN and creatinine), phosphorus deviations direct attention to some kind of abnormality in the endocrine system or bone metabolism.

NURSING ACTION

1. Instruct the patient that he or she may not eat and drink, except for water, for 8 hours before collection of the specimen. (Carbohydrates lower serum phosphorus levels because the phosphate goes into the cells with the glucose.)
2. Explain to the patient that this test measures blood phosphorus levels.
3. Collect 5 to 10 ml of venous blood in a red-top tube and transport to the laboratory immediately. Handle the specimen gently to prevent hemolysis.
4. List on the laboratory slip any medications being taken by the patient.

INTERFERING FACTORS

Drugs causing increased levels: methicillin, tetracyclines, phenytoin (Dilantin), heparin, Lipomul, laxatives with phosphate
Drugs causing decreased levels: aluminum hydroxide (Amphojel), epinephrine (adrenalin), insulin, mannitol
Carbohydrates by diet or intravenously (lowers phosphorus level)
Hemolysis (increases phosphorus level)
Delay of more than 30 minutes in processing the specimen (increases phosphorus level), since phosphorus is released from the cells.

CLINICAL IMPLICATIONS

Hypophosphatemia

Hypophosphatemia may be the result of one of the following:

Hyperparathyroidism, the hallmark of which is hypophosphatemia in association with hypercalcemia. Although possibly not the most common cause of decreased phosphate concentration, this combination in the absence of significant renal disease is clinically characteristic of hyperparathyroidism.

Childhood rickets or adult osteomalacia, particularly if the alkaline phosphatase level is elevated. In either of these conditions, the serum calcium level may be low or normal.

Certain types of renal tubular acidosis, which is relatively rare and may represent a single defect of phosphate reabsorption from the distal tubules (that is, phosphate diabetes) or multiple defects (Fanconi's syndrome and the aminoacidurias). These diseases may be associated with other abnormalities of amino acid metabolism, distal tubular acidosis, and acid-base abnormalities.

Rapid correction of hyperglycemia and diabetic ketoacidosis.

Chronic use of antacids containing aluminum hydroxide, which binds phosphate.

In the absence of the above conditions, hypophosphatemia may be an indication of malabsorption syndromes and hyperinsulinism. Most severe cases are associated with parenteral hyperalimentation, diabetic acidosis, alcohol withdrawal, severe metabolic or respiratory alkalosis, and chronic use of antacids containing aluminum hydroxide, which binds phosphate. Hypophosphatemia is also associated with hypomagnesemia, especially in alcoholics.

Hyperphosphatemia

Chronic glomerular disease (the most common cause of hyperphosphatemia)

Hypoparathyroidism (hyperphosphatemia associated with hypocalcemia and normal renal function (BUN and creatinine clearance). Herein lies the value of measuring phosphorus and calcium levels.

Hyperthyroidism

- Increased growth hormone secretion
- Pseudohypoparathyroidism
- Fractures that are in the healing stage
- Malignant hyperpyrexia (following anesthesia)
- Newborns who have been fed unadapted cow's milk, which is much higher in phosphate content than human milk

Hypervitaminosis D
Severe muscle injury
Increased phosphate intake during therapy with phosphate-containing laxatives

Normal or increased phosphate level

This is the case in both milk-alkali syndrome and in sarcoidosis; in both disorders normal renal function is associated with primary abnormal calcium metabolism. In milk-alkali syndrome there is a history of peptic ulcer, and sarcoidosis may be suggested by hypergammaglobulinemia and the clinical picture.

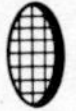

POTASSIUM (K), SERUM

Adult reference range

3.5-5.0 mEq/L (SI units: 3.5-5.0 mmol/L)

Pediatric reference range

Infant: 3.6-5.8 mEq/L
Child: 3.5-5.5 mEq/L

PHYSIOLOGY

Potassium is the major cation of the intracellular fluid. It is necessary for the transmission of normal muscle and nerve impulse, and influences acid-base balance, osmotic pressure, and cellular membrane potential. Serum potassium levels are profoundly affected by momentary acid-base changes.

VALUE OF THE TEST

Detection of high or low potassium levels, which can cause cardiac toxicity
Assessment of changes in water and electrolyte balance in patients with certain endocrine disorders
Monitoring of potassium levels in patients receiving intravenous potassium

NURSING ACTION

1. Unless the test is part of the SMAC or SMA12, instruct the patient that he or she may eat and drink before collection of the specimen.

2. Explain to the patient that this test measures blood potassium levels.
3. Collect 5 to 10 ml of venous blood in a red-top tube without using a tourniquet. If a tourniquet is needed, release it 1 to 2 minutes before drawing blood (potassium values increase 10% to 20% if the patient opens and closes the hand after the tourniquet is applied).
4. Handle the specimen gently to prevent hemolysis, which increases potassium values considerably.
5. List on the laboratory slip any medications being taken by the patient.
6. If the patient is found to be hypokalemic, encourage the eating of foods high in potassium (for example, prunes, cauliflower, tomatoes, potatoes, bananas, orange juice, peaches).
7. If the patient is being monitored with an ECG, observe for signs of hyperkalemia and hypokalemia.

INTERFERING FACTORS

Use of a tourniquet (increased level)
Overhydration (decreased level)
Dehydration (increased level)
Hemolysis of the specimen (increased level)
Drugs causing increased levels: potassium-sparing diuretics (Aldactone, Dyrenium), penicillin G potassium, cephaloridine (Loridin), heparin, epinephrine, intravenous histamine, marijuana, isoniazid
Drugs causing decreased levels: potassium-wasting diuretics, steroids, gentamicin, amphotericin, polymyxin B, bicarbonate, insulin, laxatives, lithium carbonate, sodium polystyrene sulfonate (Kayexalate), salicylates
High WBC counts (increased level)
High platelet counts (increased level)

CLINICAL IMPLICATIONS

Normokalemia with normal or decreased total body potassium

Chronic diuretic use with inadequate potassium chloride supplementation (the most commonly encountered clinical cause).

Hypokalemia

Most often, significant hypokalemia reflects total body depletion of potassium, which may have profound metabolic consequences.

Causes of hypokalemia are as follows:

1. Iatrogenic causes
   a. Diuretic therapy without potassium and chloride supplementation
   b. Diuretic therapy with supplementation of potassium and not chloride, causing a continual alkalosis with only a partial correction of the hypokalemia
2. Hypomagnesemia. This is frequently associated with hypokalemia. In this case there is continuous renal loss of potassium until the hypomagnesemia is corrected.
3. Endocrine causes
   a. Cushing's syndrome
   b. Primary or secondary hyperaldosteronism
   c. Liver disease with ascites
   d. Excessive ingestion of licorice, which contains a chemical very similar to aldosterone. The symptoms are therefore those of primary aldosteronism.
   e. Antiinflammatory drugs, indomethacin, phenylbutazone, and steroids and sex hormones, particularly estrogens
   f. Conditions associated with hyperreninemia, in which an excessive amount of renin introduced into the system can cause a secondary aldosteronemia. Such conditions include malignant hypertension, hypertensive disease, and (occasionally) unilateral renal vascular hypertension.
4. Poor dietary habits and crash diets with inadequate intake of potassium
5. Chronic stress
6. Excessive loss of potassium without adequate replacement
   a. Gastrointestinal tract (chronic diarrhea, malabsorption syndrome)
   b. Perspiration and chronic fever
7. Renal losses of potassium associated with either potassium-losing nephropathy or other kinds of renal tubular acidosis, which typically involve hypokalemia in association with acidosis and hyperchloremia and sometimes are also associated with aminoacidurias

Hyperkalemia

Renal failure (the most frequent cause). Ingestion of potassium chloride by a person with normal kidneys and normal creatinine clearance rarely results in hyperkalemia.

Addison's disease accompanied by hypovolemia and retention of blood urea nitrogen (second most common cause).

Massive tissue trauma, particularly destruction of muscle tissue, because of leakage of intracellular potassium into the serum.

Any causes of significant metabolic acidosis such as lactic acidosis and diabetic ketoacidosis.

Pseudohyperkalemia, a relatively rare condition that suggests a myeloproliferative disease such as thrombocytosis. Pseudohyperkalemia is suspected when there is hyperkalemia without ECG evidence; a true potassium level is obtained by measuring it in the plasma instead of the serum.

NURSING ALERT

Serum potassium levels of less than 3 mEq/L or more than 6.5 mEq/L should be reported to the physician.

Be aware of the clues to total body potassium depletion (the serum potassium levels may be normal):

Alkalosis. This can be verified directly by arterial blood pH, or indirectly by an elevated CO_2 content in the absence of chronic obstructive lung disease.

Hypochloremia and alkalosis.

Hyponatremia. In the face of gradual cellular potassium depletion, sodium enters the cells.

Prominent U waves or an apparent QT prolongation on the ECG.

PROTEIN (SERUM)

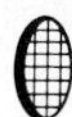

Adult reference range (total protein)

Total protein: 6.0-8.4 g/dl (SI units 60-84 g/L)

Albumin: 3.5-5.0 g/dl (SI units 35-50 g/L)

Globulin: 2.3-3.5 g/dl (SI units 23-35 g/L)

Pediatric reference range (total protein)

Newborn: 4.6-7.4 g/dl
Infant: 6.0-6.7 g/dl
Child: 6.2-8.0 g/dl

PROTEIN ELECTROPHORESIS (SERUM)

Adult reference range (protein electrophoresis)

	% of total protein
Albumin	52-68
Globulin:	
Alpha-1	2-5
Alpha-2	7-13
Beta	8-14
Gamma	12-22

Pediatric reference range (protein electrophoresis)

	Albumin	*Alpha-1*	*Alpha-2*	*Beta*	*Gamma*
Premature	3.0-4.2	0.11-0.5	0.3-0.7	0.3-1.2	0.3-1.4
Newborn	3.5-5.4	0.1-0.3	0.3-0.5	0.2-0.6	0.2-1.2
Infant	4.4-5.4	0.2-0.4	0.5-0.8	0.5-0.9	0.3-0.8
Child	4.0-5.8	0.1-0.4	0.4-1.0	0.5-1.0	0.3-1.0

PHYSIOLOGY

Serum protein is composed of albumin and globulin, free or bound to various substances that they carry.

Albumin is mostly produced by the liver and accounts for about 80% of the plasma oncotic pressure and also transports protein for some drugs and other substances.

Globulin molecules are generally larger than albumin and have been found to include glycoproteins, lipoproteins, and immunoglobulins. They are produced by the liver, the reticuloendothelial system, and other tissues, and their functions are more varied than those of albumin. They transport various substances, and are the antibody system, clotting proteins, complement, and acute phase reactant proteins. Globulins are divided according to their electrophoretic mobility into alpha-1, alpha-2, beta, and gamma globulins.

VALUE OF THE TEST

Chemical methods: Used as a screening test for hypoglobulinemia or hyperglobulinemia. Electrophoresis is more accurate.

Electrophoresis: The most commonly used screening test for serum protein abnormalities. Used to partially separate globulins, which assume certain patterns that can pinpoint areas where globulin abnormalities may be found (Fig. 1-1).

Immunoelectrophoresis: Used to detect abnormal proteins and their components (myeloma proteins, Bence Jones protein). Unable to quantitate accurately.

Albumin to globulin ratio: Should no longer be ordered since electrophoresis is now readily available, which provides the same and much more specific information about globulin abnormalities.

NURSING ACTION

1. Instruct the patient that he or she may not eat or drink, except for water, for 8 hours before collection of the specimen.
2. Explain to the patient that this test measures blood protein levels.
3. Collect 5 to 10 ml of venous blood in a red-top tube.
4. Handle the specimen gently to prevent hemolysis.
5. List on the laboratory slip any medications being taken by the patient.
6. Record vaccinations, immunizations, including toxins that the patient has received in the past 6 months.
7. Record blood transfusions, blood component therapy, or passive antisera (tetanus antitoxin, gamma globulin) the patient has received in the past 6 weeks.

INTERFERING FACTORS

Hemolysis of specimen
BSP test within 48 hours before test for protein

CLINICAL IMPLICATIONS OF SERUM PROTEIN ELECTROPHORETIC PATTERNS

1. *REFERENCE RANGE PATTERN.*
2. *ACUTE REACTION PATTERN:* Decreased albumin and elevated alpha-2 globulin. Seen in early stages of acute infection and in some cases of tissue necrosis (including myocardial in-

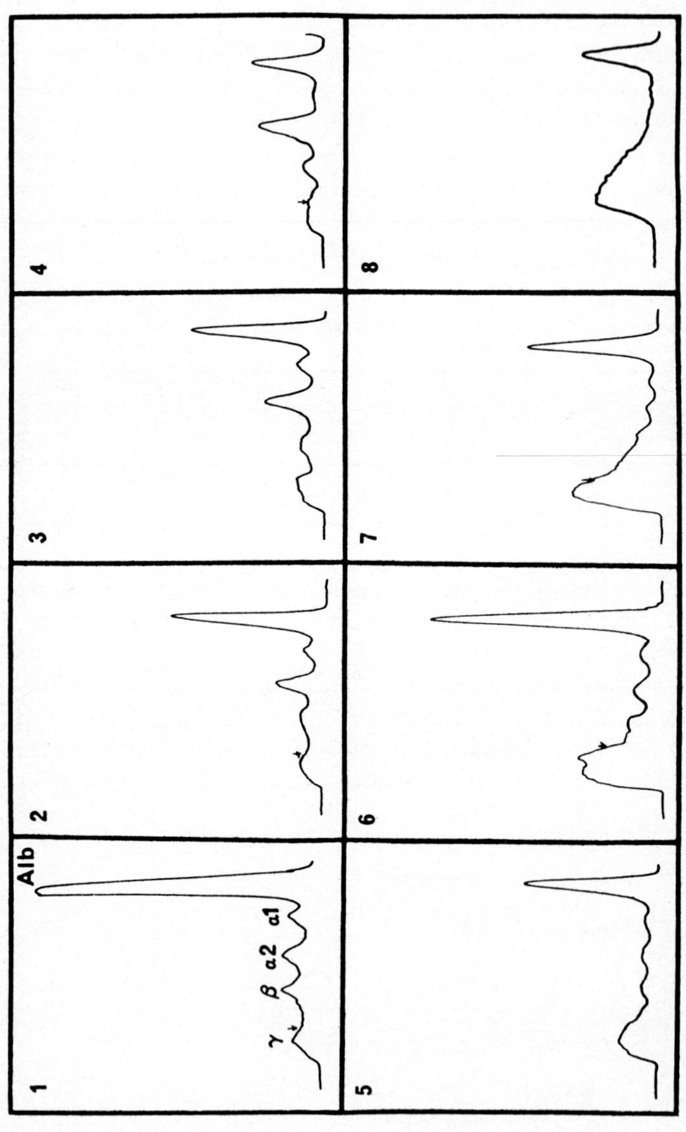
1
Alb
γ
β
a2
a1
2
3
4
5
6
7
8

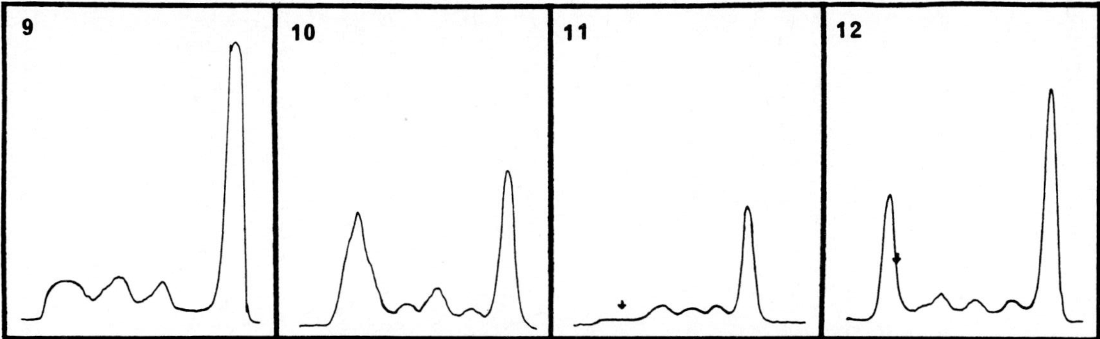

Fig. 1-1. *Typical serum protein electrophoretic patterns.*
1. Normal (arrow near gamma region indicates serum application point). 2. Acute reaction pattern. 3. Acute reaction or nephrotic syndrome. 4. Nephrotic syndrome. 5. Chronic inflammation, cirrhosis,1 granulomatous diseases, rheumatoid-collagen group. 6. Same as 5, but gamma elevation is more pronounced and there is partial (but not complete) beta-gamma fusion. 7. Suggestive of cirrhosis, but could be found in the granulomatous diseases or the rheumatoid-collagen group. 8. Characteristic pattern of cirrhosis. 9. Alpha-1 antitrypsin deficiency with mild gamma elevation suggesting concurrent chronic disease. 10. Sames as 5, but the gamma elevation is marked and the configuration of the gamma peak superficially mimics that of myeloma, but is more broad-based. 11. Hypogammaglobulinemia or light-chain myeloma. 12. Myeloma, Waldenstrom's macroglobulinemia, idiopathic or secondary monoclonal gammopathy. (Reproduced with permission from Ravel, R.: Clinical laboratory medicine, 4th edition, Chicago 1984, Year Book Medical Publishers, Inc.)

farction), severe burns, surgery and other stress conditions, and some rheumatoid diseases with acute onset.

3. *ACUTE REACTION OR NEPHROTIC SYNDROME.*
4. *NEPHROTIC SYNDROME:* Decreased albumin and increased alpha-2 globulin that are more marked than in the acute reaction pattern, with or without increased beta globulin.
5. *CHRONIC INFLAMMATION* (granulomatous diseases, cirrhosis, rheumatoid-collagen diseases): Slightly or moderately decreased albumin, slightly or moderately elevated gamma globulin, and slightly elevated or normal alpha-2 globulin.
6. *CHRONIC INFLAMMATION* with the gamma globulin elevation *more pronounced* than in no. 5.
7. *CIRRHOSIS, GRANULOMATOUS DISEASES* (sarcoidosis, far advanced pulmonary tuberculosis), *SUBACUTE BACTERIAL ENDOCARDITIS*, and certain *COLLAGEN DISEASES* (systemic lupus erythematosus, polyarteritis nodosa): Increase of the entire gamma globulin zone; the beta globulin peak does not entirely disappear.
8. *ADVANCED CIRRHOSIS:* Decreased albumin, increased gamma globulin, and incorporation of the beta globulin peak into the gamma.
9. *ALPHA-1 ANTITRYPSIN DEFICIENCY* with mild gamma globulin elevation suggesting concurrent chronic disease.
10. Same as no. 5 but the gamma globulin elevation is more marked, and the configuration of the gamma globulin peak superficially mimics that of myeloma, but is more broad-based.
11. *HYPOGAMMAGLOBULINEMIA AND LIGHT-CHAIN MYELOMA:* Decreased gamma globulin, usually without marked changes elsewhere.
12. *MYELOMA, WALDENSTRÖM'S MACROGLOBULINEMIA, IDIOPATHIC OR SECONDARY MONOCLONAL GAMMOPATHY:* High thin spike in the gamma, less frequently in the beta, or rarely in the alpha globulin area.

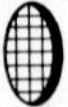

SODIUM (Na), SERUM

Adult reference range

135-145 mEq/L (SI units: 135-145 mmol/L)

Pediatric reference range

Infant: 134-150 mEq/L *Child:* 135-145 mEq/L

PHYSIOLOGY

Sodium is the major cation of the extracellular fluid. It plays an important part in regulating acid-base equilibrium, protecting the body against excessive fluid loss, and preserving the normal function of muscle tissue.

VALUE OF THE TEST

Detection of changes in water and sodium balance in certain endocrine disorders

Monitoring fluid balance in patients receiving intravenous electrolytes

NURSING ACTION

1. Unless the test is part of the SMAC and SMA12, instruct the patient that he or she may eat and drink before collection of the specimen.
2. Explain to the patient that this test measures blood sodium levels.
3. Collect 5 to 10 ml of venous blood in red-top or green-top tube and transport to the laboratory immediately. Handle the specimen gently to prevent hemolysis.
4. List drugs being taken by the patient on the laboratory slip.

INTERFERING FACTORS

Drugs causing increased levels: cough medicines, cortisone preparations, antibiotics, laxatives, methyldopa (Aldomet), hydralazine (Apresoline), reserpine (Serpasil)

Drugs causing decreased levels: potent diuretics

CLINICAL IMPLICATIONS

Hypernatremia

Hypernatremia in a normally functioning individual is very uncommon. The condition most frequently occurs secondary to dehydration (deficient water intake or excessive output, severe protracted vomiting or diarrhea, or loss of antidiuretic hormone [ADH] control).

Administration of intravenous sodium solutions to an unconscious patient is another cause. Serum sodium levels have a strong influence on the body's osmoreceptors, and in a conscious individual this initiates the thirst mechanism. The individual then drinks water until the serum sodium level is back to normal.

Hyperglycemia is associated with hypernatremia in some rare hypothalamic lesions, in head trauma, and in hyperosmolar states. Other causes of hypernatremia are dehydration and steroid (mineralocorticoid) administration or excess.

Hyponatremia

Hyponatremia is more frequently encountered clinically than is hypernatremia. In ambulatory patients and in those seen in a physician's office, hyponatremia may be associated with (1) diminution of total body sodium, (2) normal body sodium, or (3) excess body sodium.

Hyponatremia associated with an absolute sodium loss. Hyponatremia is associated with absolute sodium loss in the following conditions:

Addison's disease. In the absence of adrenal steroids, sodium reabsorption is impaired and the clinical picture is that of hyponatremia, hyperkalemia, and mild dehydration, reflected by a slight BUN elevation.

Chronic sodium-losing nephropathy. This is probably a more frequent cause than Addison's disease, and may be a stage in chronic glomerulonephritis or pyelonephritis, either of which is manifested by abnormal results of renal function tests and by an elevated BUN level.

Loss of gastrointestinal secretions because of vomiting, diarrhea, or tube drainage, with replacement of fluid but not electrolytes.

Loss of sodium from the skin through diaphoresis or burns, with replacement of fluids but not electrolytes.

Loss of sodium from the kidneys as a result of the use of diuretics (mercurial, chlorothiazide) or as a result of chronic renal insufficiency with acidosis

Metabolic loss of sodium through starvation with acidosis and diabetic acidosis.

Loss of sodium from serous cavities through paracentesis or thoracentesis.

Dilutional hyponatremia. Hyponatremia resulting from excessive water is associated with either normal or even excess total body sodium concentration and is found in the following conditions or situations:

Chronic diuretic use with sodium restriction
Secondary hyperaldosteronemia
Hepatic failure with ascites
Congestive heart failure
Excessive water administration
Acute or chronic renal insufficiency (oliguria)
Diabetic acidosis (therapy without adequate sodium replacement)

Inappropriate antidiuretic hormone syndrome. In this condition the patient continues reabsorbing water from the distal tubules and excreting a concentrated urine in spite of serum hypoosmolality. Inappropriate antidiuretic hormone syndrome has been described in association with various other diseases such as bronchogenic carcinoma (releasing ADH-like chemicals), pulmonary infections, and metabolic diseases such as porphyria, and diuretic-induced hypokalemia.

Intracellular potassium depletion. When potassium is lost from the cell sodium enters and the excess extracellular potassium is excreted in the urine, leaving the patient with a normal serum potassium level and a low serum sodium.

TRIGLYCERIDES

Adult reference range

40-150 mg/dl (SI units: 0.4-1.5 g/L)

PHYSIOLOGY

Triglycerides are found in very-low-density lipoproteins and in chylomicrons. The compound is a neutral fat synthesized from carbohydrates and stored in adipose tissue to provide energy to skeletal and cardiac muscle.

VALUE OF THE TEST

Screening tool for hyperlipidemia and establishing lipoprotein phenotypes.

Provides a good estimate of very-low-density lipoprotein levels.

Provides a rough estimate of high-density lipoprotein levels, since there is an inverse relationship.
Triglyceride levels as an indicator of atherosclerotic risk is controversial.

NURSING ACTION

1. Instruct the patient not to eat or drink, except for water, after 6 PM the night before the test.
2. Explain to the patient that this test helps to evaluate fat metabolism.
3. Collect 5 to 10 ml of venous blood in a red-top tube and transport to the laboratory immediately.
4. Hold medications until blood is drawn.
5. List drugs being taken by the patient on the laboratory slip. Do not draw blood if the patient has ingested alcohol in the past 24 hours.

INTERFERING FACTORS

A high carbohydrate diet can cause levels to be elevated.
Nonfasting specimen causes levels to be elevated.
Emotional stress
Drugs
Drugs causing increased levels: estrogen, oral contraceptives, cholestyramine resin (Questran)

CLINICAL IMPLICATIONS
Elevated triglyceride level

Lipid metabolic disorders (hyperlipoproteinemias). Additional tests for a definitive diagnosis are serum cholesterol and lipoprotein electrophoresis.
Faulty glucose metabolism (usually associated with the ketosis of uncontrolled diabetes mellitus). In this case fatty acids are released from adipose tissue to provide energy when glucose is not available.
Acute pancreatitis
Nephrotic syndrome
Uremia
Alcoholism

BLOOD UREA NITROGEN (BUN)

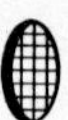

Adult reference range

8-25 mg/dl (SI units: 2.9-8.9 mmol/L)

Pediatric reference range

Infant: 5-15 mg/dl *Child:* 5-20 mg/dl

PHYSIOLOGY

Urea is the end product of protein metabolism. Its formation, which takes place in the liver by means of the deamination of amino acids, is the primary method of nitrogen excretion. After synthesis, urea travels through the blood and is excreted in the urine. When the kidneys are unable to excrete urea normally, it accumulates in the blood. Since urea itself is difficult to measure, urea nitrogen is measured because nitrogen contained in the urea is easy to analyze. An increase in the BUN is referred to as azotemia. Causes may be:

1. *Prerenal* (excessive urea in the blood or decreased renal blood flow, which interferes with glomerular filtration)
2. *Renal* (intrinsic renal disease, which could affect glomerular filtration or tubular function)
3. *Postrenal* (urinary obstruction)

There are two methods for determining BUN (Urograph and Azostix) that are useful for emergency and office screening. They will separate the individual with normal BUN from those with mild azotemia and those with marked azotemia.

VALUE OF THE TEST

A screening test for prerenal, renal, and postrenal disease

NURSING ACTION

1. Instruct the patient regarding fasting according to the rules of your laboratory. Some laboratories prefer that the patient not eat or drink for 8 hours before collection of the specimen.
2. Explain to the patient that this test evaluates kidney function.

3. Collect 10 ml of venous blood in a grey-top tube and transport it to the laboratory immediately. Handle the specimen gently to prevent hemolysis.
4. Make a list of all drugs being taken by the patient on the laboratory slip.

INTERFERING FACTORS

Drugs causing increased levels: antibiotics, diuretics, and antihypertensive agents

Overhydration may give a false low result and dehydration a false high result.

CLINICAL IMPLICATIONS

Elevated BUN

Renal failure. Acute or chronic renal failure is the most common cause of elevated BUN levels. Damage to the nephrons, particularly as in glomerular nephritis or pyelonephritis, leads to decreased glomerular filtration and excretion. As a result, the BUN value begins to rise when the glomerular filtration rate falls below 50 ml/min (the normal in an average-size man is approximately 125 ml/min).

Prerenal failure. In this case a diminished renal blood supply, such as occurs in congestive heart failure, leads to reduced glomerular filtration and an elevated BUN level.

Postrenal failure. Urinary tract obstruction can also cause uremia. Prostatic enlargement is a common cause in elderly men.

Borderline elevation of BUN

Unusually high protein intake

Excessive body protein catabolism such as occurs with sepsis or fever and gastrointestinal bleeding.

NURSING ALERT

Serum BUN levels of more than 75 mg/dl should be immediately reported to the physician.

URIC ACID (SERUM)

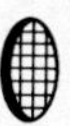

Adult reference range

Men: 4.0-8.5 mg/dl (SI units: 0.24-0.5 mmol/L)
Women: 2.7-7.3 mg/dl (SI units: 0.16-0.43 mmol/L)

Pediatric reference range

2.5-5.5 mg/dl

PHYSIOLOGY

Uric acid is the end product of purine metabolism; it is cleared from the plasma by glomerular filtration and perhaps by tubular secretion. One very rarely encounters a uric acid level significantly below the normal ranges. Therefore, we do not consider hypouricemia except to state that in malabsorption states and in very rare conditions, such as Wilson's disease or Franconi's syndrome, the uric acid level may be low.

Most of the conditions associated with the excessive production of uric acid belong to the lymphoproliferative or myeloproliferative diseases, such as acute or chronic leukemia, both leukocytic and granulocytic, multiple myeloma, or any other malignancy associated with rapid destruction of nucleic acid and purine products. Chemotherapy or radiotherapy in these disorders may further elevate the uric acid level.

VALUE OF THE TEST

A screening test for kidney disease and an indicator of disorders of nucleic acid metabolism (for example, gout).

NURSING ACTION

1. Unless the test is part of the SMAC or SMA12, instruct the patient that he or she may eat and drink before collection of the specimen.
2. Explain to the patient that this test helps to evaluate kidney function and measures substances responsible for gout.
3. Collect 5 to 10 ml of venous blood in a red-top tube and transport to the laboratory immediately. Handle the specimen gently to prevent hemolysis.

4. List drugs being taken by the patient on the laboratory slip.

INTERFERING FACTORS

Drugs causing increased levels: thiazide diuretics (impair uric acid clearance by the kidneys).

Excessive stress and fasting cause elevations in uric acid.

Foods high in purine.

CLINICAL IMPLICATIONS

Mild hyperuricemia

Idiopathic. In this case the patient is asymptomatic. It is an unfortunate mistake to label every hyperuricemia "gout" and treat the hyperuricemia rather than the patient. Usually the blood uric acid level reflects the balance between uric acid production and excretion. The association of idiopathic hyperuricemia with hyperlipidemia and coronary artery disease is of clinical importance, although the reason for the association is unclear.

Hyperuricemia

Gout. Hyperuricemia is usually equated with gout, in which there is a clinical picture of either tophi or acute arthritis with significant hyperuricemia.

Chronic renal failure. This condition can be ascertained quickly by correlating the uric acid elevation with the creatinine and BUN levels, both of which will be elevated.

Other causes include:

- Congestive heart failure with decreased creatinine clearance
- Starvation (particularly absolute starvation of obese persons for weight reduction purposes)
- Glycogen storage diseases (von Gierke's disease of Lesch-Nyhan syndrome)
- Tangier disease (α-lipoprotein deficiency)
- Hypoparathyroidism
- Primary hyperoxaluria
- Lead poisoning resulting from ingestion of moonshine whiskey (saturnine gout)
- Excessive ethyl alcohol intake

2

The complete blood count (CBC)

ANATOMY AND PHYSIOLOGY OF BLOOD

The blood consists of two major parts, plasma and blood cells. The plasma is the fluid portion consisting of mostly water in which are dissolved proteins and electrolytes, along with other organic and inorganic substances. The blood cells are suspended in the plasma and constitute about 45% of the total blood volume. They are red blood cells (RBC) or erythrocytes, white blood cells (WBC) or leukocytes, and platelets or thrombocytes.

Some of the functions of the blood include:

1. To carry oxygen from lungs to tissues and carbon dioxide from tissues to lungs.
2. To carry nutrients from the gastrointestinal tract to the tissues and waste products from the tissues to the kidneys and liver.
3. To maintain fluid and electrolyte balance throughout the body.
4. To carry phagocytic blood cells and antibodies to a point of infection.
5. To carry blood-clotting substances to a point of trauma.
6. To carry hormones from endocrine glands to target organs.
7. To help to regulate body temperature by carrying excess heat from the body core to the skin.

A CBC consists of a WBC count and differential, RBC count, hematocrit, hemoglobin, erythrocyte indices, and an inspection of the peripheral blood smear.

With accurate determinations of these values, the majority of the hematologic diagnoses can be made and a significant amount of information can be gathered for the purpose of either evaluating the stages of a particular disease or diagnosing disease entities not directly related to the hematopoietic system.

NURSING ACTION FOR THE CBC

1. Instruct the patient that he or she may eat and drink before collection of the specimen.
2. Explain to the patient that this test evaluates the blood for the presence or absence of infection in the body, the body's defense against infection, the number and condition of red blood cells in the body, and the presence or absence of anemia.
3. Collect 7 ml of venous blood in a lavender-top tube. Fill the tube completely and invert it several times to mix the anticoagulant with the blood.
4. Do not use a hand or arm receiving intravenous fluid; this causes hemodilution. Do not leave the tourniquet on more than 1 minute, because doing so causes hemoconcentration.
5. For babies or very young children collect capillary blood. Fill a capillary tube completely. Do not squeeze the tissue to get the capillary blood, since this adds tissue fluids.
6. Handle the specimen gently to prevent hemolysis.
7. List drugs being taken by the patient on the laboratory slip.

WBC COUNT

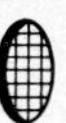

Adult reference range

Adults: 4.5-11.0 × 10^3/µl (SI units: 4.5-11 × 10^9/L)

Pediatric reference range

Newborn:	9000-30,000/µl
2 weeks:	5000-20,000/µl
1 year:	6000-18,000/µl
4 years:	5500-17,500/µl
10 years:	4500-13,500/µl

EXPLANATION OF THE TEST

A WBC count is a count of the number of white blood cells per unit volume in a sample of venous blood. The white blood cells or leukocytes are the body's first defense against infection. They are nucleated cells that are either granulocytic or nongranulocytic. The granulocytes become smaller as they mature, with the nucleus taking up less and less of the cell space. Most of them are in the bone marrow both as immature and mature WBCs; they are also in the lining of capillary walls and in the extravascular spaces of the lungs, liver, and spleen. Less than 1% are in the peripheral blood.

The granular leukocytes—neutrophils, eosinophils, and basophils—are formed from stem cells in the bone marrow (Fig. 2-1). Since nuclei of neutrophils have two to five or more lobes (as opposed to the monolobulated lymphocytes and monocytes), they are called polymorphonuclear (or segmented) leukocytes.

When bacteria invade the body, neutrophils migrate to the area of inflammation to phagocytize the invading organisms, and the bone marrow is stimulated to produce and release large numbers of mature neutrophils as well as immature forms (band cells), which appear in the peripheral circulation.

The basophils along with mast cells from tissue mediate immediate hypersensitivity reactions such as anaphylaxis, brochial asthma, and urticaria.

Eosinophils phagocytize antigen-antibody complexes and foreign particles and appear to defend against helminthic parasites. Therefore, in patients with allergic diseases the circulating eosinophil level is often elevated.

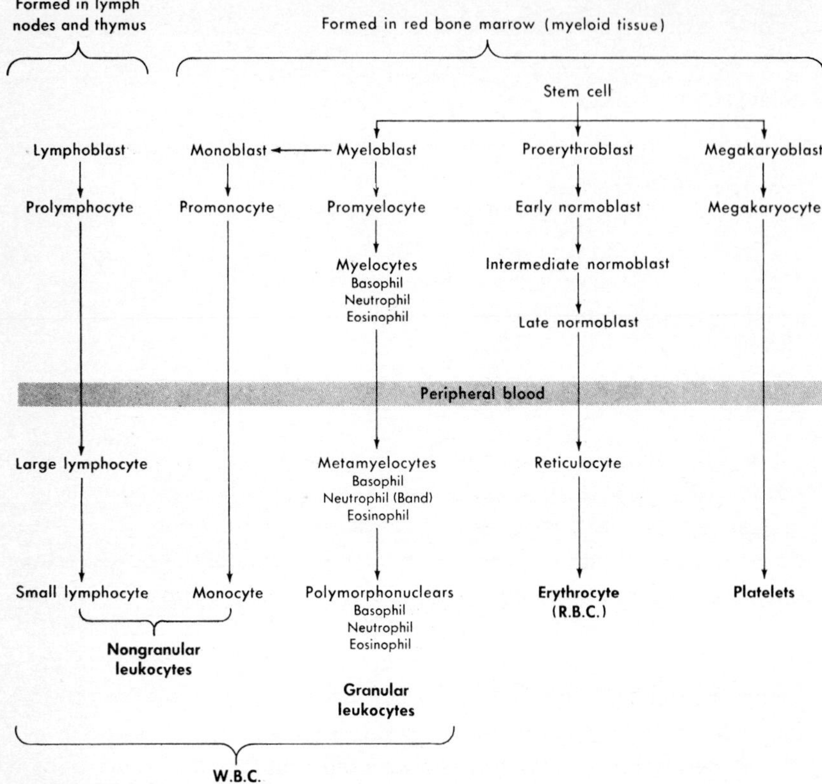

Fig. 2-1. *The development of the various formed elements of the blood. In the adult, red blood cells, the granular white blood cells, monocytes, and platelets are formed in the bone marrow. The lymphocytes are formed mainly in the lymph nodes and the thymus.*

Monocytes are leukocytes that are formed in the bone marrow and migrate into inflammatory exudates to actively phagocytize bacteria, viruses, antibody-antigen complexes, inorganic substances, and erythrocytes. Monocytes may transform into macrophages and multinucleated giant cells. Monocytosis is seen in chronic inflammatory disorders.

Lymphocytes compose 20% to 35% of circulating leukocytes. They are formed in the bone marrow from a lymphoblast stage and enter the circulation to continuously pass through lymphoid and connective tissue, their primary responsibility being antibody production, immunologic memory, and cell-mediated immunity. They are designated either B or T. T-lymphocytes are influenced in their development by the thymus, thus the "T." Both classes are derived from the bone marrow, but the T-lymphocyte matures and differentiates in the thymus. The B-lymphocyte migrates to tissue without being influenced by the thymus (the "B" stands for bursa of Fabricius, a lymphoid organ in fowls that, like the thymus, is embryologically derived from the gut). The fundamental distinction is that T-lymphocytes are involved in cell-mediated immunity, while the B-lymphocytes are devoted to antibody production.

VALUE AND LIMITATIONS OF THE TEST

A valuable indicator of the presence and cause of disease.

Absolute determination of the number of leukocytes (total white blood cells) gives only partial information. Unless an accurate differential white cell count is done, significant information or pathologic states can be missed. For example, a WBC count without a differential WBC count may be normal, even in the presence of severe sepsis. In such a case, a differential WBC count would reveal a sharp increase in the number of neutrophils and band cells.

INTERFERING FACTORS

Strenuous exercise and stress (an increased count)

Bone marrow depressants (a decreased count)

CLINICAL IMPLICATIONS

The WBC count may vary in a particular individual at different times of the day. A minor variation outside the normal range is not significant as long as the differential count and the peripheral blood smear are both normal. However, an early stage of some disorders, whether infectious or myeloproliferative, is not necessarily ruled out by a normal WBC count and a normal differential count.

Leukocytosis

Leukocytosis is defined as an absolute net increase in the number of white blood cells, resulting from various causes and taking the form of neutrophilia, eosinophilia, basophilia, or lymphocytosis (or any combination).

Mild to moderate leukocytosis (11,000 to 17,000/μl) usually indicates infectious disease, mainly of bacterial etiology. Usually the leukocytosis increases with the severity of the infection, except in elderly or debilitated patients, in whom severe sepsis can coexist with only a modest leukocytosis.

Leukemoid reaction is a marked nonleukemic leukocytosis with immaturity of one or more cell lines. Occasionally, such massive leukocytosis accompanies a systemic disease (viral infections, miliary tuberculosis, an inflammatory reaction, or growth and infiltration by metastatic neoplasms) in which the blood picture of chronic myelogenous leukemia is simulated.

Leukopenia

A *low absolute WBC count* (leukopenia) can be mild (3000-5000 cells/µl), moderate (1500-3000/µl), or extremely severe (<1500/µl) and may be associated with diminution of the WBC count as a whole, decreases in the number of neutrophils (neutropenia), eosinophils (eosinopenia), or may also be associated with low levels of all the blood particles (pancytopenia).

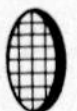

DIFFERENTIAL WHITE BLOOD CELL COUNT

Adult reference range

Cell type	*Mean %*	*Range of absolute counts*
Segmented neutrophils	56	2500-7000/µl
Bands	3	0-700/µl
Lymphocytes	21-35	1000-4800/µl
Monocytes	4	0-800/µl
Eosinophils	2.7	0-450/µl
Basophils	0.3	0-150/µl

Pediatric reference range

Newborns: Same as the adult

4 weeks: Neutrophils drop to 40%
Lymphocytes rise to 45%

10 months-20 years: A gradual return to adult ratio

EXPLANATION OF THE TEST

Visual examination of a stained slide of peripheral blood (the peripheral smear) permits an estimation of alterations in size, shape, and structure of individual WBCs and RBCs, as well as the amount of hemoglobin in the RBCs. An evaluation of the WBCs is called the differential WBC count.

Normal findings are neutrophils, lymphocytes, monocytes, basophils, and eosinophils. Under pathologic conditions other types are found such as immature forms of granulocytes, lymphocytes, and monocytes.

The differential count is reported in percentages; an increase in the percentage of one type means a decrease in another type even though the absolute number does not decrease. These percentages can be converted into absolute numbers by multiplying the percentage value for each cell type by the total WBC count. In some automated differential counters the absolute numbers are determined directly.

VALUE OF THE TEST

The differential WBC count directs the attention of the clinician to a particular disease. It is also used to monitor the patient's progress and the effects of chemotherapy.

INTERFERING FACTORS

Drugs that decrease the eosinophil count: corticosteroids.

Drugs that decrease the lymphocyte count: corticosteroids, chemotherapeutic agents.

Drugs that increase the neutrophil count: epinephrine, digitalis, heparin, and corticosteroids.

Time of drawing blood sample affects eosinophil count (low in the morning, high in the afternoon).

CLINICAL IMPLICATIONS

When leukocytosis is reported, one should very carefully inspect the peripheral smear. An accurate differential count may be enough to make a diagnosis of chronic myelocytic leukemia or chronic lymphocytic leukemia.

A thorough examination of the peripheral blood smear should routinely include a diligent search for:

Abnormal lymphocytes and monocytes that may indicate some specific disease such as infectious mononucleosis. This disease is suspected when Downey cells are found.

WBCs in early developmental stages. A "shift to the left" implies a significant number of early neutrophilic precursors and band forms rather than neutrophils. This shift indicates some kind of acute stress on the bone marrow or severe bacterial disease that is causing the release of early elements of the granulocytic series and may, at the same time, give the interpreter some indication of the stage and severity of the disease.

Abnormal granulations in the leukocytes may provide an index of the toxicity generated by a specific disease (toxic granulations).

Hypersegmentation (from three to six lobes) of neutrophil nuclei is suggestive of vitamin B_{12} deficiency or folate deficiency.

Atypical lymphocytosis indicates the possibility of infectious mononucleosis.

Decreased numbers of neutrophils and an increased proportion of lymphocytes suggest agranulocytosis.

Eosinophilia usually suggests an allergic reaction.

Blast (primitive) forms indicate the possibility of acute leukemia.

Abnormalities in basophils

Basophilia. An increased number of basophils in the peripheral blood (>150/μl).

Such a condition is uncommon and most frequently suggests some kind of myeloproliferative disease such as myelofibrosis, agnogenic myeloid metaplasia, or polycythemia rubra vera.

Abnormalities in eosinophils

Eosinophilia. An accumulation of a large number of eosinophils in the blood (characteristically >450/μl).

The most common causes of eosinophilia are allergic disorders of nearly any kind, such as hay fever, asthma, angioneurotic edema, and serum sickness.

The second most common cause is parasitic disease. *Trichinella* is predominant in the United States. Malaria and amebiasis are also possibilities, particularly if the individual has traveled widely. *Ascaris* is the most common parasite in Middle Eastern countries. Other parasites associated with eosinophilia are *Schistosoma* and *Toxoplasma*.

Other rarer conditions associated with mild to moderate eosinophilia are malignant disorders such as mycosis fungoides, brain tumors, Hodgkin's disease, and other lymphomas. Gastrointestinal causes include colitis and protein-losing enteropathy. In hypoadrenocorticism, eosinophilia may suggest the diagnosis of Addison's disease.

An extremely high eosinophil count (in the range of 80% to 90%) usually indicates pulmonary infiltrates with eosinophilia or hypereosinophilic syndrome.

Eosinopenia. Does not have diagnostic usefulness since the normal adult range is 0 to 450/μl.

Abnormalities in granulocytes

Neutropenia. The reduction of neutrophilic polymorphonuclear leukocytes in peripheral blood below 2500/μl (this figure varies, especially with race). Neutropenia in the absence of any other sign of disease should indicate that the condition is benign (hereditary, familial) or may be related to debilitation.

When the level falls below 1000/μl there is an increased risk of infection, and levels below 500/μl are almost always followed by bacterial infection unless prophylactic treatment is initiated.

Causes of neutropenia

Drugs that suppress granulocytopoiesis in the marrow (most common cause).

Severe gram-negative infection (may be transient during the onset of many infectious diseases)

Peripheral destruction of leukocytes by antibodies against the cells or against drug-modified cells (rare)

Primary and secondary splenic neutropenia associated with Felty's syndrome, portal hypertension, lymphoma, and some specific bacterial and protozoal infections

Drug-induced neutropenia, with the following drugs implicated: phenothiazines (thorazine group), antithyroid drugs, sulfonamides, phenylbutazone, chloramphenicol, phenindione, and aminophylline, or their derivatives

Excessive ingestion of alcohol

Attachment of drug-antibody complexes to the leukocytes and their subsequent destruction by complement

Abnormalities in lymphocytes

Lymphocytosis. An increase of well-differentiated lymphocytes in the peripheral blood. It may be mild or severe and occurs in two varieties: relative, in which the total number of circulating lymphocytes is unchanged but the WBC count is low because of neutropenia, and absolute, in which the number of circulating lymphocytes increases. Relative lymphocytosis often accompanies most conditions mentioned in the section on leukopenia associated with neutropenia.

Severe lymphocytosis. The most common cause of severe lymphocytosis (80% to 90% mature lymphocytes) is chronic lymphocytic leukemia. This is associated with a marked elevation of the leukocyte count.

Marked lymphocytosis with moderate leukocytosis. Found in infectious diseases, particularly pertussis, infectious mononucleosis, and acute infectious lymphocytosis.

Mild to moderate relative lymphocytosis. Seen mainly in viral infections that involve exanthema, such as measles, rubella, chickenpox, and roseola infantum.

Mild to moderate lymphocytosis and mild to moderate leukocytosis. In bacterial infections such a combination of results may indicate a chronic infectious state. In addition, the overall presenting picture may suggest other disorders: brucellosis, typhoid or paratyphoid fever, or chronic granulomatous diseases such as tuberculosis.

Moderate lymphocytosis. Thyrotoxicosis and adrenal insufficiency (Addison's disease) are associated with mild to moderate lymphocytosis.

Decreases in lymphocytes. This is associated with Hodgkin's disease, lupus erythematosus, burns, trauma, and the administration of corticosteroids.

Abnormalities in neutrophils

Neutrophilia. An increase in the number of neutrophils in the blood; this represents the most common form of leukocytosis.

Common causes of a mild to moderate neutrophilia are:

Bacterial infections
Inflammatory disorders
Tumors
Stresses
Drugs

The bacterial infections are usually moderately severe bacterial pneumonias or systemic infections.

The inflammatory but noninfectious disorders causing neutrophilia include rheumatic fever, collagen disorders, rheumatoid arthritis, vasculitis, pancreatitis, thyroiditis, and malignancies such as gastric, bronchogenic, uterine, or pancreatic carcinomas. Additional conditions are burns, crush injuries, infarctions, and poisoning with carbon monoxide or lead.

The catabolic disorders causing neutrophilia are diabetic acidosis, acute gout, thyroiditis, uremia, and Cushing's syndrome. Neutrophilia may rarely be hereditary.

RBC COUNT

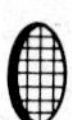

Adult reference range

Males: 4.6-6.2 million/μl
Females: 4.2-5.4 million/μl

Pediatric reference range

Newborn: 4.0-6.3 million/μl
3 months: 3.2-5.2 million/μl
1 year: 3.6-5.0 million/μl
10 years: 3.9-5.2 million/μl

EXPLANATION OF THE TEST

The RBC count is the number of red blood cells in a microliter of venous or capillary blood. Red blood cells (erythrocytes) are formed in the red bone marrow. Their production (erythropoiesis) is inhibited by a rise in the circulating red cell level and stimulated by anemia and hypoxia. The hormone erythropoietin mediates the responses to these normal and abnormal situations. Tissue hypoxia is the ultimate stimulus for erythropoietin production.

The RBCs contain a complex compound called hemoglobin, which is made up of heme, a pigmented substance containing iron, and globin, a colorless protein. Hemoglobin binds with oxygen in a reversible reaction and can also combine with carbon dioxide. Thus, RBCs function primarily to transport oxygen to the tissues and to carry carbon dioxide to the lungs, although this is not the primary transport method for the secretion of carbon dioxide.

An increased production of RBCs occurs as a physiologic response to high altitude or as a compensatory response to a pathologic condition such as hypoxia secondary to respiratory or cardiac disease. It may also be secondary to increased erythropoietin, such as would occur with kidney tumors.

Erythropoietin is a hormone synthesized principally in the kidneys and released into the blood in response to hypoxia. Its normal function in the bone marrow is to regulate the rate of erythropoiesis by inducing stem cells to differentiate into developing erythrocytes. The concentration or erythropoietin increases in response to a decrease in hemoglobin concentration in the blood, arterial hemoglobin saturation, or an increase in hemoglobin affinity for oxygen.

A decrease in production of RBCs occurs in response to deficits of erythropoietin secondary to kidney disease or because of endocrine disorders such as hypothyroidism.

VALUE OF THE TEST

RBC counts are necessary for the calculation of red cell indices and are occasionally helpful in the diagnosis of anemias.

INTERFERING FACTORS

A temporary increase in RBC count results from strong emotions, a change from recumbency to standing, diurnal variation, abdominal palpation or massage, and a cold shower. High altitude causes a moderate elevation in RBC count.

CLINICAL IMPLICATIONS

Polycythemia. Any condition in which the number of circulating RBCs rises above normal; the hemoglobin concentration and hematocrit are usually also above normal. This condition is either relative or absolute.

Relative polycythemia is the increase in RBC concentration caused by a reduction in plasma volume, such as would occur secondary to dehydration or stress. This is not a true hematologic disorder.

Absolute polycythemia is an increase in RBC concentration owing to an increase in RBC numbers; it is a true hematologic disorder characterized by marrow hyperactivity and may be associated with an increase in reticulocyte count, serum iron turnover, blood volume, and blood viscosity. It is either primary (polycythemia vera) or secondary.

Polycythemia rubra vera (primary polycythemia) is a myeloproliferative disorder that may rarely terminate as a leukemia. This is a true hematologic disorder characterized by an increase in RBC concentration caused by an increase in RBC numbers and, frequently but not invariably, WBCs and platelets. The bone marrow is hyperactive, there is a depression of erythropoietein concentration and there is an elevation in RBC mass, hemoglobin concentration, and hematocrit.

Secondary polycythemia is characterized by increased erythropoietin as a result of either appropriate or inappropriate stimuli and is found in the following conditions:

As an adaptive response (high altitudes)
Erythropoietin-secreting tumors, such as hypernephroma, renal cysts, and hepatic carcinoma
Chronic obstructive or fibrotic pulmonary disease
Cyanotic congenital heart disease with hypoxemia

The differential diagnosis may require ^{51}Cr determination of RBC volume, ^{131}I-labeled albumin determination of plasma volume, determinations of arterial oxygenation saturation and determination of splenomegaly, absolute basophil counts, leukocyte alkaline phosphatase measurements, and bioassay of urinary erythropoietin excretion.

A diagnosis of polycythemia rubra vera is suspected when there is an elevated hematocrit, unless the individual is taking testosterone or diuretics, has congestive heart failure, or lives above 7000 ft.

RBC EXAMINATION (THE PERIPHERAL SMEAR)

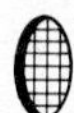

Reference range

Size: 6-8 μm in diameter.
Shape: Biconcave disks with a donut-shaped appearance, because of the fact that there is more hemoglobin in the outer portion, which stains more deeply than the center.
Color: Reddish-orange when stained; there is deeper coloring around the perimeter.
Structure: No nuclei, nuclear remnants, or cellular inclusions.

VALUE AND LIMITATION OF THE TEST

The peripheral smear permits visualization of the amount of RBC hemoglobin and size, shape, and structure of individual RBCs and platelets. This information differentiates various anemias and blood dyscrasias and may indicate the need for additional diagnostic laboratory tests.

The peripheral smear cannot demonstrate the presence of anemia; this is done by the hemoglobin, hematocrit, or RBC count. Even if the peripheral smear is highly suggestive in the later stages of the anemia, it may not be in the early stages.

CLINICAL IMPLICATIONS

Acanthocytes: Small and spherical erythrocytes with several irregular fingerlike projections that are slightly thickened on their ends. Large numbers are associated with hereditary abetalipoproteinemia; small numbers are associated with liver disease.

Chistocyte (and "helmet" cells): Fragmented, triangular, or helmet-shaped erythrocytes seen in association with hemolytic anemias, disseminated intravascular coagulation, hemolytic-uremic syndrome, uremia, and in some cases of widespread malignancy.

Echinocytes ("burr" cells): Normal RBCs with uniform small triangular projections; may also be seen with uremia; artifacts that occasionally must be distinguished from acanthocytes.

Elliptocytes: Oval RBCs found in congenital elliptocytosis, as well as several acquired anemias.

Howell-Jolly bodies: Small, round, single or multiple, blue-black RBC inclusions composed of nuclear chromatin; associated with severe hemolytic anemia and splenectomy.

Hyperchromic: More than normal color (increased hemoglobin content). This is typical of erythrocytes in congenital spherocytosis.

Hypochromic: Less than normal color (decreased hemoglobin content). There is an increase in the central clear area of the RBC, which suggests chronic iron deficiency.

Macrocytic: Larger than normal cell size; when present in considerable number, they suggest megaloblastic anemia or reticulocytosis.

Microcytic: Smaller than normal cell size; suggests a differential diagnosis between chronic iron deficiency and other etiologies, especially thalassemia minor.

Normochromic: Normal color (normal hemoglobin content).

Normocytic: Normal cell size.

Pappenheimer bodies: Hemosiderin granules (blue on Wright's stain). Seen following splenectomy and with sideroblastic anemia and severe hemolytic anemia (occasionally).

Polychromatophilic: Suggestive of reticulocytosis. This feature is indicative of homogeneous faint blue-gray staining of erythrocytes and markedly increased RBC production. May be associated with acute bleeding, hemolytic processes, leukemia, leukoerythroblastic disease secondary to metastatic tumor of the bone marrow, myeloproliferative disorders, factor-deficiency anemia responding to therapy, and the like.

Sickle cell: Crescent-shaped cell; associated with sickle cell anemia.

Spherocytes: Round cells without a central clear area; found in congenital spherocytosis and in some hemolytic diseases associated with antigen-antibody reaction (e.g., ABO incompatibility).

Target cells: A peripheral ring and a central disk of hemoglobin; found in large numbers in Hb C disease; in lesser numbers associated with abnormal hemoglobins, chronic liver disease.

Teardrop cells: Associated with myeloid metaplasia and, in lesser numbers, in other myeloproliferative diseases. Also seen in metastatic malignancy in the bone marrow.

Clinical significance of a normal peripheral smear for RBCs, a normal absolute RBC count, and other laboratory findings

Findings on the blood film may suggest a disorder even when the absolute RBC count is normal.

Significant spherocytosis and polychromatophilia suggest compensated, acquired hemolytic anemia.

Spherocytosis with polychromatophilia is suggestive of hereditary spherocytosis.

Marked hypochromia associated with target cells is suggestive of thalassemia major or minor.

Erythrocytes with basophilic stippling are characteristic of lead poisoning.

Macrocytosis in association with hypersegmented neutrophils suggests vitamin B_{12} and/or folic acid deficiency.

Rouleaux formation (an aggregate of RBCs stacked like a pile of coins) suggests multiple myeloma or macroglobulinemia.

Parasites in RBCs are the distinguishing characteristic of various types of malaria.

Schistocytes and helmet cells in association with a decreased platelet count suggest consumption coagulopathy.

Clinical significance of platelet abnormalities on the peripheral smear

The absolute absence of platelets from a peripheral smear is extremely significant, often indicating risk of hemorrhage. Decreased numbers of platelets (thrombocytopenia) may be caused by various conditions.

Sometimes, careful observation of a peripheral smear can provide a better indication of the platelet status than can an absolute count. If an abnormality is noted in the shape and character of the platelets, thrombocytopathy (abnormal-looking thrombocytes) is said to exist.

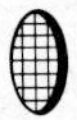

ERYTHROCYTE INDICES

Adult reference range

	MCV	*MCHC*	*MCH*
Adult	82-98 μm^3	32%-36%	27-31 pg

Pediatric reference range

	MCV	*MCHC*	*MCH*
3 months	92-115 μm^3	27%-34%	24-38 pg
1 year	87-100 μm^3	27%-33%	22-32 pg
10 years	80-96 μm^3	27%-31%	23-34 pg

EXPLANATION OF THE TEST

The erythrocyte indices are measurements of mean cell volume (MCV), mean cell hemoglobin concentration (MCHC), and mean cell hemoglobin (MCH), and detect deviations of red cell populations from the normal. When the test is done by the automated cell counters it is more sensitive than is the manual method.

Mean corpuscular volume (MCV) is the average volume of an individual cell. This value is usually given from the automated system. However, it can also be calculated by dividing the volume of packed cells (hematocrit) by the number of RBCs. The result is expressed in cubic micrometers.

Mean corpuscular hemoglobin concentration (MCHC) is the amount of hemoglobin/dl of RBCs. This value can be calculated by dividing the hemoglobin level, in grams, by the hematocrit and multiplying the result by 100 to produce a percentage. If a manual counting method is used, the MCHC is often a more reliable index of RBC hemoglobin than is the MCV.

Mean corpuscular hemoglobin (MCH) is the average hemoglobin content (weight) of each individual RBC. It is calculated by dividing the hemoglobin value by the red blood cell count. The result is expressed in picograms (micromicrograms) of hemoglobin per RBC. MCH is increased in macrocytosis and decreased in microcytosis and hypochromia, although there is some variation because a larger RBC with normal hemoglobin concentration contains a greater weight of hemoglobin than does a smaller cell with normal hemoglobin.

VALUE AND LIMITATIONS OF THE TEST

Complements a careful examination of the peripheral blood smear. Although much of the same information is gleaned from both, one test may uncover some abnormalities when the other does not.

The MCV helps to identify anemias as normocytic, microcytic, or macrocytic and when evaluated along with reticulocyte count and red cell distribution width (RDW) helps to differentiate among the anemias (see Table 2-1); the MCH and MCHC identifies anemias as normochromic or hypochromic.

Gives only an average value of deviations from normal, and may miss abnormalities in blood having mixed or second red cell populations.

CLINICAL IMPLICATIONS (See also Table 2-1)
Erythrocyte indices in anemia

Adult reference range

	MCV	*MCHC*
Normocytic, normochromic	76-100 μm^3	30%-38%
Microcytic, hypochromic	60-76 μm^3	20%-30%
Microcytic, normochromic	60-76 μm^3	30%-38%
Macrocytic, normochromic	100-160 μm^3	30%-38%

MCV increased

Folic acid deficiency (dietary, malabsorption, pregnancy)
Vitamin B_{12} deficiency (pernicious anemia, malabsorption)
Reticulocytosis, marked (acute bleeding, hemolytic anemia)
Cirrhosis

Chronic alcoholism

Less common causes of increased MCV include: malignancy, phenytoin or cytotoxic drugs, myxedema, sideroblastic anemia, or aplastic anemia

MCV decreased

Chronic iron deficiency

Alpha- or beta-thalassemia

Anemia of chronic disease (uremia, rheumatoid-collagen diseases, severe chronic infection, and so on)

Less common causes of decreased MCV include: polycythemia, lead poisoning, congenital spherocytosis, and some abnormal hemoglobins (Hb E, Hb Lepore)

MCHC increased

Spherocytosis

Free plasma hemoglobin (intravascular hemolysis)

High titer of cold agglutinins

MCHC decreased

Chronic iron deficiency

Sideroblastic anemia

Anemia of chronic disease

HEMATOCRIT (Hct)

Adult reference range

Adult males:	40%-54%
Adult females:	38%-47%

Pediatric reference range

Newborn:	42%-62%
3 months:	29%-54%
1 year:	29%-41%
10 years:	36%-40%

EXPLANATION OF THE TEST

Hematocrit is the volume of red blood cells (packed cell volume) found in 100 ml of blood. For example, a value of 46% means that there are 46 ml of red blood cells in 100 ml of blood. Hematocrit may also be determined by the automated method, in which case the mean corpuscular volume (MCV) is multiplied by RBC.

VALUE OF THE TEST

Hematocrit is a combined measure of the size, capacity, and number of cells present in the blood and, along with the hemoglobin value, establishes the presence and severity of anemia.

INTERFERING FACTORS

The Hct may be low if blood is collected from an extremity with an intravenous line.

CLINICAL IMPLICATIONS

Decrease in hematocrit is seen in:

Massive or prolonged blood loss
Anemia
Leukemia
Excessive rapid intravenous fluid administration

Increase in hematocrit is seen in conditions that cause hemoconcentration such as:

Severe burns
Surgery
Shock
Severe dehydration (vomiting, diarrhea, diaphoresis, and so on)
Loss of plasma into interstitial fluid
Polycythemia vera
Chronic obstructive pulmonary disease

HEMOGLOBIN (Hgb)

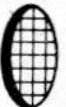

Adult reference range

Males:	14-18 g/dl
Females:	12-16 g/dl

Pediatric reference range

Newborn:	14-20 g/dl
1 year:	11.2-14 g/dl
3 years:	11.2-12.5 g/dl
10 years:	12.5-13 g/dl

EXPLANATION OF THE TEST

Hemoglobin is the oxygen-carrying pigment and main component of the red blood cells. It combines with and transports oxygen to body tissues and helps to carry carbon dioxide to the lungs. Its level is reported in grams per deciliter. For example, a value of 15.5 means that there are 15.5 g of hemoglobin in each deciliter (100 ml) of blood.

VALUE OF THE TEST

Establishes the presence of anemia and evaluates the effectiveness of therapy.

INTERFERING FACTORS

Taking blood from an extremity receiving intravenous fluids
Leaving tourniquet on more than 1 minute (results elevated because of hemostasis)
Living in high altitudes (increased hemoglobin)
Overhydration or dehydration

CLINICAL IMPLICATIONS

Hemoglobin concentrations below normal indicate an anemic condition (see Chapter 10). The hemoglobin usually parallels the hematocrit and the RBC count.

Anemia

Anemia is a reduction below normal in the quantity of hemoglobin or in the volume of packed red cells per dl of blood; it can result from many disorders. Anemias are usually classified into three broad categories:

1. Hypochromic microcytic anemia
2. Normochromic normocytic anemia
3. Macrocytic anemia, which may be normochromic, hypochromic, or hyperchromic

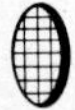

RED CELL DISTRIBUTION WIDTH (RDW)

Adult reference range

8.5-11.5 (S-Plus I)
11.5-14.5 (Coulter S-Plus II)

EXPLANATION OF THE TEST

Commercial automated blood counts now provide not only the mean red cell volume (MCV) but also a histogram of the distribution of red cell volume, reported as red cell distribution width (RDW), which may be normal or high. Red cells produce pulses when measured by automated electronic instruments. The height of these pulses is proportional to the size, and the width of the size distribution curve can be measured, giving the RDW.

VALUE OF THE TEST

When evaluated along with MCV and reticulocytes, it helps to distinguish among the anemias.

CLINICAL IMPLICATIONS

A high RDW with a normal MCV points to early iron deficiency, as well as vitamin B_{12} deficiency and/or folate deficiency. These two findings should be followed by transferrin saturation and serum ferritin determinations.

RETICULOCYTE COUNT

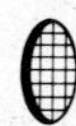

Reference range

0.5%-1.5%; 25,000 to 75,000 cells/µl (SI units: 25-75 10^9/L)

EXPLANATION OF THE TEST

Reticulocytes are immature RBCs, being larger than mature erythrocytes yet nonnucleated, that circulate in the blood for 1 to 2 days while maturing. Their numbers are generally reported as a percentage of mature RBCs. This figure is used as a measure of bone marrow activity. When bone marrow activity and hemoglobin levels are normal the reticulocyte count is between 0.5% to 1.5%. If the bone marrow has the usual capacity for erythropoiesis and normal stores of iron and other nutrients, the amount of reticulocytosis will be determined by the degree of blood loss or RBC destruction. Thus, if the bone marrow is normally responsive, the reticulocyte count will rise following blood loss or during effective therapy for certain kinds of anemia.

VALUE OF THE TEST

Helps to differentiate between hypoproliferative and hyperproliferative anemias.
Assesses blood loss, bone marrow response to anemia, and therapy for anemia.
When evaluated along with MCV and RDW, helps to distinguish among the anemias.
List drugs being taken by the patient on the laboratory slip.

CLINICAL IMPLICATIONS

Reticulocyte counts reflect bone marrow activity and can be diagnostic if evaluated along with MCV and RDW. This is done for various disorders in Table 2-1 below.

OTHER ROUTINE HEMATOLOGIC SCREENING TESTS

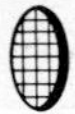

ERYTHROCYTE SEDIMENTATION RATE (SED RATE OR ESR)

Adult reference range

Westergren method:
Men under 50 years: <15 mm/hr
Men over 50 years: <20 mm/hr
Women under 50 years: <20 mm/hr
Women over 50 years: <30 mm/hr

Pediatric reference range

Newborn: 0-2 mm/hr
Neonatal to puberty: 3-13 mm/hr

EXPLANATION OF THE TEST

The erythrocyte sedimentation rate is the speed at which RBCs settle in well-mixed venous blood. This rate is increased when the negative charge on the RBC membrane decreases so that there is an increased rouleaux formation. Such would be the case in conditions where there is elevated fibrinogen and globulin levels.

The sedimentation rate of macrocytes is more rapid than that of normocytes, which in turn have a more rapid sedimentation rate than do microcytes.

Table 2-1 MCV, RDW, and reticulocyte count in the diagnosis of anemias

Disorder	MCV	RDW	Reticulocytes
Heterozygous thalassemia	L	N	H
Chronic disease	L	N	L
Iron deficiency	L	H	N or sl H
Hb S beta-thalassemia	L	H	H
Hemoglobin H	L	H	H
Red cell fragmentation	L	H	H
Normal	N	N	N
Chronic liver disease	N	N	L
Nonanemic hemoglobinopathy	N	N	H
Transfusion	N	N	N
Chemotherapy	N	N	L
Chronic lymphocytic leukemia	N	N	N or sl H
Chronic myelocytic leukemia	N	N	N or sl H
Hemorrhage	N	N	H
Hereditary spherocytosis	N	N	H
Mixed deficiency	N	H	N or L
Early iron deficiency	N	H	N or H
Early folate deficiency	N	H	N or L
Anemic hemoglobinopathy	N	H	sl H
Myelofibrosis	N	H	L
Sideroblastic anemia	N	H	L
Aplastic anemia	H	N	L
Preleukemia	H	N	L
Folate deficiency	H	H	L
Vitamin B_{12} deficiency	H	H	L
Immune hemolytic anemia	H	H	H
Cold agglutinins	H	H	H
Chronic lymphocytic leukemia (high count)	H	H	H/L

Adapted from Bessman, J.D., Gilmer, P.R., and Gardner, F.H.: Improved classification of anemias by MCV and RDW, Am. J. Clin. Pathol. **80**(3):322, 1983.
N = normal; H = high; L = low; sl = slightly

VALUE OF THE TEST

Monitors inflammatory or malignant disease
Aids in the detection and diagnosis of occult disease (tuberculosis, tissue necrosis, or connective tissue disease)

INTERFERING FACTORS

Prolonged standing of the specimen decreases ESR.

CLINICAL IMPLICATIONS

Marked elevation

Monoclonal gammopathies
Hyperfibrinogenemias

Moderate elevation

Rheumatoid arthritis
Chronic inflammations
Neoplasia

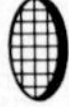

PLATELET COUNT

Adult reference range

150,000-400,000/μl (SI units: 0.15-0.4 10^{12}/L)

Pediatric reference range

Newborns-1 week: 150,000-250,000/μl

EXPLANATION OF THE TEST

Platelets (thrombocytes) are disk-shaped nonnucleated cells that help to form the hemostatic plug and are visible on stained blood smears. The bleeding time, as a measure of the clotting process, is not prolonged until there are 80,000 to 100,000 platelets/μl. However with idiopathic thrombocytic purpura, the bleeding time is generally not prolonged even with markedly low platelet counts.

VALUE OF THE TEST

Indicated when the peripheral smear reveals a lower than normal number of platelets
A screening test for disorders involving platelet factors
Valuable in the diagnosis of thrombocytopenia
Vital in the diagnosis and treatment of hemorrhagic diseases

CLINICAL IMPLICATIONS

Thrombocytosis is the elevation of the platelet count above normal levels. This condition is seen in:

Polycythemia
Essential thrombocytosis

Following splenectomy
Infections
Anemia
Iron deficiency
Malignant lymphoma
Hemorrhage
Response to exercise

3

Routine urinalysis

FORMATION OF URINE

The formation of urine begins in the glomerulus of the kidney with an ultrafiltrate of plasma. In the proximal tubules up to 85% of sodium and chloride is reabsorbed; water passively reenters the circulation with these ions. In the ascending loop of Henle, sodium is reabsorbed without water (the membrane here is impermeable to water). In the distal and collecting tubules, water reabsorption is under the control of antidiuretic hormone. From the collecting tubules, where acidification takes place and concentration is at its maximum, the urine proceeds down the ureters to the bladder unchanged.

EXPLANATION OF THE TEST

Routine urinalysis includes observation of the specimen for color and odor, determination of pH, specific gravity, protein or albumin, glucose, ketone bodies, and microscopic examination of the urinary sediment. Quick chemical screening can be performed with reagent tablets or multiple-reagent strips.

VALUE AND LIMITATION OF THE TEST

A complete urinalysis, with careful attention to microscopic examination of the sediment, remains one of the most important tests in the diagnosis of renal disease.

An abnormal urinalysis along with reduced creatinine clearance is diagnostic of some form of renal disease, although it does not reveal the severity of the disease.

NURSING ACTION

1. Instruct the patient that the first morning specimen is desirable because it is usually more concentrated than those voided during the course of the day.
2. Instruct the patient to void into a clean, dry container or bedpan; a minimum of 20 ml is needed. The specimen should be free of feces or vaginal discharge. Instruct the female patient that it is necessary to cleanse the external genitalia before voiding.
3. Send the specimen to the laboratory as soon as possible. If there is a delay, refrigerate the specimen. However, the urine should be examined within 1 hour because the white and red blood cells degenerate after that time span.

CLINICAL IMPLICATIONS

The urinary constituents evaluated and the conditions screened for are*:

Constituent	Condition screened for
Specific gravity	Kidney function test
Color/appearance	Blood/pus
Albumin	Kidney disease
Sugar/acetone	Diabetes
Hemoglobin	Blood
Microscopic findings	
RBCs	Tumor, stone, glomerulonephritis
WBCs	Infection
Casts	Kidney disease
Crystals	Stones
Squamous epithelial cells	Index of contamination

*From Ravel, R.: *Clinical laboratory medicine*, Chicago, 1984, Year Book Medical Publishers.

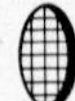

COLOR AND ODOR OF URINE

NORMAL

Normal urine is golden yellow (ranging from pale yellow to deep gold, depending on concentration). This is due to the presence of urochrome and other pigments. The color of the urine is not usually reported in a routine urinalysis unless it is abnormal.

VALUE OF THE OBSERVATION

The routine urinalysis directs the clinician's attention toward the presence of hematuria, infection, obstructive jaundice, or porphyria.

INTERFERING FACTORS

Red urine can be produced by porphyria, phenazopyridine, or ingestion of beets.

Asparagus produces a characteristic odor, and with time urine standing at room temperature will eventually smell of ammonia as a result of bacterial activity and decomposing urea.

CLINICAL IMPLICATIONS

A darker color suggests hematuria, hemoglobinuria, bilirubinuria, urobilinuria, or porphyria. Tests specifically directed toward the cause of these entities should be ordered. If the urine is red or brown it should be centrifuged. If the sediment is red and the supernatant clear, hematuria is present. If the supernatant is red to brown, test it with a Hematest tablet or dipstick (Hemastix); these will turn blue in the presence of heme. If the heme test is positive and microscopic examination shows no red cells, myoglobinuria (rhabdomyolysis) or hemoglobinuria (hemolysis) may be suspected.

Urine that changes to bright burgundy when exposed to the light is highly suggestive of porphyria.

Tea-colored urine that stains the underwear suggests the presence of urobilinogen (obstructive jaundice).

Heavily infected urine has an unpleasant odor. The fruity aroma of the urine of an individual with diabetic ketosis and the dark orange discoloration of urine from patients taking Pyridium are well-known diagnostic clues commonly encountered in the emergency room.

NURSING ALERT

If the urine is bright red, check the urine hemoglobin. This is assumed to be due to hemorrhage until proven otherwise.

Intact red cells suggest lower urinary tract bleeding, whereas cells that are crenated or abnormal suggest upper urinary tract bleeding (interstitial disease).

GLUCOSE

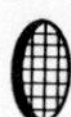

Normal

Negative

EXPLANATION OF THE TEST

The normal renal plasma threshold for glucose is approximately 160 to 180 mg/dl serum glucose level. Normally, this amount of glucose may be filtered through the glomerulus and be reabsorbed in the proximal tubule. If the serum glucose level exceeds this, it cannot all be reabsorbed by the tubules and remains in the urine (glycosuria). In diabetes mellitus there is hyperglycemia and glucosuria. However, in some individuals the renal tubular threshold for glucose is normally lower, producing glucosuria without hyperglycemia. In other individuals, glucose spills into the urine because of faulty tubular transport mechanism, such as in nephrotic syndrome or Fanconi's syndrome.

VALUE OF THE TEST

Detection and monitoring of diabetes mellitus

NURSING ACTION

The dipstick procedure. Be sure to use a freshly voided specimen and shake off excess after dipping in urine. The glucose test becomes positive at a glucose concentration of 40-100 mg/dl, depending on which reagent strip is used.

Note: Glucose oxidase enzyme paper dipsticks (Tes-Tape, Clinistix, multiple-test strips) are specific for glucose; however, the Clinitest is not and has been reported to give equivocal results or be falsely negative.

INTERFERING FACTORS

Large amounts of vitamin C (false-negative results with glucose oxidase method; false-positive results with reducing substance methods)
Reaction with cleaning compounds containing hydrogen peroxide and hypochlorites (false-positive)
Homogentisic acid, levodopa, and large doses of aspirin (false-negative Clinistix)

CLINICAL IMPLICATIONS (a partial list)
Glycosuria with hyperglycemia

Diabetes mellitus
Alimentary glucosuria (transient hyperglycemia)
Increased intracranial pressure
Cushing's syndrome
Pheochromocytoma
Hyperthyroidism (occasionally)

Glycosuria without hyperglycemia

Pregnancy (lactosuria and glucosuria)
Renal glucosuria
Fanconi's syndrome
Carbon monoxide, lead, or mercuric chloride poisoning

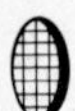

PROTEIN

Reference range

Protein excretion: <150 mg/24 hr (SI units: <0.15 g/24 hr)

EXPLANATION OF THE TEST

In health the large protein molecules are not filtered by the glomerulus. A fraction of the smaller molecules that are filtered are reabsorbed by the tubules. The remainder is excreted. Protein excretion above 150 mg/24 hr is almost always significant and is usually due to selective glomerular leakage of the smaller molecules (albumin). When the larger molecules pass through the glomerulus a greater degree of damage is indicated.

Detection of protein in the urine is usually done with the dipstick method, although in very dilute urine or in myeloma, the dipstick may not detect significant proteinuria. However, the amount of protein excretion may accurately be quantitated by a 24-hour urine collection, and this measurement is more important than the measurement of the concentration of protein in the urine by the dipstick method. The normal 24-hour urine protein excretion is less than 150 mg.

In some types of glomerular disease, large amounts of albumin may be excreted, causing hypoalbuminemia and edema. Electrophoresis and immunoelectrophoresis of the protein in the urine make possible the recognition of various immunoglobins that are seen in disease states, such as multiple myeloma, lymphoma, and amyloidosis.

VALUE AND LIMITATIONS OF THE TEST

The dipstick method can be used in the detection of abnormal proteinuria.

The results of the dipstick method are always partially subjective, depending as they do on the individual's interpretation of color change and intake of fluids.

When there is marked proteinuria there tends to be a wide variation in readings.

The dipstick may or may not react to the presence of Bence Jones protein and is not reliable for less than 20 to 30 mg/dl.

INTERFERING FACTORS

Dehydration

Contamination with vaginal secretions

Salt depletion

Very alkaline urine (false-positive results with dipstick)

Dipstick left in the urine for a prolonged time (false-negative results)

Proteinuria can be the result of severe exercise, fever, congestive heart failure, and jaundice.

CLINICAL IMPLICATIONS

The absence of protein in the urine rules out significant renal glomerular disease, whereas its presence is a reliable indicator of renal disease and is followed by an evaluation of a *24-hour specimen* to detect the degree of proteinuria and *electrophoresis* to detect the kinds of protein present.

Functional proteinuria

Severe muscular exertion
Upright position (orthostatic proteinuria)
Fever
Venous congestion and heart failure
Hypertension

MICROSCOPIC EXAMINATION OF SEDIMENT

Reference range

White cells: 0-5/HPF
Red cells: 0-5/HPF
Casts: One every 10-20/LPF

EXPLANATION OF THE TEST

Urinary sediment is the substance that separates from freshly voided urine upon standing or following light centrifugation. If examined within 3 hours of voiding, it represents bladder contents and a sampling of urinary tract morphology.

VALUE OF THE TEST

Detects renal and/or urinary tract disease

INTERFERING FACTORS

Excessive time lapse from specimen collection to testing
Inadequate cleansing of the meatus
Contamination (yeast may stimulate RBCs; menstrual blood)

CLINICAL IMPLICATIONS

RBCs

Gross bleeding: stones, tumor, tuberculosis, acute glomerulonephritis

Significant microscopic hematuria: bleeding and clotting disorders, blood dyscrasias, renal infarction, malignant hypertension, subacute bacterial endocarditis, collagen diseases, Weil's disease, bladder, urethral, and prostatic conditions

WBCs

Pyuria with significant proteinuria: renal origin
Pyuria with slight proteinuria: lower urinary tract origin
Pyuria without bacteriuria but with hematuria: tuberculosis of the kidney or collagen disease
WBCs in clumps: renal origin suggested
WBC casts: renal origin (pyelonephritis) definitely indicated

Casts

Casts are formed in the distal and collecting renal tubules as a result of the agglutination of protein cells or cellular debris. They take the shape of the renal tubules in which they form, and because they are cylindrical structures, their occurrence in the urine is sometimes called cylindruria. Protein is necessary for cast formation and proteinuria often accompanies cylindruria. Factors involved in their formation include urinary pH, concentration, protein, and stasis. Note that hyaline casts are seen with concentrated urine or after diuretic use and are not indicative of renal disease.

WBC casts, RBC casts, epithelial cell casts, and fatty casts (and oval fat bodies) are always clinically significant. Granular casts suggest renal disease because they are breakdown products of RBCs, WBCs, or fatty cell casts.

WBC casts with pyuria suggest a tubulointerstitial disorder such as pyelonephritis and also may be found in glomerular diseases.

RBC casts may appear colorless if only a few RBCs are present. However, they are often yellow. Their presence indicates glomerulonephritis or vasculitis.

Fatty casts are found in glomerular disease associated with moderate to heavy proteinuria.

Epithelial cell casts are associated with tubular damage in acute tubular necrosis, other tubulointerstitial diseases, or exudative glomerulonephritis.

Waxy and broad casts indicate advanced renal failure.

Oval fat bodies float free in the urine and have the same significance as fatty casts. They are the fatty degeneration of renal epithelial cells and have a "Maltese cross" appearance in polarized light, such as in nephrotic syndrome.

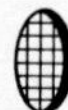

pH

Reference range

4.5-8

EXPLANATION OF THE TEST

Normal fresh urine is slightly acid when an acid-residue diet is consumed, and with good renal function the urine pH usually reflects plasma pH. If the specimen has not been standing too long, the pH will reflect the patient's acid-base balance. The processes by which the kidneys acidify urine include reabsorption and reconstitution of the bicarbonate ion, ammonium ion excretion, and titratable or phosphate buffers.

VALUE OF THE TEST

Reflects acid-base balance
Alerts the clinician to the possibilities of tubular diseases and urinary tract infection
Monitors the urinary alkalosis by which the body eliminates excess drugs (e.g., aspirin) in the treatment of drug overdose

NURSING ACTION

Send the freshly voided specimen to the laboratory, where the pH is measured to within 0.1 of a unit with a pH electrode or it may be determined with a reagent strip (accuracy to within 0.5 of a unit).

INTERFERING FACTORS

Urine standing at room temperature will slowly become alkaline because of the activity of ammonia-splitting bacteria.

Following a meal, urine becomes more alkaline as gastric acid is secreted into the stomach.

A diet disproportionately high in fruits and vegetables and low in meat protein may produce alkaline urine, as can alkalinizing drugs that may be given to prevent kidney stones.

High meat diets and acidifying drugs cause persistently acid urine.

CLINICAL IMPLICATIONS

Alkalinity. If the specimen is freshly voided, a urinary pH greater than 7 suggests urinary tract infection with a urea-splitting organism (i.e., *Proteus mirabilis*). Alkaline urine is also seen in metabolic alkalosis, except for long-standing hypokalemic chloremic alkalosis, and renal tubular acidosis.

Acidity. Acid urine is associated with renal tuberculosis, pyrexia, phenylketonuria, and alkaptonuria. Strongly acid urine is associated with all forms of acidosis. In hypokalemic hypochloremic alkalosis the urine is paradoxically acid because hydrogen ions are excreted in lieu of the potassium, which is severely depleted. Uric acid crystallizes in acid urine, and calcium crystals acidify mostly in alkaline urine.

SPECIFIC GRAVITY (SG)

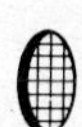

Adult and child reference range

1.016-1.022 (normal fluid intake)
1.001-1.035 (range)

Neonate reference range

1.012

EXPLANATION OF THE TEST

Specific gravity of urine represents the ratio of its density (dissolved substances) as compared to that of water at a specified temperature. This value is measured by a urinometer, which is a hydrometer calibrated for measuring the specific gravity of urine. The concentration of the urine influences the depth to which the instrument sinks.

VALUE AND LIMITATIONS OF THE TEST

Reflects only the major deviations from normal.

Although this measurement is not as precise and informative as that of osmolality, it is a quick and simple procedure and provides information about the concentrating and diluting ability of the renal tubules.

NURSING ACTION

1. Instruct the patient to abstain from water for 16 to 17 hours. This may be impossible in patients with cardiac disease, renal failure, electrolyte problems, or in the aged.
2. Ensure that the specimen is at room temperature before making the measurement.

INTERFERING FACTORS

Specific gravity is elevated in the presence of:

Radiocontrast material (effect lasts 1 to 2 days following administration)
Dextran
Dehydration
Glucose in large amounts

CLINICAL IMPLICATIONS

Normal specific gravity. Although a normal specific gravity definitely rules out chronic severe diffuse renal disease, it does not rule out many other types of active renal disease.

Low specific gravity. In the absence of abnormal urinary substances such as protein or glucose, the specific gravity of a fasting patient should be over 1.025 and at least as high as 1.020. Anything below this value reflects distal renal tubular disease and inability of the kidney to concentrate urine to the maximum. If there is protein present in the urine, the clinician must subtract .003 for 10 g protein/L and .004 for 1% glucose.

Failure to concentrate urine may exist without the presence of irreversible renal tubular damage, such as in diabetes insipidus, the diuretic phase of acute tubular necrosis, hyperthyroidism (occasionally), salt-restricted diets, and sickle cell anemia.

Fixed specific gravity. Chronic diffuse bilateral renal disease is associated with a fixed specific gravity as the disease progresses (there will also be a decrease in creatinine clearance). A fixed specific gravity is usually accompanied by nocturia and polyuria, especially in the clinical setting of nephrogenic diabetes insipidus. The polyuric state can also occur without renal disease (e.g., diabetes mellitus, infusion of mannitol, hypercalcemia, psychogenic polydipsia, diabetes insipidus). Renal diseases can occur secondary to any interstitial disease; they are most commonly seen in amyloidosis, hypothalemic nephropathy, and hypercalcemic nephropathy.

UNIT 2

Evaluative and Diagnostic Laboratory Tests for Specific Diseases

Unit 1 dealt with the routine laboratory tests for screening of patients. In Unit 2 guidelines are provided for ordering and understanding the tests that lead to a definitive diagnosis when an abnormality is detected in a routine screening examination.

The anatomy and physiology of the organ or system that is involved in a disease process are discussed first. This is followed by a short description of major disorders; then the diagnostic laboratory tests are listed in sequence of performance. Each laboratory test is then described along with its clinical value and clinical implications. Nursing action is discussed as it relates to patient preparation, the test itself, and immediate aftercare. Interfering factors are listed and complications are mentioned under Nursing Action and Nursing Alert.

4

Diagnostic tests for cardiac disorders

ANATOMY AND PHYSIOLOGY

The heart is a muscular pump that contains four chambers and four valves. The heart is innervated by the autonomic nervous system, it receives its blood supply from the coronary arteries, and it possesses a marvelous conduction system.

The course of the blood through the four chambers of the heart, the valves, and the great vessels is shown in Fig. 4-1. The blood enters the two atria simultaneously, unimpeded by valves. The right atrium receives venous blood through the inferior and superior venae cavae. The left atrium receives arterial blood through the four pulmonary veins. During diastole both the atria and the ventricles fill. During atrial systole an extra complement of blood is pushed into the ventricles. When ventricular systole begins, the two valves (mitral and tricuspid) guarding the atria close (S_1), and blood is pumped to the lungs from the right ventricle (via the pulmonary artery) and to the systemic circulation from the left ventricle (via the aorta). When diastole begins, the valves (pulmonary and aortic) guarding the two ventricles close (S_2).

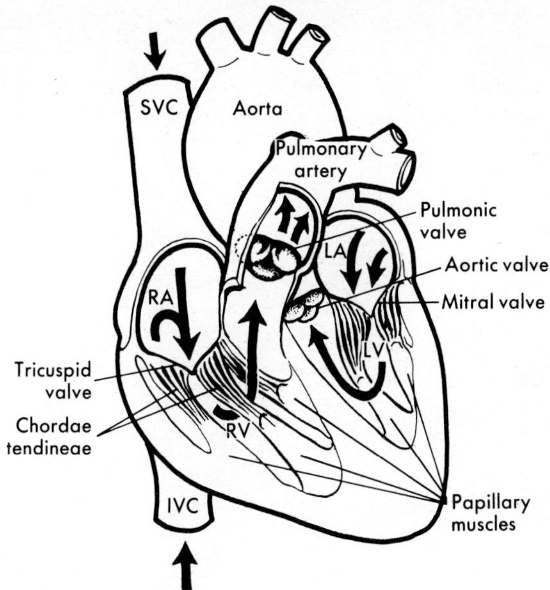

Fig. 4-1. *Heart chambers, valves, papillary muscles, and course of blood flow. (From Tilkian, A., and Conover, M.: Understanding heart sounds and murmurs, 2d ed., Philadelphia, 1984, W.B. Saunders Co.)*

The two coronary arteries (right and left) spring from the root of the aorta. During diastole the coronary arteries fill, supplying the myocardium with oxygenated blood.

The conduction system of the heart is shown in Fig. 4-2. The sinus node, which paces the heart, lies in the superior portion of the right atrium. The atrioventricular (AV) node lies in the lower posterior part of the right atrium. Its function is to receive the impulse from the sinus node and delay it slightly so that the atria will have time to pump their contents into the ventricles before they contract, thus complementing cardiac output.

Since there is a fibrous ring separating the atria from the ventricles, the bundle of His is the sole muscular connection between these two parts of the heart. The impulse enters the AV node and is conducted down the bundle of His, the bundle branches, and the Purkinje fibers to the ventricular myocardium. The right bundle branch serves the right side of the heart, and the left bundle branch, which is divided into an anterior division and a posterior division, serves the left side.

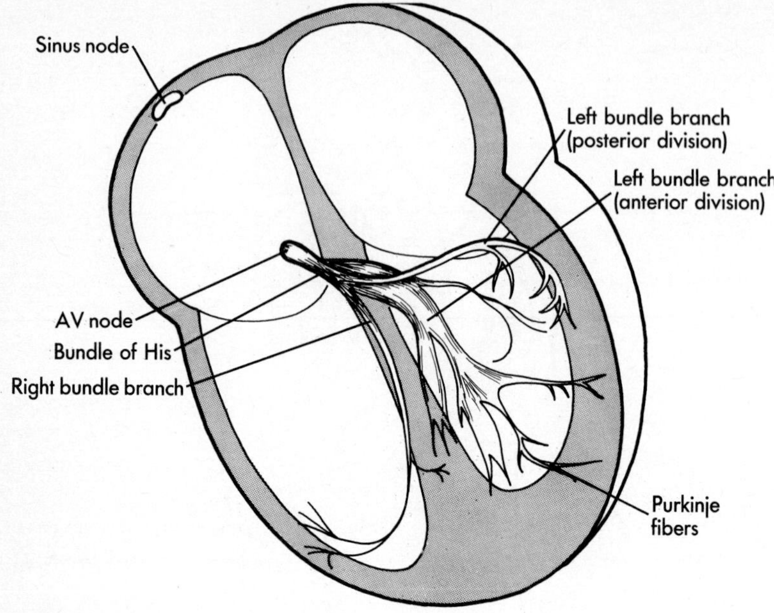

Fig. 4-2. *The conduction system.*

The conduction system of the heart enables the impulse to travel six times faster than would be possible without it.

GENERAL DIAGNOSTIC TESTS

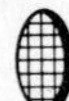

THE ELECTROCARDIOGRAM (ECG)

EXPLANATION OF THE TEST

The electrocardiograph is the instrument that records the electrical activity of the heart and the electrocardiogram (ECG) is the record of that activity. Three bipolar and nine unipolar leads constitute the standard 12 lead ECG. Leads I, II, III, aV_R, aV_L, and aV_F are limb leads; leads V_1 to V_6 are precordial leads. Although the ECG is used in almost all types of heart disease, this section will emphasize those areas in which the test has been found most useful.

VALUE OF THE TEST

Indispensable in the diagnosis and monitoring the treatment of coronary artery disease

Aids in the diagnosis of myocardial infarction, valvular heart disease, and some cases of congenital heart disease

A simple and accurate method of diagnosing arrhythmias, bundle branch block, and Wolff-Parkinson-White (WPW) syndrome and of monitoring drug therapy and electrolyte status

NURSING ACTION

1. Instruct the patient that he or she may eat and drink before the test.
2. Rub the electrode sites with gauze to break down the skin's resistance.
3. Ask the patient to lie still, relax, and breathe normally during the procedure. Make sure that the patient understands that you are merely making a record of the electrical activity of the heart and that the procedure is painless and harmless.
4. When assessing the mechanism and location of arrhythmias, record at least leads I, II, III, V_1, and V_6. These should be simultaneously recorded if possible.

CLINICAL IMPLICATIONS

Coronary artery disease

ECG changes in coronary artery disease include nonspecific ST-T abnormalities, ST depression or elevation, T-wave inversion, and QRS changes.

Nonspecific ST- or T-wave abnormalities is a vague but common electrocardiographic interpretation that can frustrate the beginner or one who expects a diagnostic label to result from every ECG. Such abnormalities are what the term implies—changes of the ST segment or T waves that are outside the range of what is considered normal, and this renders the ECG abnormal. They can be seen in a variety of disorders, cardiac or noncardiac, and do not necessarily signify heart disease. Still, these deviations may be the earliest manifestation of coronary artery disease.

ST depression that is horizontal or downsloping 1 mm or more is frequently seen in myocardial ischemia. Although not diagnostic of coronary artery disease, ST depression can be suggestive of this disorder. Digitalis and electrolyte abnormalities can accentuate or mimic these changes.

Marked *ST elevations* in well-localized leads in a 45-year-old man clutching his chest in an emergency room characterize the onset of acute myocardial infarction. But an unqualified diagnosis of acute myocardial infarction would be incorrect. Such a tracing may reflect early changes in acute myocardial infarction ("hyperacute") or may revert to normal in a matter of minutes, at which time the tracing would be characteristic of variant (Prinzmetal's) angina, reflecting reversible myocardial ischemia secondary to reversible coronary artery spasm. Thus an unqualified diagnosis of myocardial infarction, either acute or chronic, cannot be based upon an abnormality of ST-T waves, regardless of the severity of the changes. ST elevations that remain unchanged over many weeks following an acute myocardial infarction may point to a ventricular aneurysm.

Prominent or giant *T inversions* may reflect diffuse myocardial ischemia or possibly subendocardial infarction but are by no means specific. Central nervous system lesions, usually caused by massive damage or subarachnoid hemorrhage, can produce marked T-wave inversions that can easily be confused with those of severe coronary artery disease.

Changes of the QRS complex are commonly seen in coronary artery disease. Abnormal Q waves are the hallmark of myocardial infarction. By also observing the associated changes in the ST-T segment, one can make a reasonable estimate of the infarction—whether it is recent or old. It is generally accepted that the more leads in which the Q waves are seen, the larger the infarction. Also, most Q waves persist indefinitely, but it is not uncommon for an electrocardiogram with diagnostic Q waves to lose the Q waves or even revert to normal months or years following an infarction. Pathologic Q waves do not necessarily signify coronary artery disease or myocardial infarction. They can also be seen in infiltrative myocardial disorders, such as amyloidosis.

The diagnostic usefulness of the *P waves* in coronary artery disease is limited. In patients who have atrial infarctions or who have heart failure accompanied by elevated pressures in the left atrium, P waves may become abnormal.

U waves are seen in normal people and are of the same polarity as the T wave. They become more prominent in electrolyte disorders (hypokalemia), and may be inverted in myocardial ischemia.

The *PR segment* is commonly normal in coronary artery disease.

A prolonged PR segment (first-degree heart block) is frequently seen in patients with myocardial infarction, especially of the inferior wall, and may also be the result of digitalis excess.

The *Q-T interval* in coronary artery disease with myocardial ischemia may be prolonged. This fact is helpful in differentiating the ST-T abnormalities caused by ischemia (which is accompanied by Q-T prolongation) from those caused by digitalis (which is commonly accompanied by Q-T shortening). The Q-T interval may also be prolonged as a result of the administration of cardiac drugs (quinidine and others) or as a result of brain damage. Marked Q-T prolongation can lead to torsades de pointes or ventricular fibrillation.

Valvular heart disease

The ECG commonly reflects valvular heart disease by either increased QRS voltage or ST-T abnormalities, indicating enlargement or hypertrophy of the affected cardiac chambers. Common examples include aortic stenosis or insufficiency, mitral stenosis, and hypertension. *Aortic stenosis* or *aortic insufficiency* can cause left ventricular hypertrophy and enlargement, reflected in the ECG by increased voltage and ST-T abnormalities. *Mitral stenosis* produces increased pressure in the left atrium, causing this chamber to hypertrophy and dilate, and the result is reflected as a broad-notched P wave in leads II and III (P mitrale), indicating left atrial enlargement. Similar examples can be extended to all other valvular lesions. *Hypertension* acts in a manner that is similar to that of aortic stenosis, since it also causes a pressure overload of the left ventricle, producing left ventricular hypertrophy. It should be noted that left ventricular hypertrophy identified by the ECG does not necessarily mean a fixed increase of the muscle mass of the left ventricle, since treating the hypertension may improve the electrocardiogram, and in some cases may cause it to revert to normal.

Congenital heart disease

An abnormal ECG commonly accompanies congenital heart disease in infants as well as in adults. The ECG is characteristic but leads to an exact diagnosis in only a few conditions, such as endocardial cushion defect, atrial septal defect of the ostium primum type, and transposition of the great vessels with ventricular inversion. More frequently, the abnormality helps in localizing the disease to the right or the left side of the heart. Of course, in infants and children the set of criteria used for normal values is different from that used in adults.

Arrhythmias

The ECG is the simplest and most accurate method of arrhythmia diagnosis, although an astute examiner can sometimes make a specific diagnosis of a rhythm disorder by examining the radial pulse, the jugular venous pulsations, and the quality of the heart sound. In some cases, further investigations, by intracardiac electrophysiologic studies, may be necessary before a definite diagnosis can be established. Any deviation from the arbitrarily set sinus rhythm of 60 to 100 beats/min is considered to be an arrhythmia; however, some arrhythmias are considered to be usual elements of a normal heart, such as sinus arrhythmia or sinus tachycardia.

Atrial premature beats can be seen in an otherwise normal heart. If they are frequent, they may indicate atrial disease, electrolyte imbalance, pulmonary disease, or congestive heart failure, and may precipitate atrial fibrillation.

Junctional premature beats, when seen in normal individuals, have no clinical significance. Frequent junctional premature beats may be associated with digitalis toxicity, myocardial infarction, or the mechanical stimulation of the bundle of His by a prosthetic tricuspid valve. Occasionally, junctional extrasystoles are concealed and may cause unexpected conduction prolongation or nonconduction, mimicking first-degree AV block or second-degree AV block, types I and II.

Ventricular premature beats may be considered benign if they are seen in a healthy young individual without other evidence of cardiac disease. They may herald ventricular tachycardia or fibrillation, especially if they are seen in a setting of myocardial ischemia, severe heart disease, or acute myocardial infarction, in all of which the ventricular fibrillatory threshold is lowered. When three or more ventricular extrasystoles are present, the condition is commonly designated ventricular tachycardia. In the presence of organic heart disease, usually coronary artery disease, any of these arrhythmias increases the risk of sudden death.

Atrial tachycardia. In this arrhythmia an atrial ectopic focus beats at a rate of 100 to 250 beats/min. When the rhythm is the result of digitalis toxicity, triggered activity is thought to be the mechanism and the ECG is typical: P waves that are similar to those in sinus rhythm (P axis superior-inferior), 2:1 block, and ventriculophasic PP intervals. In chronic pulmonary disease the atrial tachycardia is commonly multifocal (chaotic atrial tachycardia).

Atrial fibrillation is the most common sustained atrial arrhythmia. Its presence frequently indicates organic heart disease, usually mitral valve disease or coronary artery disease. Although the diagnosis can be suspected because of an irregular pulse, an electrocardiogram is essential for an accurate diagnosis. Frequent premature beats can mimic the pulse of atrial fibrillation, while a regular pulse may be seen in atrial fibrillation with a high degree of AV block. This latter condition may indicate digitalis excess. See discussion later in the chapter of atrial fibrillation in WPW syndrome.

Atrial flutter is another common atrial arrhythmia that usually indicates the presence of organic heart disease. It is frequently seen in acute pericarditis.

Paroxysmal supraventricular tachycardia (PSVT) is sometimes referred to as "reciprocating"; it may be initiated by a premature atrial, junctional, or even ventricular beat. This form of tachycardia is commonly sustained by a reentry mechanism within the AV node (AV nodal reentry) or by an AV reentry mechanism using two anatomically separate pathways—the AV node and an accessory pathway (circus movement tachycardia). AV nodal reentry may be seen in otherwise healthy young people who are free of significant heart disease. However, when an accessory pathway forms part of the reentry circuit, recurring, persistent tachycardia may develop; this condition may be very debilitating and may precipitate atrial fibrillation or flutter. If the effective refractory period of the accessory pathway is short, the resulting rapid ventricular response to the atrial fibrillation may deteriorate into ventricular fibrillation.

Junctional rhythms that exceed 60 beats/min but are less than 100 beats/min are referred to as accelerated rhythms, which are one of the common causes of AV dissociation, especially in the clinical setting of acute myocardial infarction, acute myocarditis, or digitalis excess. If this ectopic rhythm exceeds 100 beats/min, the condition is called junctional tachycardia. This condition, the result of enhanced automaticity, must be differentiated from PSVT, which results from a reentry mechanism.

Ventricular tachycardia is rarely seen in an otherwise normal heart. Since it usually indicates severe heart disease, it requires prompt and accurate diagnosis and treatment. Occasionally, ventricular tachycardia cannot be distinguished from supraventricular tachycardia on the surface electrocardiogram, especially when there is preexisting bundle branch block or concealed WPW syndrome. In such a situation, if permitted by the clinical setting, an intracardiac ECG provides a definitive diagnosis.

Ventricular fibrillation is the end stage of severe organic heart disease, but it can also be induced by drugs (such as digitalis), electrolyte abnormalities (marked hypokalemia and marked hypomagnesemia), or electrocution. Ventricular fibrillation is the most common immediate cause of sudden death. This extreme rhythm disorder permits no effective cardiac output. Irreversible brain damage and subsequent death result if effective resuscitative measures are not instituted in 3 to 5 minutes. As a rule, one should not wait to make an electrocardiographic diagnosis of ventricular fibrillation *before* instituting such measures.

Sinoatrial (SA) block and sinus arrest are relatively rare arrhythmias. A marked increase in vagal tone can cause sinus arrest and prolonged asystole. Extreme fright, a hypersensitive carotid sinus, and an exaggerated diving reflex are some of the causes of this increase. Atropine administration is effective therapy, but in recurrent cases pacing may be a necessity. Airway obstruction and hypoxia—as in sleep apnea syndrome (see Chapter 14)—are another cause of SA block and sinus arrest. Inflammatory or ischemic involvement of the SA node can cause SA block, but in such a setting an escape junctional or ventricular rhythm frequently emerges.

Atrioventricular (AV) block

The ECG can be diagnostic of AV block as long as certain considerations are observed. Care should be taken not to confuse physiologic refractoriness with pathologic AV block and thus run the risk of overdiagnosing and overtreating the patient. Before nonconduction is diagnosed, one should make sure that the opportunity to conduct is present, by noting the R-P intervals, heart rate, and the possibility of concealed junctional or fascicular extrasystoles.

First-degree AV block may be secondary to increased parasympathetic tone, or may reflect digitalis excess, myocarditis, or infiltration of the myocardium by tumor or amyloid. By itself, first-degree

AV block causes no hemodynamic compromise and warrants no treatment.

Second-degree AV block is present when one or more, but not all, atrial impulses fail to reach the ventricles because of impaired conduction. Second-degree AV block can be of two types. In type I (Wenckebach) there is progressive prolongation of the P-R interval preceding a nonconducted P wave; in type II the P-R interval is constant.

Type I second-degree AV block can be benign, resulting from a marked increase in parasympathetic tone. When seen in trained athletes or only during sleep, it can be a normal finding. Digitalis excess and diaphragmatic myocardial infarction are common pathologic causes.

Type II second-degree AV block is indicative of organic heart disease; frequently it indicates involvement of the His-Purkinje system. Common causes are anteroseptal myocardial infarction and degenerative or infiltrative disease of the myocardium. Pacemakers are commonly necessary.

Third-degree or complete AV block is present when the opportunity for conduction exists but conduction does not take place. Thus, before this diagnosis can be made numerous factors must be taken into consideration, including the refractoriness of the AV junction, autonomic influences, drugs, the atrial rate, the ventricular rate, and the level of the escape pacemaker.

Complete AV block is usually caused by degenerative disease of the conduction system. Coronary artery disease is the second most common cause, and it can also be seen in traumatic or inflammatory disease or drug toxicity. Newly acquired complete AV block in adults usually causes significant hemodynamic impairment and can cause syncope (Stokes-Adams syndrome) or death. As a rule, dual chamber pacemakers are used in all adult patients. In congenital complete heart block with stable, narrow QRS complexes and an adequate ventricular rate, a pacemaker may not be necessary if close follow-up care is available.

Bundle-branch block

The ECG is diagnostic of right bundle-branch block and hemiblock. In the presence of left bundle-branch block, a diagnosis of myocardial infarction or ventricular hypertrophy may be difficult or impossible to make. Right bundle-branch block does not mask a diagnosis of myocardial infarction and may be the clue to silent coronary artery disease. It is commonly seen postoperatively, especially after repair of ventricular septal defect, or in the presence of atrial septal defect. Bifascicular block (right bundle-branch block and left anterior hemiblock or left posterior hemiblock) in the presence of acute myocardial infarction usually indicates massive myocardial damage with a poor prognosis. Although pacemakers have been used electively (or prophylactically) in these patients, their use has not substantially improved survival. In chronic bifascicular block, pacemakers are effective in preventing recurrences of syncope caused by intermittent second-degree or complete heart block.

Wolff-Parkinson-White (WPW) syndrome

The ECG is diagnostic of overt WPW syndrome during sinus rhythm. However, the diagnosis of a concealed or a latent accessory pathway is only made during arrhythmias or with electrophysiologic studies. In this condition congenital defects exist in the form of extra muscular tracts (accessory pathways) between the atria and the ventricles. Such tracts provide an anatomic link for AV reentry tachycardia, which may be precipitated by either atrial or ventricular premature beats. If conduction during atrial fibrillation occurs exclusively over an accessory pathway with a short refractory period, the ventricular rates can be very high (160-300 beats/min) and the rhythm may degenerate into ventricular fibrillation. The classical ECG features of the originally described syndrome are a short PR interval and a broad QRS complex. Other features are a delta wave (the initial slurring of the QRS), secondary T-wave changes, and abnormal Q waves. It is important to note, however, that the ECG may be completely normal, or show only minimal preexcitation, in the presence of an accessory pathway, and yet the patient may be subject to the same life-threatening arrhythmias as in the overt syndrome.

Effects of drugs and electrolytes on the electrocardiogram (see Table 4-1)

Digitalis, which is commonly used in patients with heart disease, can mimic many of the diagnostic changes of the ECG. It is important to be familiar with the usual electrocardiographic abnormalities produced by this drug. In usual therapeutic doses digitalis causes sagging

Table 4-1 Effects of drugs and electrolytes on the electrocardiogram

Drug or electrolyte	PR	QRS	Q-T_c	Sinus rate	Waveform changes
Amiodarone	0	0	+	—	
Aprindine	+	+	+	−	
Atropine	−	0	0	+	T changes
Bretylium tosylate	Sl+	0	0	—	
Daunomycin	0	0	0	0	−QRS voltage; ST-T changes
Digitalis	+	0	−	−	ST sags; T flattens
Diltiazem	+	0	0	−	
Disopyramide	0	Sl+	+	Sl+	
Doxorubicin HCl	0	0	0	0	−QRS voltage
Encainide	+	+	Sl+	0	
Ethmozin	Sl+	Sl+	Sl−	Sl−	
Excess calcium	Sl+	Sl+	−	0	T widens and rounds
Excess potassium	+	+	0	0	P widens; ST depresses; T wave, tall and peaked
Deficient calcium	0	0	+	0	
Deficient potassium	0	Sl+	0	0	U prominent; ST sags; T notches, then inverts
Imipramine HCl	Sl+	Sl+	Sl+	Sl+	T changes
Lithium	0	0	0	*	T flattens
Minoxidil	0	0	0	0	T changes; +QRS voltage
Phenothiazines	0	0	+	0	T changes
Phenytoin	Sl−	Sl−	Sl−	0	
Procainamide	Sl+/−	+	+	0	ST-T changes
Propranolol (and other beta blockers)	Sl+	0	Sl−	−	T changes
Quinidine	Sl+/−	+	+	0	ST depresses; T flattens or inverts; U wave
Tocainide	0	0	0	Sl−	
Verapamil	+	0	0	−	

0 = no significant change; + = increase; − = decrease; Sl+ = slight increase; Sl− = slight decrease; * = rarely, sinus arrest.

of the ST segment with flattening of the T waves, shortening of the Q-T interval, and slight prolongation of the P-R interval (Table 4-1). In the presence of atrial fibrillation, digitalis also slows the ventricular rate. In digitalis excess the following arrhythmias are commonly noted: marked P-R prolongation, second- and third-degree AV block, junctional extrasystoles, sinus bradycardia, accelerated junctional rhythm, and atrial tachycardia with AV block. Digitalis toxicity should be strongly suspected in the presence of bigeminal ventricular extrasystoles, multifocal ventricular extrasystoles, pairs of ventricular extrasystoles, or runs of ventricular tachycardia. In the presence of atrial fibrillation, digitalis excess may produce a regular pulse because of high-degree AV block and/or an accelerated junctional focus. Arrhythmias suggesting digitalis toxicity appear earlier if there is concurrent potassium and/or magnesium depletion.

Quinidine in therapeutic doses can cause prolongation of the Q-T interval, with widening and notching of the P waves. There could be some depression of the ST segment and flattening or inversion of the T waves. When therapeutic levels in the blood are exceeded, the toxic effects noted are varying degrees of AV block, widening of the QRS complexes over 50% of normal, and ventricular arrhythmias, including ventricular tachycardia (torsades de pointes) or fibrillation. Ventricular tachycardia or fibrillation can occur in the absence of drug toxicity. Usually, marked Q-T prolongation or U waves precede the onset of the characteristic arrhythmias ("torsades de pointes"). Ventricular tachycardia or fibrillation secondary to marked Q-T prolongation can also be caused by procainamide (Pronestyl), disopyramide (Norpace), and amiodarone (Cordarone).

Propranolol (Inderal), metoprolol (Lopressor), nadolol (Corgard), and atenolol (Tenormin) belong to the group of drugs known as *beta blockers*. These drugs slow the sinus rate, producing sinus bradycardia with slight PR prolongation. The Q-T interval is shortened, and the T wave may remain normal or be slightly higher (Table 4-1). In atrial fibrillation, beta blockers slow the ventricular response.

Phenytoin (Dilantin) is used in the treatment of digitalis toxicity. This drug shortens the P-R and Q-T intervals without having a significant effect on the QRS complex (Table 4-1). This characteristic of phenytoin makes it the drug of choice in the treatment of digitalis toxicity in the presence of prolongation of the P-R interval or first- or second-degree AV block.

Disopyramide (Norpace), like quinidine, in high doses may cause prolongation of the P wave, QRS complex, and P-R interval.

Lidocaine has little effect on the ECG. Studies have shown increased conduction delay in ischemic tissue without any effect on normal tissue.

Verapamil (Isoptin, Calan) is a calcium channel blocking agent with important antiarrhythmic properties. Verapamil produces a dose-related block at the AV node; it is therefore used in the treatment of paroxysmal supraventricular tachycardia. Verapamil also slows the ventricular rate in atrial fibrillation in the absence of WPW syndrome and can cause various degrees of AV block. It does not alter the rest of the ECG. *Diltiazem (Cardizem)* is another calcium channel blocking agent; its action on the AV node is similar to that of verapamil.

Lithium in therapeutic doses can cause flattening and inversion of the T waves. Sinus node dysfunction with SA block can result from lithium treatment, usually when a lithium compound is given in toxic doses.

Hyperkalemia is reflected in the electrocardiogram in the following manner: The first electrocardiographic manifestation of hyperkalemia occurs when blood concentrations of potassium enter the range of 5.5 to 6.5 mEq/L. At this level the T waves become characteristically tall and peaked. With further elevations in the plasma potassium concentration, there is a decreased amplitude of the R waves, with increased S waves, S-T depressions, and prolongation of the QRS duration and the P-R interval. When the plasma potassium concentration exceeds 7.5 mEq/L, intraatrial conduction disturbances develop and are reflected in broad, low-amplitude P waves and P-R interval prolongation. At still higher potassium levels, the P wave disappears altogether, and the QRS becomes markedly widened and moves into a smooth diphasic (sine) wave. The final stage, if the hyperkalemia is untreated, consists of ventricular tachycardia, flutter, fibrillation, and standstill.

Hypokalemia initially causes an apparent prolongation of the Q-T interval. This results from the appearance of a U wave that merges with the T wave and may cause notching of the T wave. T-wave inversion follows, and then sagging of the ST segment. Ventricular arrhythmias—premature beats, torsades de pointes, and fibrillation—may occur. The administration of potassium reverses these changes rapidly.

Hypercalcemia characteristically shortens the ST segment of the Q-T interval and may also widen and cause a rounding of the T waves.

Hypocalcemia causes a prolongation of the Q-T interval.

Hypermagnesemia can cause P-R prolongation and intraventricular conduction delay, with QRS widening. These changes may occur at magnesium levels of 10 mEq/L. Complete heart block, cardiac arrest, and asystole may occur if the plasma magnesium concentration exceeds 15 mEq/L. Such elevations are rarely seen in clinical medicine.

Hypomagnesemia can cause P-R prolongation, broadening and lowering of T waves, and Q-T prolongation. These changes may resemble the changes of hypokalemia and may be secondary to intracellular potassium depletion. Ventricular premature beats, ventricular tachycardia (torsades de pointes), and ventricular fibrillation can also occur.

Computer interpretation of the electrocardiogram

Computer assistance in the interpretation of electrocardiograms is available. Several programs now in use provide immediate interpretation and facilitate preparation of final written reports. Computer programs are excellent in differentiating normal from abnormal tracings and in listing the abnormalities present in a tracing. The limitations of these programs include difficulty in recognizing artifacts, generally poor performance in the diagnosis of complex arrhythmias, and the ability to do serial comparisons easily. Improvements in these areas are expected. Computer ECG interpretations are always checked by physicians.

NURSING ALERT

A *normal electrocardiogram does not rule out severe organic heart disease*. Severe obstructive disease of all major coronary arteries without myocardial infarction or active ischemia of the heart is one situation that could exist in spite of a perfectly normal electrocardiogram.

A *definitely abnormal electrocardiogram does not necessarily signify heart disease*. Many abnormalities, even pronounced, can result from CNS lesions or autonomic influences, or can be produced by drugs, electrolytes, or other causes.

Electrocardiographic interpretations should be made in the context of the clinical situation. Serious errors will be made if the clinical data are not used in interpreting an electrocardiogram.

The limitations of the standard resting electrocardiogram should be recognized. It is at most a 1-minute record of the heart's electrical activity, and it is recorded at rest, without stressing the heart. Whenever necessary, further tests should be used, such as the Holter monitor for arrhythmia diagnosis or stress electrocardiography for diagnosis of coronary artery disease. These will be discussed in the following sections.

AMBULATORY ELECTROCARDIOGRAPHY (HOLTER MONITORING)

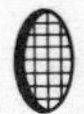

EXPLANATION OF THE TEST

Ambulatory electrocardiography is an extension of the resting electrocardiogram. A portable recorder is worn by the patient, and the electrocardiogram is recorded continuously on magnetic tape during unrestricted activity. The tapes are scanned rapidly by electrocardioscanners, and abnormalities or selected areas of interest are printed out in real time. Computers and microprocessors are utilized in the rapid processing of tapes. This permits detailed and quantitative analysis of the data.

This technique can be extended to prolonged monitoring of patients from their homes, using telemetry transmissions and telephone lines. Such technical advances now permit continuous ECG monitoring of patients for days and weeks while they are at home and engaged in unrestricted activity.

VALUE AND LIMITATIONS OF THE TEST

Permits a much larger sample of the heart's electrical activity to be recorded than is possible with the usual resting ECG. This procedure samples 50,000 to 100,000 beats on a 10- to 24-hour record.

Records resting, unrestricted activity, and sleep recordings.

Arrhythmias, as well as episodes of ischemia (ST segment shifts), can be diagnosed, even if the patient is totally asymptomatic.

An invaluable diagnostic tool when a patient is complaining of dizziness, syncope, or palpitations. If the rhythm disorder and the symptoms are shown to be coincident, an exact diagnosis can be made.

Especially useful in monitoring a patient discharged from the hospital soon after a complicated myocardial infarction.

An excellent means of detecting adverse effects of antiarrhythmic agents as well as confirming if the agent is effective in suppressing a given arrhythmia. Antiarrhythmic agents can aggravate preexisting arrhythmias or precipitate new arrhythmias.

Useful in the diagnosis of ischemic heart disease and the evaluation of the effectiveness of therapy.

The record is generally not available to the physician for 24 hours. A system has recently been developed to permit earlier or real-time transmission of the ECG signal to a monitoring station, using telephone lines.

There is a potential for misdiagnosis (failure to recognize artifacts) or overdiagnosis (detection of benign arrhythmias) with the subsequent initiation of unnecessary and potentially hazardous therapy.

NURSING ACTION

1. Explain the procedure to the patient and demonstrate how to wear the recorder and how to position it during sleep.
2. Apply the electrodes and attach the electrode cables to the monitor tape recorder (make sure there is a fully charged battery in the unit).
3. Test the unit by connecting the recorder to a standard electrocardiograph and observe for artifacts while the patient sits, stands, etc.
4. Instruct the patient in the use of the diary and demonstrate a sample one. Instruct him or her in correlating symptoms with the arrhythmias.
5. Show the patient how to use the marker button.
6. Encourage the patient to pursue all the usual daily activities *except* bathing, showering, or swimming. The monitor must not get wet.

7. Instruct the patient to avoid magnets, metal detectors, and high voltage areas. Tell the patient how to check the recorder for proper functioning and how to reattach loose electrodes.
8. Note in the diary if electrical gadgets such as blankets, toothbrushes, and the like are being used. They produce artifacts on the ECG tape.

INTERFERING FACTORS

Electric blankets
Electric toothbrushes

CLINICAL IMPLICATIONS

Clinical implications are the same as for the standard ECG (p. 101).

EXERCISE ELECTROCARDIOGRAPHY

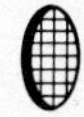

EXPLANATION OF THE TEST

This test consists of gradual increments of the level of exercise on a motorized treadmill or bicycle ergometer while the ECG is being monitored. Various investigators have proposed protocols for gradually increasing the workload. The most widely used is that of Robert Bruce. In addition to monitoring heart rate, blood pressure, and heart electrical activity during exercise, expired gases can be collected, oxygen consumption and saturation monitored, and samples collected for blood gas determinations at key points during exercise in an attempt to physiologically define the causes of the patient's symptoms.

VALUE AND LIMITATIONS OF THE TEST

Aids in the diagnosis of coronary artery disease when the resting ECG is normal.
Permits suspected arrhythmias to be safely provoked during exercise in a controlled setting.
Useful in the evaluation of a patient's functional capacity or "physical fitness."
Useful in evaluating the effectiveness of therapy, including drugs or surgery (e.g., coronary artery angioplasty or bypass surgery), and in prescribing rehabilitative exercise.

Obtains an objective evaluation of a patient's disability when the history is confusing or difficult to obtain.

A combined cardiopulmonary exercise test is valuable in patients with heart and lung disease or when the presenting problem is effort dyspnea or fatigue with no clear cause.

The value of the test is limited by the frequency of false-positive and false-negative ECGs in the diagnosis of ischemic heart disease. This frequency is reduced by myocardial perfusion imaging using thallium 201a following exercise (see discussion later in the chapter). Also, computer analysis of an exercise ECG may improve its diagnostic accuracy.

NURSING ACTION

1. Take all the steps necessary before and during the test to reduce risks (1 death in 10,000 tests) by assuring that (a) a history and physical examination has been performed before the test, (b) a recent resting ECG has been done and is on the patient's chart, (c) the test is carefully monitored, and (d) all personnel are familiar with resuscitative equipment.
2. Instruct the patient that he or she may have a light meal, and should not smoke or drink beverages with caffeine or alcohol for 2 hours before the test.
3. Advise the patient to wear loose clothing and comfortable shoes.
4. Explain the nature of the test to the patient and make sure that the patient understands that he or she may stop the test if extreme fatigue or chest pain develops.
5. Informed consent is not routinely obtained but is advisable in high-risk patients.
6. Tell the patient to continue medications unless otherwise specified by the physician ordering the test.
7. Note the patient's drug history immediately before testing, since nitroglycerin and other coronary dilators enable a patient with coronary artery disease to perform at a higher level of exercise and may result in the production of fewer arrhythmias. The decision to stop some or all medications for a stress test must be individualized.

INTERFERING FACTORS

Digitalis and electrolyte abnormalities (may mimic an abnormal response)

Nitroglycerin and other coronary dilators (may mask an ischemic response)

Beta blockers (prevent maximal heart rate and may mask an underlying ischemic response)

CLINICAL IMPLICATIONS

Maximal oxygen consumption. This can be estimated from the minutes of exercise (given a standard load).

Myocardial work. The heart rate and blood pressure achieved at each stage of exercise are multiplied to provide a good approximation of myocardial work. An inappropriate increase or decrease in heart rate or blood pressure during exercise can be important clues to cardiac dysfunction.

Myocardial ischemia. The degree and duration of ST depression relate to myocardial ischemia.

Arrhythmias. Those provoked during exercise or during the recovery period can be evaluated.

Patients commonly perform better on a second test because of familiarity with the procedure. Usually this learning does not progress from a second to a third test.

NURSING ALERT

Discontinue the test for any of the following reasons:

1. Systolic blood pressure of over 220 to 230 mm Hg.
2. Fall in systolic blood pressure of 10 mm Hg or more during exercise.
3. Appearance of certain arrhythmias such as ventricular tachycardia, bradycardia, or heart block.
4. ST depression or elevation of 2 mm or more.
5. Loss of consciousness, angina, vertigo, syncope, inappropriate shortness of breath, muscle weakness, fatigue, or intermittent claudication.

Be alert to the following complications:

Be alert to the development of complications that may necessitate hospitalization (0.2%) such as myocardial infarction, prolonged bouts of chest pain, severe arrhythmias, and hypotensive and hypertensive episodes.

Be aware that false-negative results, even when maximal heart rate is achieved, may be seen in 25% of patients with coronary artery disease. Coronary occlusion and myocardial infarction can occur in patients whose maximal exercise ECG was normal days or weeks before the insult.

Be alert to the ECG effect of digitalis, electrolyte abnormalities, cardiomyopathies, left ventricular hypertrophy, and left bundle-branch block, since these may result in a false-positive test.

Be aware that the test is contraindicated in patients with acute cardiac illness (e.g., acute myocardial infarction or myocarditis), severe uncontrolled arrhythmias, uncompensated congestive heart failure, critical aortic stenosis, and drug toxicity.

Be aware that the physician will avoid ordering the test for patients with acute coronary insufficiency or unstable angina. (In such cases where the diagnosis is in doubt, coronary arteriography may be the diagnostic test of choice.)

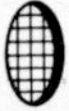

VECTORCARDIOGRAPHY

EXPLANATION OF THE TEST

The vectorcardiogram displays all of the electrical forces generated in the heart at any given instant, plotting voltage against voltage in three dimensions.

VALUE OF THE TEST

Reinforces our understanding of the scalar ECG.

Determines the cause of slowing of electrical waveforms.

Establishes the differential diagnosis between inferior wall myocardial infarction and left anterior hemiblock.

Differentiates right bundle-branch block from right ventricular hypertrophy.

Helpful in detecting left ventricular hypertrophy in the presence of left bundle-branch block.

NURSING ACTION

1. Instruct the patient that he or she may eat and drink before the test.

2. Explain the procedure to the patient. Make sure that the patient understands that the test is similar to a routine ECG and is safe and painless.
3. Explain that the electrodes will be applied to the back as well as to positions on the precordium.

INTERFERING FACTORS

Incorrect placement of electrodes

Excessive patient movement during the test

Heavy body build, which may simulate right ventricular hypertrophy

PACEMAKER EVALUATION

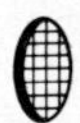

EXPLANATION OF THE TEST

The purpose of pacemaker evaluation is to assess the electrical function of the unit and detect malfunctions and imminent power-source depletion. This is done by means of an electrocardiograph equipped with an electronic interval counter, which measures the pulse interval and duration. The pulse interval or the pulse generator rate can be transmitted over the telephone.

VALUE OF THE TEST

Obtains the longest possible use of a pacemaker pulse generator without exposing the patient to the risk of pacemaker failure.

Detects early failure of a pacemaker battery and avoids unnecessary replacement of a well-functioning unit.

NURSING ACTION

1. See the section on electrocardiography for nursing implications of the test.
2. Inform the patient regarding the following:
   a. Identification should be worn at all times.
   b. Pressure over the insertion area should be avoided.
   c. Clothing should fit loosely over the implant.
   d. Medical proof of an implanted pacemaker needs to be shown when passing through monitoring devices, such as those in airports.

ROUTINE RADIOGRAPHIC EXAMINATION OF THE HEART

EXPLANATION OF THE TEST

Routine radiographic examination of the heart constitutes four projections—posterior-anterior (PA), lateral, and right and left oblique (Figs. 4-3 to 4-6).

VALUE AND LIMITATIONS OF THE TEST

The chest x-ray examination and the cardiac series are used almost as extensions of the physical examination.

Valuable when calcification of various parts of the heart is suspected.

Provides valuable information about the size and contour of the cardiac chambers.

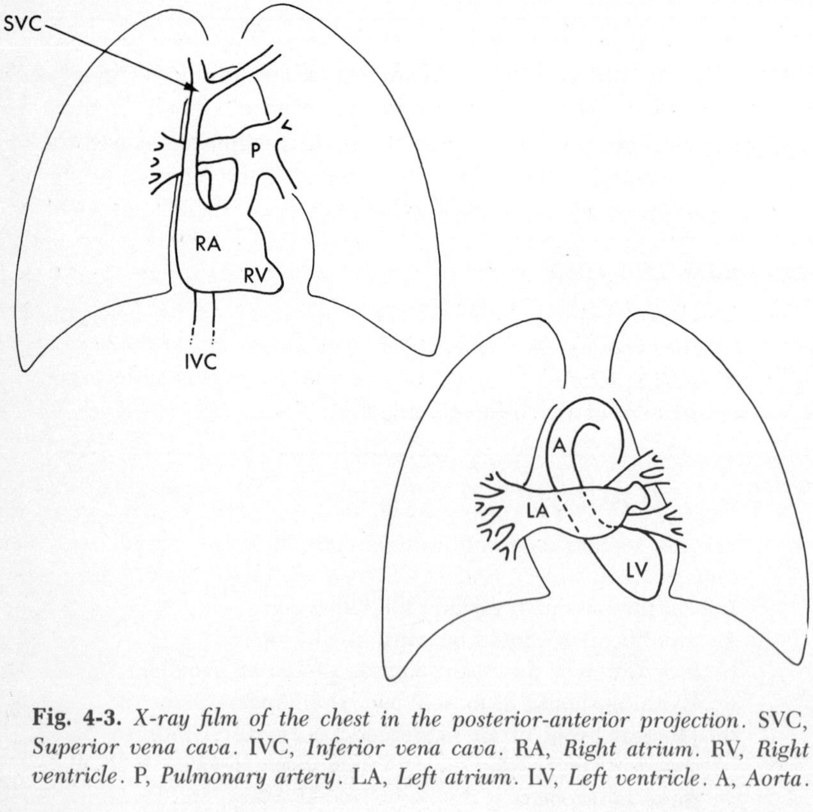

Fig. 4-3. *X-ray film of the chest in the posterior-anterior projection.* SVC, *Superior vena cava.* IVC, *Inferior vena cava.* RA, *Right atrium.* RV, *Right ventricle.* P, *Pulmonary artery.* LA, *Left atrium.* LV, *Left ventricle.* A, *Aorta.*

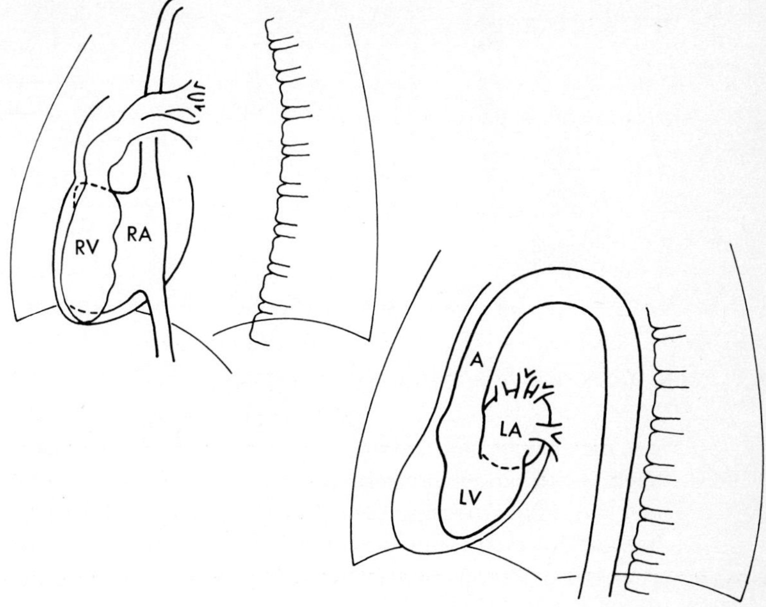

Fig. 4-4. *X-ray film of the chest in the left lateral projection.*

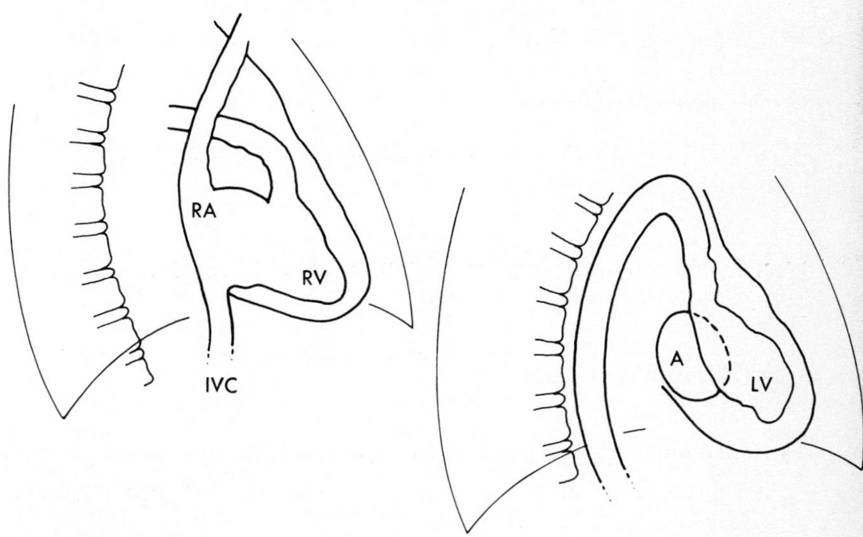

Fig. 4-5. *X-ray film of the chest in the right anterior oblique projection.*

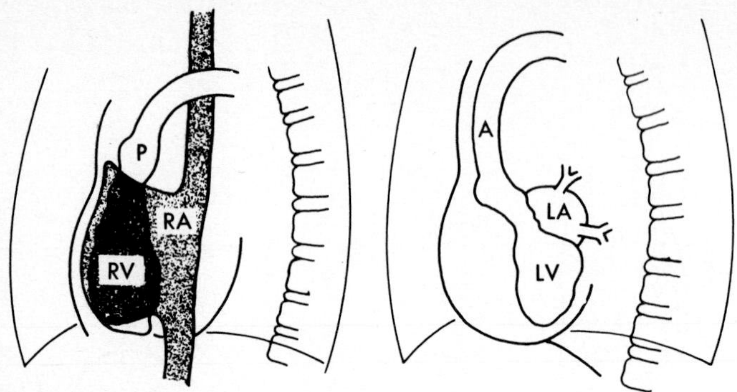

Fig. 4-6. *X-ray film of the chest in the left anterior oblique projection.*

Anatomic changes and enlargement of individual chambers can be seen in the various projections.

The test is limited because the dynamic aspects of the working heart are not detected. Thus the heart can appear perfectly normal on chest x-ray examination in the presence of severe organic heart disease.

The accuracy of x-ray detection of cardiac enlargement is diminished by variations of heart size in systole as compared with diastole.

Diagnostic errors can result either from the recording technique or from the interpretation of the information.

A portable chest x-ray examination cannot be used to assess cardiac size, although it can be helpful in assessing the degree of pulmonary congestion.

NURSING ACTION

1. Instruct patient to remove jewelry and other metal objects and don a hospital gown, removing other clothing above the waist.
2. No other special preparation is necessary.

INTERFERING FACTORS

Films exposed during expiration may produce a false impression of an enlarged heart and pulmonary vascular congestion.

Films of obese persons may also give the impression of an enlarged heart; the diaphragm is high and there is excessive pericardial fat.

Overpenetration of x-rays may cause the disappearance of pulmonary vascular markings.

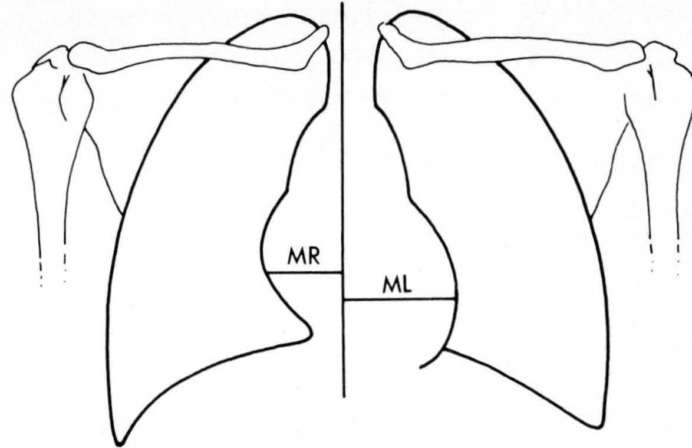

Fig. 4-7. *The cardiothoracic ratio, which is derived by adding the midright (MR) and midleft (ML) measurements. The sum is then divided by the longest transverse diameter of the chest.*

Rotation of a patient may produce a false appearance of enlargement or may result in the magnification of various vessels.

In the presence of pectus excavatum deformity of the chest, the heart may be displaced posteriorly, producing a false impression of cardiomegaly.

In pectus carinatum deformity of the chest, the anterior-posterior diameter is increased and possible enlargement of the right ventricle may go undetected.

Patients with a straight dorsal spine may appear to have cardiomegaly, especially in a lateral projection.

In patients with severe kyphoscoliosis, accurate assessment of cardiac size and pulmonary vasculature may be impossible.

CLINICAL IMPLICATIONS

The cardiothoracic ratio

The simplest and most frequently used measurement of the heart is the cardiothoracic ratio. This ratio is obtained by first adding the longest distance from the midline of the chest to the right side of the heart and the longest distance from the midline to the left side of the heart (Fig. 4-7). This transverse diameter of the heart is then divided by the longest transverse diameter of the chest to arrive at a cardiothoracic ratio. This is a relatively crude way of assessing cardiac size, but because the cardiothoracic ratio is easily obtained, it is commonly used. Generally, a cardiothoracic ratio over 50% is considered indicative of cardiac enlargement. Some reasonable assessment of individual chamber enlargement can be made from inspection of the plain chest film in the PA and lateral projections.

Inspection of the lung fields

One looks for overcirculation or undercirculation, pulmonary vein patterns, and edema.

An observation of overcirculation or undercirculation of the lung fields is most helpful in the differential diagnosis of congenital heart diseases. In the presence of a left-to-right shunt there are signs of increased circulation in the pulmonary vessels; in the presence of a right-to-left shunt there is evidence of undercirculation.

The patterns of the pulmonary veins, their size and prominence, as well as the presence or absence of pulmonary lymphatic markings, help in the diagnosis of elevated pulmonary venous pressure, which is a common sign of congestive heart failure.

Pulmonary edema can be of two kinds, alveolar and interstitial. Alveolar edema is characteristic of acute left-sided heart failure and is manifested by bilateral confluent densities that start centrally and spread peripherally. This is commonly referred to as the *butterfly-wing pattern*. In interstitial edema, fluid accumulates in the interstitial tissues of the lungs and produces a generalized haziness and clouding of the vascular shadows. When such fluid collects in the interlobular septa of the lung, septal lines are formed that are referred to as *Kerley's lines*.

Inspection of the pleural spaces

Approximately 250 ml of pleural effusion is necessary for an accurate radiologic diagnosis. Pleural effusion is usually manifested as blunting of the costophrenic angle. Larger effusions, 1 liter or more, can also accumulate; such an effusion may be an accompaniment of congestive heart failure, or it may be independent of heart disease and indicate the presence of lung disease. Occasionally, pleural effusions are hidden under the lung (subpulmonic effusion) and therefore do not obliterate the costophrenic angle. Such effusions can be detected by obtaining film with the patient in the lateral position (lateral decubitus film). Pleural fluid examination is discussed in Chapter 6.

Inspection of the rib cage

Inspection of the rib cage may provide a clue to the existence of coarctation of the aorta, in which condition collateral circulation from enlarged intercostal arteries would produce characteristic deformity or notching of the rib margins.

Cardiac series

The ability to make an accurate diagnosis of the enlargement of a specific chamber is enhanced by obtaining a cardiac series, in which a bolus of barium is swallowed by the patient, opacifying the posterior-lying esophagus. In addition to the PA and lateral films, two oblique films are obtained. In a cardiac series an enlarged left atrium or even an enlarged aorta could be noted because it would displace the barium-filled esophagus (Fig. 4-8). This, along with additional projections, would aid in the diagnosis of left or right ventricular enlargement.

Cardiac fluoroscopy

Cardiac fluoroscopy is most useful in detecting calcifications of various parts of the heart. Introduction of image intensifiers has decreased the overall radiation hazard of this test and has improved the quality of the images. Cardiac fluoroscopy is also useful in detecting calcification in the coronary artery system. Although the diagnostic method of choice for detection and semiquantitation of coronary artery disease is selective coronary arteriography, cardiac fluoroscopy is a useful *screening* tool for this purpose. Approximately 75% of patients with coronary artery disease have calcification of the coronary artery system, but 20% of patients (especially older patients) with no obstructive coronary disease also have calcification of the coronary arteries. Calcification of the various valves of the heart, specifically the aortic and mitral valves, is unequivocal evidence of disease of these valves. Although heavy calcification suggests more advanced disease of the valves (usually narrowing), an exact correlation cannot be made. Other cardiac diseases in which calcification is helpful in the diagnosis are tumors of the heart, constrictive pericarditis (evidenced by calcification of the pericardium), and old myocardial infarction or trauma (evidenced by calcification of the myocardium).

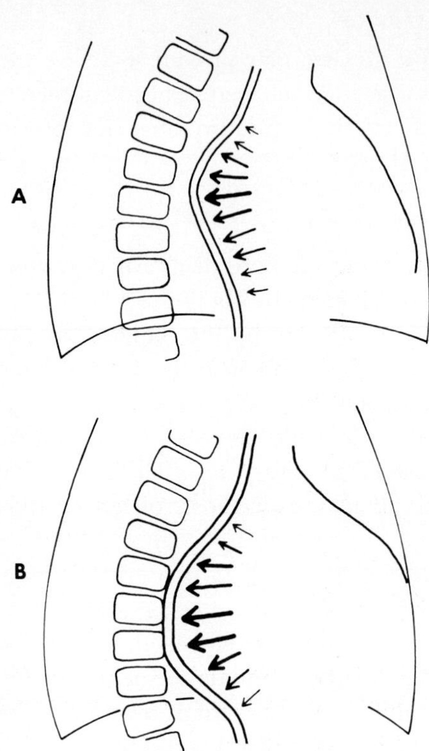

Fig. 4-8. *X-ray film of the chest obtained after a patient has swallowed barium (a "cardiac series"). Note the moderate,* **A,** *and marked,* **B,** *degrees of left atrial enlargement, which are reflected in the displacement of the atrium by the barium-filled esophagus. This is a right anterior oblique projection.*

NURSING ALERT

Protect yourself from scatter radiation since the risk of radiation increases with repeated exposures.

Be aware that this test is performed in young children and pregnant women only when absolutely necessary and should *not* be performed on pregnant women.

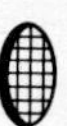

CARDIAC ENZYMES

PHYSIOLOGY

Enzymes are proteins that act as catalysts in chemical reactions. The blood levels of various enzymes are noted in the diagnosis of many pathologic states, one of which is acute myocardial infarction. Normally, these enzymes are present in the blood in small amounts. But following injury or infarction to an organ the levels of various enzymes increase in the blood, in proportion to the organ's enzyme content and the extent of injury. Different organs have different enzyme contents.

PATHOPHYSIOLOGY

Careful scrutiny of the pattern and time course of changes in enzyme levels in the blood can help to verify a diagnosis of acute myocardial infarction that is based on history and physical examination and an ECG. The pattern and time course of increases and decreases in enzyme levels following myocardial infarction are depicted in Fig. 4-9.

Enzyme level determinations also permit the diagnosis of an extension of an infarction or of a reinfarction. In addition, within certain limitations, the degree of elevation of enzyme levels correlates with the degree of myocardial injury.

Attempts have been made to use enzyme techniques in *quantitating* myocardial infarction and assessing the value of various treatment interventions. Most of these have remained research tools. Various enzymes have been used in the past in the diagnosis of myocardial infarction, but the discovery of the isoenzymes of creatine kinase (CK) and lactic dehydrogenase (LDH) has made the use of other enzymes obsolete. Work is in progress to further improve the laboratory diagnosis of acute myocardial infarction; this work involves the measurement of urinary and plasma levels of myoglobin and the use of highly sensitive assays for CK-MB and CK-BB fractions.

In the diagnosis of acute myocardial infarction, the clinical setting and time of presentation determine the significance of increases or decreases in the levels of the various enzymes. At one extreme, when the ECG shows unequivocal diagnostic features, enzyme level determinations may be superfluous. At the other extreme, when elec-

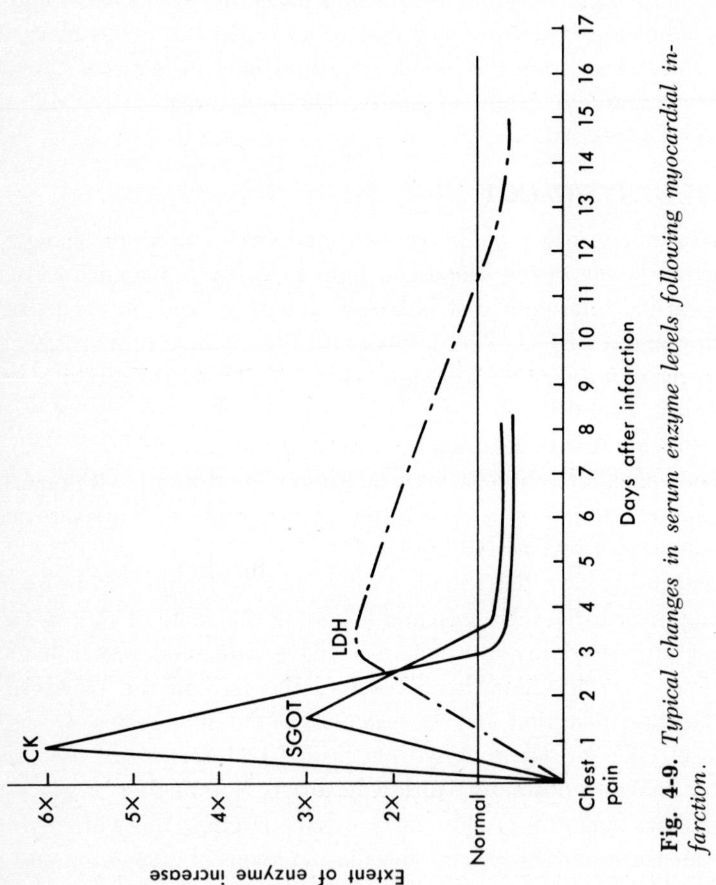

Fig. 4-9. *Typical changes in serum enzyme levels following myocardial infarction.*

trocardiographic changes are nondiagnostic, the levels of both CK and LDH isoenzymes may be monitored every 12 hours to make a specific diagnosis. In most hospitals, a cardiac enzyme *panel* includes determinations for CK and LDH and their isoenzymes.

CREATINE KINASE (CK) AND CK ISOENZYMES

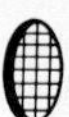

Adult normal

Male: 55-170 U/L at 37°C (SI units: 55-170 U/L at 37°C)
Female: 30-135 U/L at 37°C (SI units: 30-135 U/L at 37°C)

Pediatric

Newborn: 10-300 IU/L at 30°C
Child: Male: 0-70 IU/L at 30°C; *Female:* 0-50 IU/L at 30°C

EXPLANATION OF THE TEST

Measurement of serum levels of CK and its isoenzymes is a rapid, sensitive, and specific test for the diagnosis of acute myocardial infarction because the total CK activity in myocardial tissue is high and because one of the CK isoenzymes (MB) is found in significant amounts only in heart muscle. CK activity is greatest in skeletal muscle and second greatest in myocardium. The CK activity in brain, bladder, stomach, and colon is about half that in myocardium.

There are three known CK isoenzymes: MM, MB, and BB. Methods for measuring their levels are readily available. Heart muscle is the only tissue in which a significant fraction of the CK activity results from isoenzyme MB. The CK in skeletal muscle is over 98% MM but may contain some MB. Brain, bladder, stomach, and colon contain primarily isoenzyme BB (see Table 4-2).

Table 4-2 Tissue location of CK isoenzymes

CK isoenzyme	Tissue
BB	Brain, smooth muscle, thyroid, lung, prostate
MB	Cardiac muscle, tongue, diaphragm; trace amounts in skeletal muscle
MM	Skeletal muscle, cardiac muscle

VALUE AND LIMITATIONS OF THE TEST

Detection of early myocardial infarction and reinfarction.
Evaluation of causes of chest pain.
Monitoring for myocardial ischemia or injury after cardiac surgery, coronary angioplasty, or cardioversion.
Detection of skeletal muscular disorders and early dermatomyositis.
The CK-MM level, although sensitive to myocardial injury, is not specific for it, since the level can be elevated after trauma to any muscle.

NURSING ACTION

1. Instruct the patient that he or she may eat and drink before the test.
2. Inform the patient that this test will help to evaluate cellular function and that multiple blood samples are necessary.
3. Collect 5 ml of venous blood in a red-top tube.
4. Handle specimen gently and transport immediately to the laboratory to prevent hemolysis.

INTERFERING FACTORS

Drugs that increase CK levels: halothane, succinylcholine, alcohol, lithium, large doses of aminocaproic acid
Vigorous exercise
Intramuscular injections
Trauma: surgery, cardioversion, invasive diagnostic procedures, muscle massage, and severe coughing

CLINICAL IMPLICATIONS

Myocardial infarction

Following the onset of acute myocardial infarction, elevated CK-MB and total CK values are detected in the blood in 3 to 5 hours. At 6 to 12 hours more than 98% of patients with acute myocardial infarction will show an abnormal rise. In most of these patients, the high level will persist for about 24 hours. After 30 hours many persons who have had myocardial infarctions have no MB elevation. CK-MB levels at various hours after the onset of symptoms are shown in Fig. 4-10.

Eighty percent of myocardial CK consists of the MM fraction, which persists in the blood longer than the MB fraction. Therefore,

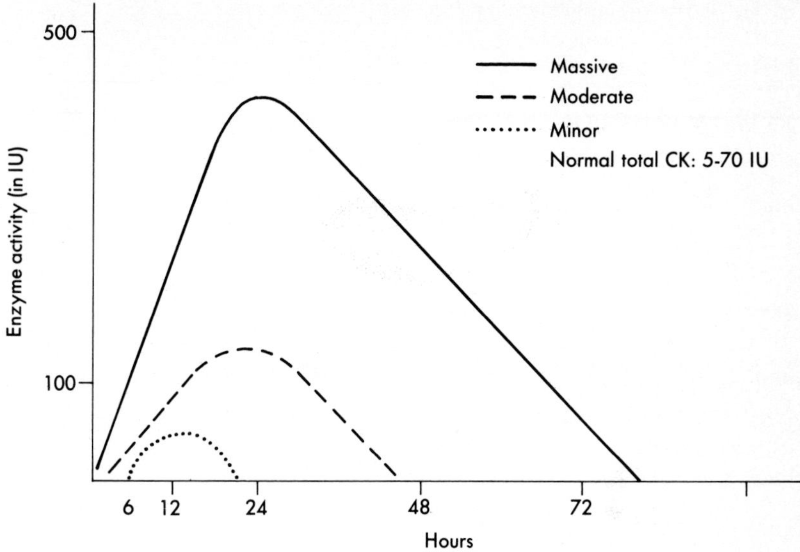

Fig. 4-10. *Typical curve of CK-MB levels after acute myocardial infarction.*

it is possible to have an elevated CK level, all MM fraction, secondary to myocardial infarction, especially if the sampling is done more than 24 hours after acute infarction.

Serial CK-MB determinations remain the best single laboratory aid to the *early* diagnosis of acute myocardial infarction. The CK-MB level may be elevated in Duchenne's muscular dystrophy, dermatomyositis, and polymyositis. The clinical distinction between acute myocardial infarction and one of these conditions should be relatively easy. Elevated CK-MB levels are occasionally seen in pericarditis, myocarditis, viral myositis, various myopathies, as well as sustained tachyarrhythmias and sustained vigorous exercise. The mechanism of elevated CK-MB in some of these conditions is not clear.

LACTIC DEHYDROGENASE (LDH) ISOENZYMES

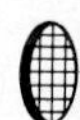

Adult reference range

LDH_1 18.1%-29% of total
LDH_2 29.4%-37.5% of total

LDH_3 18.8%-26% of total
LDH_4 9.2%-16.5% of total
LDH_5 5.3%-13.4% of total

EXPLANATION OF THE TEST

Five tissue-specific isoenzymes of LDH can be measured by heat inactivation or electrophoresis. These are designated LDH_1 through LDH_5 (see Table 4-3).

LDH_1 has the greatest activity in heart muscle, renal cortex, and erythrocytes.

LDH_2 has the greatest activity in normal serum, with LDH_1 second ($LDH_2 > LDH_1$). Following acute myocardial infarction this ratio in the serum is reversed ($LDH_1 > LDH_2$); this situation is sometimes referred to as a *flipped ratio*. LDH_5 is the major isoenzyme in liver and muscle.

VALUE OF THE TEST

Aids in the differential diagnosis of myocardial infarction, pulmonary infarction, anemias, and hepatic disease.

Supports CK-MB isoenzyme test results in diagnosing myocardial infarction.

Aids in diagnosis of myocardial infarction when blood for CK-MB test was drawn too late.

Table 4-3 Tissue location of LDH isoenzymes

Principal LDH isoenzymes	Tissue
LDH_1, LDH_2	Heart
	Kidney
	Brain
	Red blood cells
LDH_3	Thyroid
	Adrenal gland
	Lymph nodes
	Pancreas
	Thymus
	Spleen
	Leukocytes
LDH_4, LDH_5	Liver
	Skeletal muscle

NURSING ACTION

1. Unless part of a chemistry panel, instruct the patient that he or she may eat and drink before collection of the specimen.
2. Collect 5 ml of venous blood in a red-top tube. Handle the specimen gently to prevent hemolysis.
3. List on the laboratory slip narcotics or other intramuscular injections received by the patient within the previous 8 hours.

INTERFERING FACTORS

Hemolysis (elevated)
Intramuscular injections (elevated)

CLINICAL IMPLICATIONS

Acute myocardial infarction: Elevation of serum total LDH levels and a characteristic isoenzyme pattern are almost always found in patients who have had acute myocardial infarctions.

Following the onset of symptoms of acute myocardial infarction, increases in LDH level above the normal range are usually seen in 12 hours, with peak activity occurring about the third day. After 6 to 8 days values usually return to normal, but they may remain elevated for 14 days.

During the first 12 hours after an acute myocardial infarction, the LDH isoenzyme ratio usually remains normal ($LDH_2 > LDH_1$). Twelve to 24 hours after the infarction a characteristic pattern of myocardial infarction appears ($LDH_1 > LDH_2$), and may persist for about 12 days, even when total LDH values have returned to normal. Refer to Table 4-4 for a summary of LDH isoenzyme patterns in various disease states.

Injuries: To liver, skeletal muscle, kidney, lung, or erythrocytes also cause LDH elevations.

MYOGLOBIN (serum)

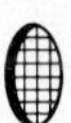

Adult normal

0-85 ng/ml

Table 4-4 LDH isoenzyme patterns in various disease states

LDH isoenzyme pattern	Disease state
LDH_1 and LDH_2 elevated generally; $LDH_1/LDH_2 > 1$	Myocardial infarct Pernicious anemia Acute renal damage Hemolysis
LDH_5 elevated	Liver damage
$LDH_1 > LDH_2$; LDH_5 elevated	Myocardial infarct with liver congestion
LDH_2 and LDH_3 elevated	Lymphoproliferative disorders Pulmonary infarct
Elevation of levels of all isoenzymes	Heart failure Crush syndrome Neoplastic disease

EXPLANATION OF THE TEST

Myoglobin is a small molecular-weight protein that is found in cardiac tissue as well as skeletal muscle. It is measured by radioimmunoassay.

VALUE OF THE TEST

Useful in the diagnosis of infarct extension or reinfarction. It is more sensitive than CK isoenzyme determinations, but not as specific, in that skeletal muscle injury or disease will cause elevations.

NURSING ACTION

1. Instruct the patient that he or she may eat and drink before the test.
2. Withdraw 5 ml of venous blood in a red-top tube. The laboratory will need 1 ml of serum.
3. Handle the specimen gently to prevent hemolysis.
4. Myoglobin is stable 4 days at room temperature.

INTERFERING FACTORS

Increased levels may occur as a result of skeletal muscle injury, inflammation, or ischemia; delirium tremens; or severe exertion. Other reported causes of a release of myoglobin are diabetic acidosis, hypokalemia, systemic infection with fever, and barbiturate poisoning. The false-positive rate (patients without myocardial infarction) has been reported to range from 0% to 22%.

CLINICAL IMPLICATIONS

Serum myoglobin levels increase very early following an acute myocardial infarction. Within 2 hours of the onset of myocardial infarction, significantly elevated levels occur. Serum myoglobin measurement for the diagnosis of acute myocardial infarction is not widely used as yet.

BLOOD LIPIDS

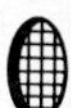

Adult reference range

Cholesterol: 120-220 mg/dl (SI units: 3.10-5.69 mmol/L)
Triglycerides: 40-150 mg/dl (SI units: 0.4-1.5 g/L)

EXPLANATION OF THE TEST

Blood lipid levels have received much attention in relation to coronary artery disease. The association between serum cholesterol level and coronary artery disease is unequivocal. Less strong is the association between triglyceride levels and coronary artery disease. The blood lipids (cholesterol, triglycerides, and phospholipids) circulate in the plasma, in which they are bound to protein; thus the term *lipoproteins*. Electrophoresis is the method used to separate the lipoproteins; from this procedure the following classification has evolved:

1. *Chylomicrons*—primarily exogenous triglycerides.
2. *Very-low-density lipoproteins (VLDL)*—primarily endogenous triglycerides
3. *Intermediate-density lipoproteins (IDL)*—transitional forms, with 30% cholesterol and 40% triglycerides
4. *Low-density lipoproteins (LDL)*—50% cholesterol
5. *High-density lipoproteins (HDL)*—may serve to remove cholesterol from tissues

LDL has a strong and direct association with coronary artery disease, while HDL has been *inversely* associated with the risk of coronary artery disease. High levels of HDL thus have a protective role. Determination of the *total cholesterol* level is therefore not sufficient for the assessment of coronary risk. It is important to determine whether elevated cholesterol levels are caused by an increase in the concentration of LDL (high risk of coronary artery disease) or the concentration of HDL (low risk of coronary artery disease). Generally accepted normal values for these lipids are listed in Table 4-5.

VALUE OF THE TEST

Useful in the determination of whether elevated cholesterol levels are caused by an increase in LDL (high risk of coronary artery disease) or HDL (low risk of coronary artery disease).

NURSING ACTION

1. Instruct the patient to eat a normal diet for 3 to 7 days and then nothing by mouth for 12 to 14 hours before the test. Explain that fasting is necessary if useful information is to be obtained from this test.
2. If blood glucose measurements are to be made, instruct the patient to have an average carbohydrate intake before the test.
3. Explain to the patient that this test helps to evaluate fat metabolism.
4. Collect 10 ml of venous blood in a red-top tube and transport to the laboratory immediately.
5. Explain to the patient that it may be necessary to draw blood more than once. Because there can be marked fluctuations from day to day in the same patient, several measurements should be made before a diagnosis of hyperlipidemia is made and dietary and/or drug therapy instituted.

Table 4-5 Normal values for plasma lipoproteins (mg/dl)

Age	Total cholesterol	Triglycerides	LDL cholesterol	HDL cholesterol
<24	125-200	50-146	73-138	32-57
25-39	140-250	60-250	90-180	32-60
40-49	161-260	70-250	100-185	33-60
50-64	170-265	75-200	105-190	34-70
>64	175-280	70-200	105-200	33-75

Adapted from Levy, E.I., and Feinleib, M.: Risk factors for coronary artery disease and their management. In Braunwald, E., editor: Heart disease, Philadelphia, 1980, W.B. Saunders Co., pp. 1254-1255.

INTERFERING FACTORS

A high-fat, high-sugar diet

Drugs causing elevated levels: aspirin, corticosteroids, oral contraceptives, epinephrine, norepinephrine, bromides, phenothiazines, trifluoperazine (Stelazine), vitamins A and D, sulfonamides, and phenytoin (Dilantin)

CLINICAL IMPLICATIONS

The association between hyperlipidemia (specifically, high levels of LDL) and coronary artery disease is well established; this association is most striking in the younger population. Furthermore, lowering abnormally elevated cholesterol levels will decrease the incidence of cardiovascular morbidity and mortality. Thus it is prudent to detect these elevations and to use dietary and, if indicated, drug measures to bring these levels within the normal range or at least to lower them. It is generally agreed that the lower the blood lipid levels, the smaller the chance of acquiring coronary artery disease. When hyperlipidemia coexists with obesity, there is commonly an abnormal glucose tolerance test (p. 393); fasting blood glucose measurements will verify the presence of diabetes. The value of detecting diabetes in an asymptomatic patient lies in recognizing the risk factor for coronary artery disease. Generally, for an asymptomatic patient no treatment is necessary except weight reduction in the obese.

NURSING ALERT

Be aware that this test should not be performed days to weeks after a myocardial infarction, since glucose levels are elevated following MI.

MEASUREMENT OF BLOOD DRUG LEVELS

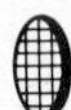

EXPLANATION OF THE TEST

This is a quantitative test to monitor the blood levels of antiarrhythmic and other cardiac drugs.

VALUE OF THE TEST

To monitor the blood levels of cardiac drugs for their successful and safe use

To check for toxicity in suggestive clinical situations

NURSING ACTION

1. Instruct the patient that there are no food or fluid restrictions.
2. Withdraw venous blood in the tube designated by the laboratory.
3. Completely fill the collection tube and gently invert it several
4. Note on the laboratory slip date and time. Usually a peak time or a steady-state sample is taken.
5. Note if the patient is taking medications. If so, notify the laboratory.
6. Handle the blood specimen gently to prevent hemolysis and transport to the laboratory immediately.

INTERFERING FACTORS

There is a potential for numerous drug interactions, for example:

Serum quinidine levels are elevated by acetazolamide, antacids, and sodium bicarbonate.

Serum lidocaine and serum quinidine levels are suppressed by barbiturates and phenytoin.

Serum digitalis levels are doubled by quinidine.

CLINICAL IMPLICATIONS

The therapeutic and potentially toxic blood levels for cardiac drugs are shown in Table 4-6. This table is intended only as a general guide. The cardiac condition, clinical context, and electrolyte status of a patient must be considered in interpreting the clinical importance of blood levels of these drugs. For example, serum digoxin levels of 1.5 ng/ml may be associated with clinical toxicity and arrhythmias in a setting of severe myocardial disease or hypokalemia, hypomagnesemia, and hypercalcemia. However, serum levels of digoxin higher than 3 ng/ml may be safe and necessary in patients with normal electrolytes and without extensive myocardial disease

Table 4-6 Therapeutic and potentially toxic blood levels of cardiac drugs

Drug	Therapeutic blood level (per ml)
Amiodarone (Cordarone)	1-2 μg
Bretylium (Bretylol)	0.8-2.4 μg
Digitoxin	20-35 ng
Digoxin (Lanoxin)	1-2 ng
Diltiazem (Cardizem)	100-200 ng
Disopyramide (Norpace)	2-4 μg
Flecainide	<1 μg
Lidocaine	1.4-5 μg
Metoprolol (Lopressor)	20-200 ng
Mexiletine	0.5-2 μg
N-Acetylprocainamide (NAPA)	2-22 μg
Nifedipine (Procardia)	50-100 ng
Phenytoin (Dilantin)	10-18 μg
Procainamide (Pronestyl)	4-8 μg
Propranolol (Inderal)	20-85 ng
Quinidine	2.5-5 μg
Theophylline	10-20 μg
Tocainide (Tonocard)	6-12 μg
Verapamil (Isoptin, Calan)	100-200 ng

NURSING ALERT

NOTIFY THE PHYSICIAN IMMEDIATELY WHEN THE FOLLOWING DRUG LEVELS ARE ENCOUNTERED.

Digitoxin	>40 ng/ml
Digoxin (Lanoxin)	>4 ng/ml
Disopyramide (Norpace)	>6 μg/ml
Lidocaine	>6 μg/ml
Mexiletine (Mexitile)	>3 μg/ml
Phenytoin (Dilantin)	>18 μg/ml
Procainamide (Pronestyl)	>10 μg/ml
Quinidine	>5 μg/ml
Theophylline	>20 μg/ml
Tocainide (Tonocard)	>14 μg/ml

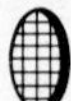

MISCELLANEOUS BLOOD TESTS

The *complete blood count (CBC)* is useful in detection of anemias, which may (1) present as angina in a patient with coronary artery disease, (2) aggravate congestive heart failure, (3) constitute a diagnostic clue in subacute bacterial endocarditis, or (4) constitute evidence of hemolysis in patients with prosthetic valves.

The *white blood cell count (WBC)* is elevated in patients with myocardial infarction, bacterial endocarditis, or the postmyocardial infarction (Dressler) syndrome.

The *sedimentation rate* is elevated in acute myocardial infarction, bacterial endocarditis, Dressler's syndrome, and in many other diseases that cause inflammation. It is considered to be characteristically low in congestive heart failure.

Abnormalities of electrolytes are common in patients with heart disease. These abnormalities can result from congestive heart failure, or they can occur as side effects of drug therapy for this condition. Chronic congestive heart failure causes total-body, as well as myocardial, potassium and magnesium depletion. Diuretics used as treatment for congestive heart failure may further increase these losses. Accurate diagnosis of an electrolyte abnormality requires determination of the tissue (intracellular) levels of these cations. Serum levels, which are routinely measured, *may* reflect intracellular deficits.

In both congestive heart failure and myocardial infarction scrupulous attention to electrolyte balance (sodium, potassium, and magnesium as well as calcium and phosphorus) will decrease the number and severity of problems with arrhythmias and drug (especially digitalis) toxicity.

In severe congestive heart failure, creatinine clearance may fall and the blood urea nitrogen and serum creatinine levels may rise.

Antistreptolysin-O (ASO) titer is elevated after streptococcal infections and can be the clue to diagnosis of acute rheumatic fever.

The *VDRL test*, discussed in Chapter 11, can be the clue to syphilitic heart disease, usually presenting as aortic insufficiency or disease of the ostia of the coronary arteries.

A test of *prothrombin time* is used in initiating and maintaining anticoagulation therapy with oral anticoagulants (drugs such as Coumadin). Usually the prothrombin time is kept within 2 to 2.5 times the control, and that is generally comparable to 20% to 30% of the normal prothrombin activity. The partial thromboplastin time (PTT) and the clotting time are used in following the cases of patients receiving heparin; 2 to 2.5 times the normal is the therapeutic range.

Anticoagulation therapy with heparin, and subsequently with Coumadin-type drugs, is used in pulmonary embolism, deep venous thrombosis, cerebral embolism, and acute peripheral arterial embolism and is felt to be beneficial in patients with acute myocardial infarction with congestive heart failure, during the period of bed rest. Many drugs interfere with the metabolism and action of the Coumadin-type anticoagulants. Frequent measurements of the prothrombin time and careful checks of the interaction of drugs are important in minimizing the risk of hemorrhage in patients receiving anticoagulant drugs.

Blood cultures are crucial in the diagnosis of infective endocarditis. It is important to obtain an adequate number of cultures. Generally, six is considered adequate. The specimens should be obtained by sterile technique, with inoculation preferably being done at the bedside. The specimens should be cultured on aerobic, anaerobic, and microaerophilic media.

Arterial blood gas determinations are discussed in Chapter 6. Patients with myocardial infarction or congestive heart failure commonly have abnormalities of the arterial blood gases. Patients who have hypoxemia or desaturation secondary to altered ventilation/perfusion ratios usually benefit from oxygen administration in an attempt to keep their oxygen saturation 90% or higher. Patients who have myocardial infarctions, especially with pulmonary congestion or edema, commonly hyperventilate, with subsequent lowering of the P_{CO_2} and mild respiratory alkalosis. In the presence of severe pulmonary edema, hypoventilation with elevation of the P_{CO_2} and mild respiratory acidosis may occur.

Some drugs used in the treatment of myocardial infarction, especially morphine, produce a predictable drop in the rate and depth of respiration and may, in excessive doses, precipitate hypoventilation with respiratory acidosis. Therefore, in patients who are receiving larger than usual doses of morphine or morphine along with other respiratory suppressants, arterial blood gas determinations are indicated to detect and/or avoid respiratory depression.

Nitroglycerine and nitroprusside may decrease arterial oxygen saturation. The mechanism is poorly understood, but it probably involves an increase in the degree of mismatch between ventilation and perfusion. In a marginally compensated patient, such a decrease in oxygen saturation may be clinically important.

The carbon monoxide level is elevated in moderate to heavy smokers, as well as in persons living in areas of heavy industrial pollution; such an elevation may precipitate or exacerbate angina pectoris in a person who has coronary artery disease. Measurement of carbon monoxide levels in the blood thus can be helpful in identifying factors that are contributing to a patient's angina pectoris.

NURSING ALERT

PT and PTT: Assure that there is not even a trace of heparin in the flush solution, because it interferes with results. Draw blood for prothrombin time and PTT by direct venipuncture and not from catheters.

Blood culture: Use special care to protect from contamination the blood drawn for culture; contamination results in a false-positive test. Note on the laboratory report if the patient is being treated with antibiotics before the blood culture; this may lead to false-negative results.

Blood gases: When blood is drawn for blood gases, the patient may be breathing room air or air enriched with oxygen. If on oxygen supplement, the amount of oxygen flow should be noted on the laboratory slip so that the interpretation can be accurate.

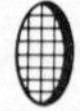

URINE EXAMINATION

Measurement of the volume of urine through 24 hours is helpful in the diagnosis of cardiac disorders, since in heart failure the night volume may be from 30% to 50% more than the day volume. Such nighttime elevation is referred to as nocturia.

The presence of red cells in the urine may be evidence of infective endocarditis or embolic disease of the kidneys.

Mild proteinuria, 1 to 2 g of protein per day in the urine, can be seen in congestive heart failure. Patients with marked elevation of venous pressure, constrictive pericarditis, or tricuspid insufficiency may present with massive proteinuria, and even with the nephrotic syndrome.

Recently, the detection of myoglobin in the urine (myoglobinuria) has been found useful as a sensitive test in the diagnosis of myocardial infarction, but clinical experience with this test remains limited.

NONINVASIVE SPECIALIZED DIAGNOSTIC METHODS IN CARDIOLOGY

The following is a discussion of the more important specialized tests used in cardiovascular diagnosis. These tests are grouped together because they are noninvasive; that is, they do not break the patient's skin or alter the events that are being observed. They pose no risk or significant discomfort to the patient and can be repeated at frequent intervals with absolute safety. Great technological advances have been made in such testing procedures over the past decade and further advances will certainly be forthcoming in the next decade.

ECHOCARDIOGRAPHY

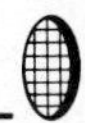

Normal

See Figure 4-11A

EXPLANATION OF THE TEST

Echocardiography (ultrasound cardiography), in the brief span of 15 years, has become an indispensable tool, being the most frequently used test after the ECG. It examines the size, shape, and motion of cardiac structures. Techniques of echocardiography include M-mode, two-dimensional, exercise, contrast, and Doppler studies. A complete study should include two-dimensional as well as M-mode recordings and Doppler study.

This is a safe procedure with no inherent risks. However, it should be remembered that a poorly performed or inadequately interpreted echocardiogram is worse than none at all. The potential exists for misdiagnosis and incorrect therapeutic decisions as a result of poor-quality echocardiograms.

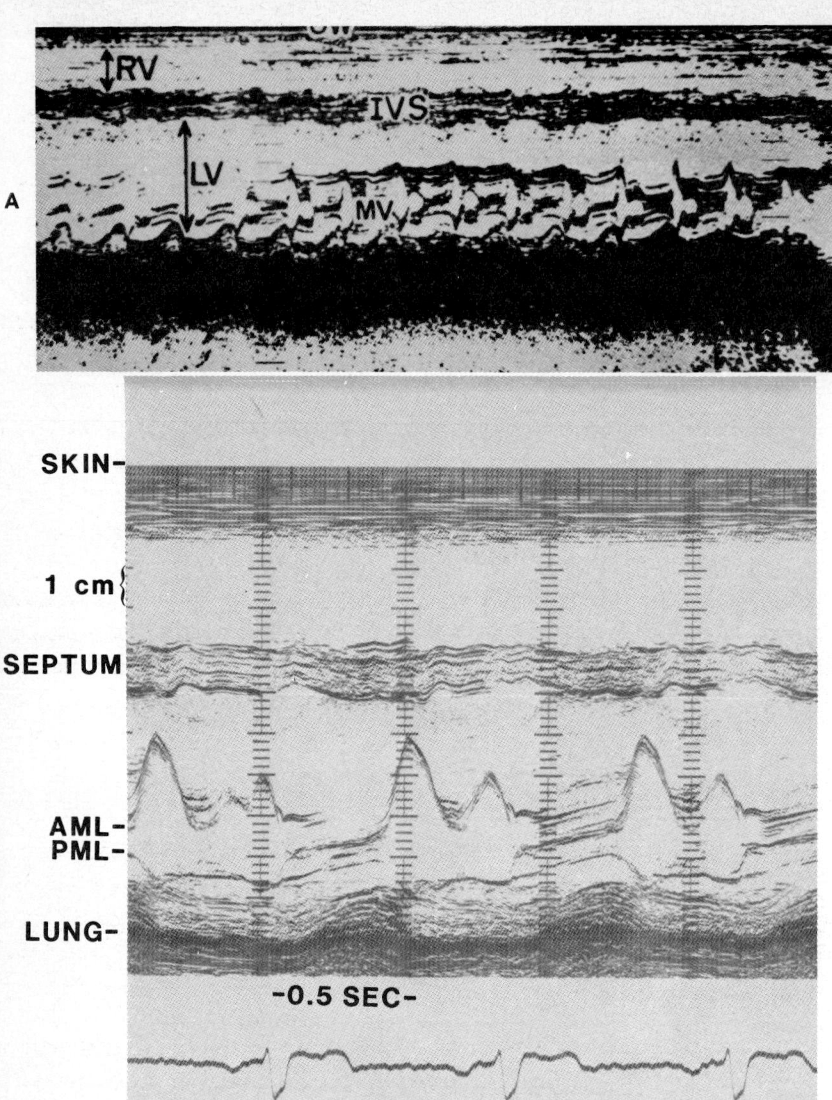

Fig. 4-11. ***A,*** *M-mode scan from the left ventricle* (LV) *to the aorta* (Ao) *and left atrium* (LA) *in a normal person.* RV, *Right ventricle.* IVS, *Interventricular septum.* CW, *Chest wall.* MV, *Mitral valve.* ***B,*** *M-mode echocardiogram of a normal mitral valve.* AML, *Anterior mitral leaflet.* PML, *Posterior mitral leaflet.* *(From Linhart, J.W., and Joyner, C.R., editors: Diagnostic echocardiography, St. Louis, 1982, The C.V. Mosby Co.)*

TYPES OF ECHOCARDIOGRAPHY

M-mode echocardiography utilizes echoes (reflected ultrasound) from pulsed high-frequency sound waves to locate and study the movements and dimensions of various cardiac structures. The technique permits direct recordings of the motion of the mitral, aortic, tricuspid, and pulmonic valve leaflets, the intraventricular septum, and the right and left ventricular walls. In addition, the technique provides accurate measurements of the size of the cardiac chambers and the changes in their dimensions during the cardiac cycle, and it allows recognition of abnormal filling defects, as in atrial tumors. Because the ultrasound beam tracks the motion of various cardiac structures over a period of time, it provides a time-motion study of the heart (hence the term M [motion]-mode echocardiography). (See Figs. 4-11 and 4-12.)

Two-dimensional echocardiography represents a further development of ultrasound technique. While in M-mode echocardiography the angle of the ultrasound beam is kept stationary, in two-dimensional echocardiography this angle is rapidly moved within a sector (usually 45 to 86 degrees), producing a "sector scan." Images produced by this technique are presented in a more familiar format, comparable to that in angiography. The ability of 2-D echo to appreciate spatial anatomic relationships makes this test more versatile than the M-mode technique. Current methods use both techniques simultaneously. The sound beam can be moved with a mechanical device (mechanical sector scanner) or by electronic systems (phased array scanner). Both types of 2-D echo scanners provide good-quality two-dimensional images of cardiac structures (chambers, walls, valves, and so on) in real time. The images, along with the electrocardiogram, are recorded on videotape to permit later viewing. All 2-D echo machines also have the capability for simultaneous M-mode recordings on strip charts. Newer recorders are compact in size, permitting bedside examinations.

A complete 2-Dimensional examination includes long- and short-axis views. Figs. 4-13 and 4-14 show the transducer in the parasternal position and apical two- and four-chamber views.

Exercise echocardiography provides valuable information about coronary artery disease and left ventricular ischemia induced by exercise. However, the technical difficulty involved in obtaining good images during or immediately following exercise (and motion) has limited its usefulness. Technical improvements in image acquisition, processing, and display are rapidly overcoming this hurdle.

Contrast echocardiography enhances the other forms of echocardiography through the use of contrast agents. Microbubbles of air, suspended in a liquid (e.g., saline, dextrose, blood), act as an effective contrast agent for echocardiography. When injected intravenously, they outline the right-sided chambers and aid in the diagnosis of intracardiac shunt and tricuspid regurgitation. These air microbubbles do not cross the pulmonary capillaries and intravenous injection does not provide contrast in the left atrium or the left ventricle. The technique is safe as long as visible macrobubbles of air are not injected in the circulation.

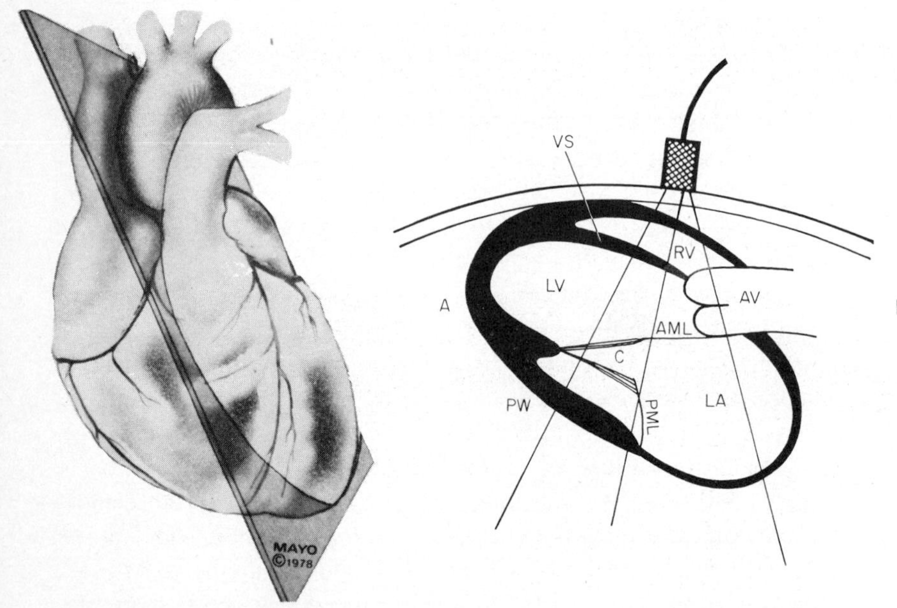

Fig. 4-12. A, *The long-axis plane of the left ventricle extends along an imaginary line from the right shoulder to the left flank. The scan begins at the base of the heart and continues toward the apex of the left ventricle (long axis of the heart).* **B,** *Diagrammatic representation of the long-axis plane of the left ventricle.* **C,** *Resultant two-dimensional ultrasonic image in the long-axis plane (parasternal, long-axis plane, left ventricle).* AV, *Aortic valve.* RV, *Right ventricle.* VS, *Ventricular septum.* LV, *Left ventricle.* LA, *Left atrium.* PW, *Posterior wall.* A, *Anterior.* P, *Posterior.* I, *Inferior.* S, *Superior.* (**A** *and* **C** *from Seward, J.B., and Tajik, A.J.: Med. Clin. North Am.* **64:**177, *March 1980.)*

Doppler echocardiography explores the blood flow patterns and measures changes in the velocity of blood flow within the heart and great vessels. This information is then used to estimate gradients across cardiac valves (evaluation of stenosis) as well as to detect valvular regurgitation. These techniques can also be used to estimate cardiac output. Advances in Doppler technique now permit the mapping of blood flow within the heart, color-coding the direction and pattern of flow, and superimposing these images on M-mode and 2-dimensional images (real time 2-D Doppler flow imaging). These techniques have revolutionized the noninvasive diagnosis of congen-

C

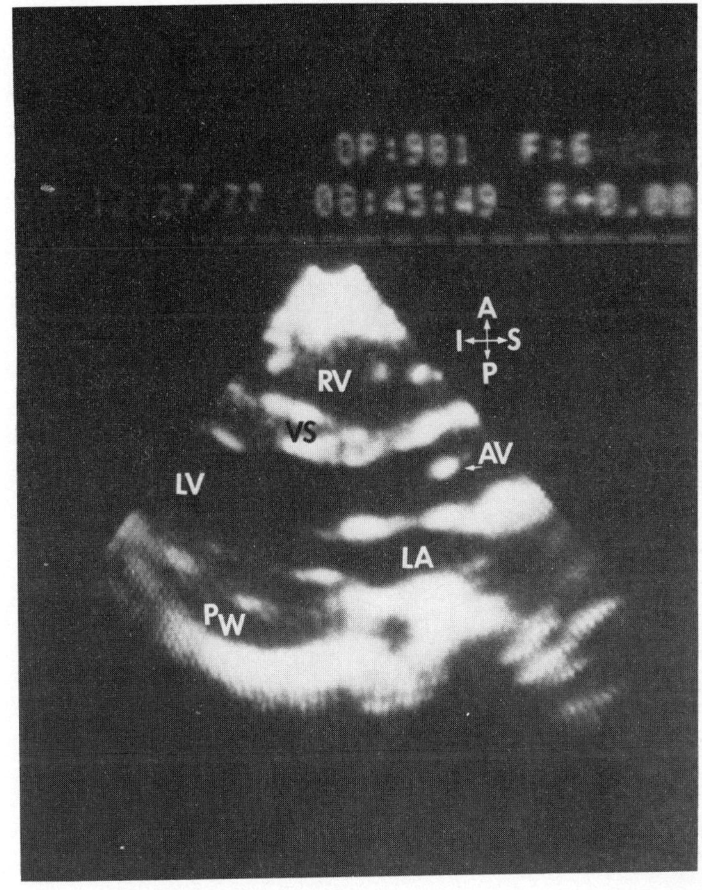

Fig. 4-12, cont'd. *For legend see opposite page.*

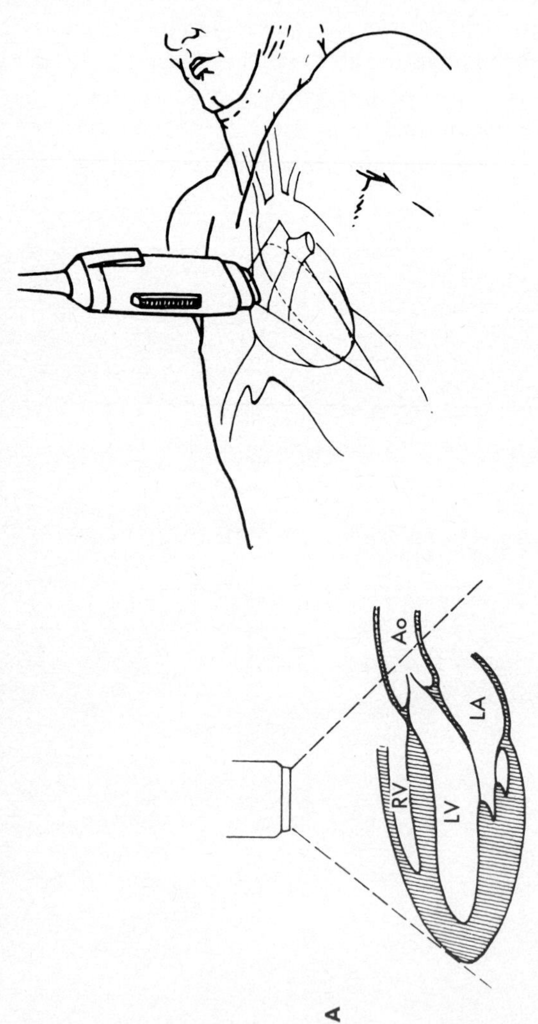
Ao
LA
RV
LV
A

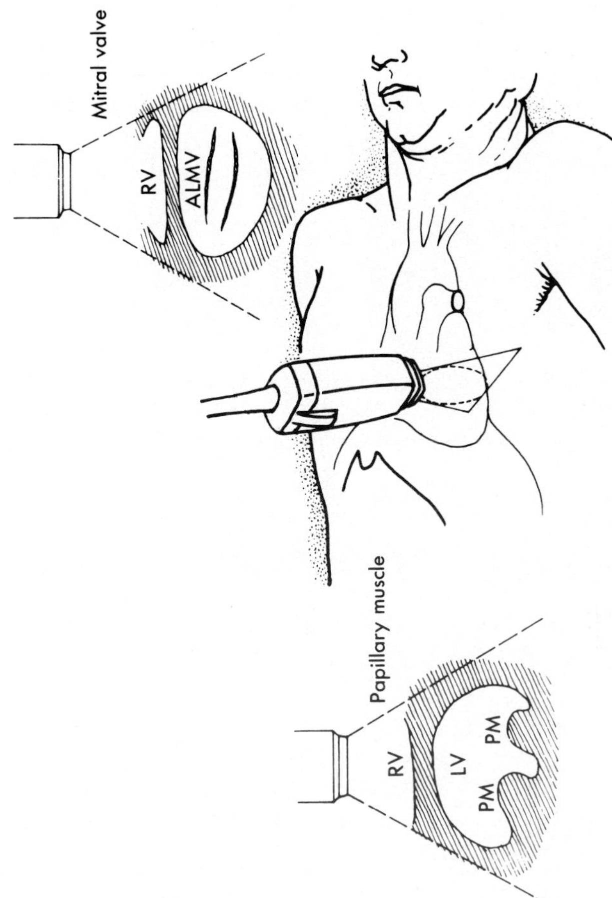

Fig. 4-13. *Two-dimensional echocardiogram.* **A,** *Conventional precordial long-axis view.* **B,** *Short-axis view.* RV, *Right ventricle.* LV, *Left ventricle.* LA, *Left atrium.* Ao, *Aorta.* ALMV, *Anterior leaflet mitral valve.* PM, *Papillary muscle.* (*From Carr, K.W., and others: Measurement of left ventricular ejection fraction by mechanical cross-sectional echocardiography,* Circulation **59:**1196-1206, 1979. *By permission of the American Heart Association, Inc.*)

ital heart disease and also aid in the evaluation of valvular heart disease in adults.

VALUE AND LIMITATIONS OF THE TEST

Permits definitive diagnosis and treatment, including surgery, of persons who have mitral stenosis, pericardial effusion, atrial tumors, or mitral valve prolapse.

Provides information valuable in the treatment of valvular heart disease, infective endocarditis, hypertrophic cardiomyopathy, congestive cardiomyopathy, congenital heart disease, coronary ar-

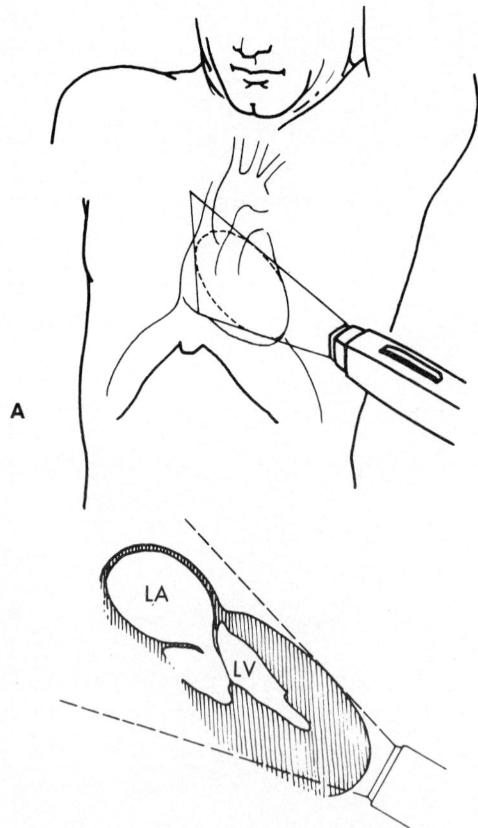

Fig. 4-14. A, *Apical two-chamber, two-dimensional echocardiogram (axial).* ***B,*** *Four-chamber view (hemiaxial). Views are obtained with the transducer located at the apex and directed toward the right shoulder.* LA, *Left atrium.* LV, *Left ventricle.* RA, *Right atrium.* RV, *Right ventricle. (From Carr, K.W.,*

tery disease with myocardial infarction, left ventricular aneurysm, and intracardiac masses or clots.

Two-dimensional echocardiography has limitations in the diagnosis of coronary artery disease because satisfactory images of the major coronary arteries cannot be regularly obtained. Exercise echocardiograpy, evaluating left ventricular wall motion abnormality during stress, attempts to overcome this limitation.

The technical quality of the images is inadequate for diagnostic purposes in approximately 5% to 10% of patients.

Equipment is costly ($60,000 to $160,000).

Quantitative data analysis (determination of ejection fraction and valve areas) is still in the developmental stage.

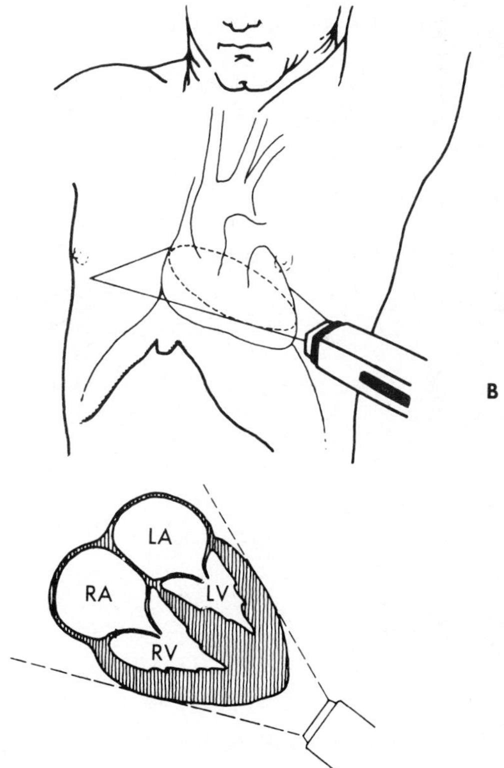

and others: Measurement of left ventricular ejection fraction by mechanical cross-sectional echocardiography, Circulation **59:***1196-1206, 1979. By permission of the American Heart Association, Inc.)*

The resolution approaches 2.5 to 3 mm. Better focusing techniques and high-frequency transducers may improve this situation.

NURSING ACTION

1. Explain the procedure to the patient. Make certain that the patient understands that the test is totally noninvasive, safe, and painless.
2. Explain to the patient that a specially trained technician will perform the procedure. Tell the patient that he or she will be placed in supine position and conductive jelly applied to different places on the chest. The transducer is angled at different parts of the heart. Explain that for different views of the heart the transducer is placed beneath the xiphoid process or above the sternum. For a left lateral view the patient is positioned on the left side.
3. Tell the patient that he or she may be asked to inhale and exhale slowly or hold the breath and that amyl nitrite inhalation may be used in special circumstances.

NURSING ALERT

Contrast echocardiography: Be sure to use a large-bore intravenous catheter to permit rapid bolus injection for providing adequate contrast; a small, slow infusion is not satisfactory.

NUCLEAR CARDIOLOGY

Radioactive tracer techniques are being used in cardiovascular diagnosis with increasing frequency. These tests generally qualify as "noninvasive" because they are safe and can be performed repeatedly. Nevertheless, they do involve the intravenous injection of a tracer material.

The general technique consists of injecting a radioactive tracer material into a vein and recording the radioactivity emitted over a specific area of the body. By using various types of tracers as well as different recording techniques, vastly different types of information can be obtained. Among the diagnostic tests employing radioactive techniques are angiocardioscanning (blood pool imaging), myocardial perfusion scanning during rest and after exercise, resting and exercise wall-motion studies of the right and left ventricles, and technetium 99m pyrophosphate imaging, which localizes the myocardial infarction.

RADIONUCLIDE ANGIOCARDIOGRAPHY

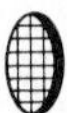

EXPLANATION OF THE TEST

This procedure obtains images of the chest as a bolus of blood-labeling agent passes through the heart and major vessels; it is also called *blood pool imaging*. Images are obtained at end-systole, end-diastole, or regular intervals during the cardiac cycle. Right and left ventricular function can be assessed, the wall motion of both ventricles can be reconstructed, and the ejection fraction (index of ventricular function) can be calculated. Such a study is called a "first pass" or "first transit" study. The technetium 99m can be tagged to albumin or to red cells, thus preventing its rapid exit from the vascular pool. This will permit "equilibrium studies," in which all cardiac chambers are visualized simultaneously. The ECG is used to time systole and diastole; multiple counts are obtained over a period of time, providing an "equilibrium blood pool study" or "equilibrium study." Such studies will give information about regional as well as overall ventricular function. Also, ventricular aneurysms and clots can be identified. Computers can generate time (systolic and diastolic) activity (count) curves for the right and left ventricles, permitting calculation of the ejection fraction.

The *ejection fraction (EF)* is calculated by dividing the stroke volume (end-diastolic volume minus end-systolic volume) by the end-diastolic volume. It is assumed that counts in the ventricle are directly proportional to the volume of blood, and therefore end-diastolic counts (EDC) and end-systolic counts (ESC) are used to estimate the ejection fraction (EF):

$$EF = \frac{EDC - ESC}{EDC}$$

The ejection fraction is a sensitive index of ventricular function. Normal hearts generally have an ejection fraction greater than 55%. Combining such a study with exercise further increases the value of the test. Normally, exercise will cause an increase in ejection fraction. A drop in ejection fraction because of exercise is abnormal and clearly reflects ventricular dysfunction.

VALUE AND LIMITATIONS OF THE TEST

Detection of abnormalities in myocardial contraction.

Detection of an intracardiac shunt or complex congenital heart disease.

Helpful in evaluating a surgically performed shunt in congenital heart disease.

Noninvasive evaluation of left ventricular function (wall-motion studies), providing a regional and global assessment at rest and during exercise. Serial evaluations are possible in myocardial infarction, cardiomyopathy, and valvular heart disease.

The success of the test may be limited by frequent ectopic beats or atrial fibrillation causing inaccurate data because of errors in the timing of systole and diastole.

In equilibrium studies, if the right and left ventricles are not separated adequately, the data may be inaccurate.

NURSING ACTION

1. Inform the patient that he or she may eat and drink before the test.
2. Secure a signed consent.
3. Explain the nature of the test to the patient and give assurances that he or she will receive a minimum of radiation. Inform the patient that ECG electrodes will be applied, an intravenous injection given, and a camera will record the passage of the injection through the circulation.
4. The radionuclide blood-labeling agent is given intravenously.
5. The camera records the first passage of the isotope through the heart and is then gated, using the ECG, for selected 60-millisecond intervals (end systole and end diastole); 500 to 1000 cardiac cycles are recorded.
6. Additional gated images may be recorded after assisting the patient into left or right anterior oblique position and administering 0.4 mg of nitroglycerin sublingually.
7. The patient may be requested to exercise while in the supine position.

MYOCARDIAL PERFUSION SCAN

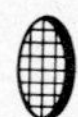

EXPLANATION OF THE TEST

This procedure evaluates myocardial tissue perfusion while the patient is at rest or exercising. A radioactive tracer (thallium 201) is injected intravenously and accumulates in the myocardium with adequate perfusion. Thus, inadequately perfused areas (e.g., coronary artery narrowing) can be identified because of the lack of accumulation of the radioactive tracer. Myocardial perfusion, and therefore indirectly coronary flow and coronary obstructive disease can be evaluated. The thallium 201 accumulates in the myocardium in direct proportion to regional myocardial blood flow and extraction of the thallium by the myocardial cells. A viable myocardial cell, with intact cell membrane function, is necessary in order for this extraction to occur.

Combining thallium 201 perfusion imaging with an exercise ECG increases the diagnostic yield of the exercise treadmill test.

VALUE AND LIMITATIONS OF THE TEST

The scan is helpful in the diagnosis of myocardial infarction (acute or chronic).

The coronary arteries are not visualized by these studies, which provide only indirect evidence of coronary artery narrowing or obstruction. Thus, if such narrowing is not very severe or if there is adequate collateral flow, a study may be normal. Quantitation of regional perfusion using computer analysis may increase the diagnostic value of a study.

NURSING ACTION FOR STRESS IMAGING

1. For stress imaging, instruct the patient that he or she may have a light meal before the test, but nothing by mouth for 3 hours prior.
2. Instruct the patient to wear loose clothing and comfortable shoes.
3. Secure a signed consent.
4. Inform patient that ECG electrodes will be in place during test.
5. Instruct the patient to report fatigue, pain, or shortness of breath.
6. Ask the patient to walk on the treadmill and inform him or her

that the pace will be gradually increased; ECG and blood pressure are monitored.

7. When the patient is at peak stress, 1.5 to 3 mCi of thallium is injected into the antecubital vein and flushed with 10 to 15 ml of normal saline solution.
8. Before assuming a supine position under the scintillation camera, the patient walks on the treadmill an additional 45 to 60 seconds to allow for uptake of the isotope.
9. The precordial leads are now removed if the patient has remained asymptomatic.
10. Scanning begins after 3 to 5 minutes and again at 3 to 6 hours. In special circumstances a third set of images is obtained 12 to 24 hours after the exercise.

NURSING ACTION FOR RESTING IMAGING

1. Instruct the patient not to have a heavy meal during the time between the end of the exercise and the beginning of resting imaging.
2. The patient receives the injection of thallium while he or she is at rest.
3. The patient assumes a supine position under the scintillation camera and scanning begins after 3 to 5 minutes.

CLINICAL IMPLICATIONS

Coronary artery disease and myocardial ischemia: An exercise thallium 201 perfusion study is more helpful than a resting test when a perfusion defect is identified during exercise but disappears over time (4 to 24 hours).

In the presence of severe coronary artery narrowing and decreased blood flow to a given region of the heart, the accumulation of thallium in that region is decreased. Such an abnormality is accentuated if the study is combined with exercise. Total occlusion of a vessel, with infarction of the left ventricular muscle supplied by that vessel, results in no uptake of thallium.

Fig. 4-15 illustrates the change in configuration of thallium 201 scintigrams with rotation of the heart. Normal images are compared with images caused by anterior myocardial infarction.

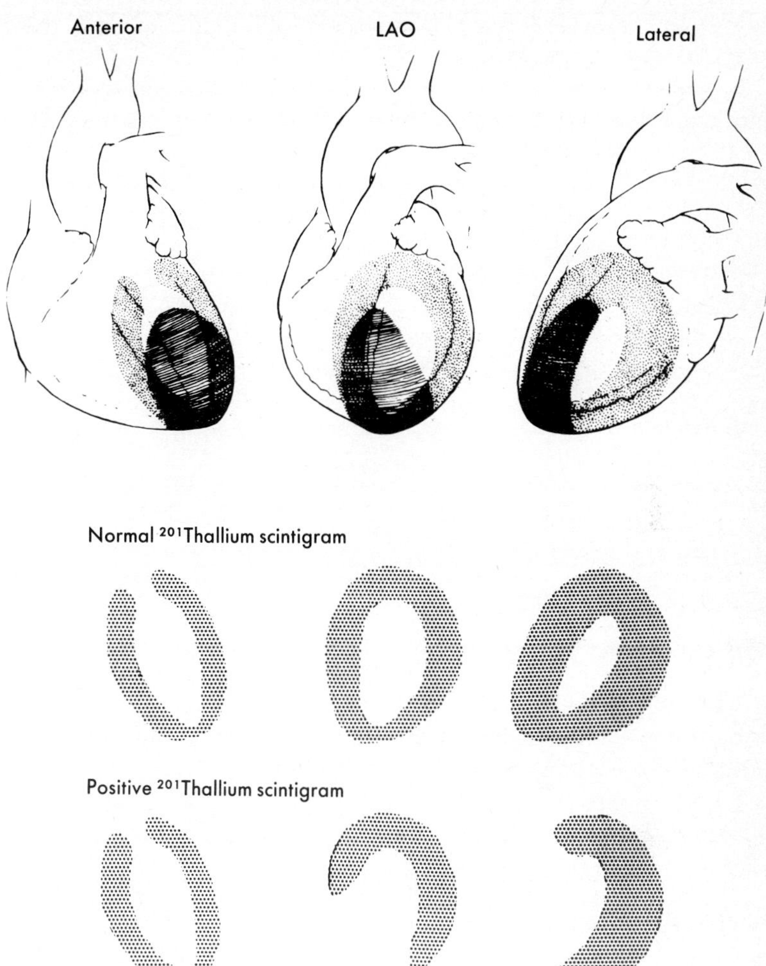

Fig. 4-15. *Change in configuration of thallium 201 scintigrams with rotation of the heart.* Top row: *Location of left ventricular myocardium* (dotted area) *in anterior, LAO, and left lateral projections. Linear shading denotes area of anterior wall infarction.* Middle row: *Normal thallium 201 images.* Bottom row: *Anterior wall defects in thallium 201 images caused by anterior myocardial infarction. (From Parkey, R.W., and others: J. Nucl. Med.* **17***:771, 1976.)*

NURSING ALERT

Imaging should be done within 5 to 10 minutes after the end of exercise. Thus it is important to record the time that exercise ends and imaging is started.

Discontinue stress testing if the patient develops chest pain, severe dyspnea or fatigue, syncope, excessive rise in blood pressure, ischemic ECG changes, or sustained arrhythmias or becomes pale, clammy, confused, or begins to stagger.

Immediately notify the nuclear cardiology department if this test is to be cancelled or rescheduled to avoid unnecessary waste of the radionuclide, since this substance is expensive (over $100 to $150) and not routinely available without prior arrangement.

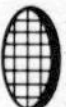

DIPYRIDAMOLE THALLIUM MYOCARDIAL PERFUSION STUDY

EXPLANATION OF THE TEST

When exercise is not possible or advisable during myocardial scintigraphy, the dipyridamole thallium myocardial perfusion study can be used as a substitute.

Dipyridamole (Persantine) is a coronary vasodilator, chemically unrelated to nitrates, and its administration followed by myocardial scintigraphy simulates the exercise phase of that test.

VALUE OF THE TEST

Simulates the exercise phase of the thallium perfusion study.

NURSING ACTION

1. Instruct the patient that he or she may have a light meal before the test, but nothing by mouth for 3 hours prior.
2. Advise the patient to wear clothing that allows easy access to the chest. Inform him or her that ECG electrodes will be in place during the test.
3. Secure a signed consent.
4. Instruct the patient to report fatigue, pain, or shortness of breath.
5. Immediately following the intravenous injection of dipyridamole,

thallium 1.5 to 3 mCi is injected into the antecubital vein and flushed with 10 to 15 ml of normal saline solution.

6. Ask the patient to then assume a supine position under the scintillation camera. Scanning begins immediately; results are comparable to the exercise thallium perfusion study. In 4 to 6 hours thallium myocardial perfusion is evaluated again (simulating the resting state).

CLINICAL IMPLICATIONS

Same as that of the thallium 201 perfusion study

NURSING ALERT

Maintain close blood pressure monitoring to avoid hypotension resulting from vasodilation.

TECHNETIUM 99m PYROPHOSPHATE IMAGING

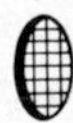

EXPLANATION OF THE TEST

In this test, a tracer isotope (technetium 99m pyrophosphate) is injected intravenously. Infarcted tissue will have an increased uptake of the isotope, aiding in the diagnosis and estimation of the size of the myocardial infarction.

VALUE OF THE TEST

Limited

NURSING ACTION

1. Inform the patient that he or she may have a light meal, but should not smoke or drink beverages with caffeine or alcohol for 3 hours before the test.
2. Advise the patient to wear loose clothing to allow for electrode placement. Inform him or her that there will be an intravenous injection 2 to 3 hours before scanning begins.
3. Intravenous technetium 99m (20 mCi) is injected 2 to 3 hours before use of the scintillation camera.

4. After this time lapse, the patient is placed in supine position, and continuous ECG monitoring is established.
5. Cardiac scanning is performed in several positions—anterior, left anterior oblique, right anterior oblique, and left lateral.

CLINICAL IMPLICATIONS

Cardiac amyloidosis may be suspected if there is diffuse uptake of the isotope by both the right and left ventricles.

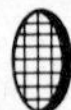

EMISSION COMPUTED TOMOGRAPHY (ECT)

EXPLANATION OF THE TEST

In this technique a radionuclide is injected intravenously and its distribution is quantitated in myocardial tissue. Thallium is a single photon-emitting radionuclide—thus the name *single photon emission computed tomography (SPECT)*. Images are obtained from many angles over 180 degrees and reconstructed using tomographic techniques, enhancing the ability to evaluate the regional myocardial blood flow.

VALUE OF THE TEST

Quantitatively assesses regional myocardial metabolism and myocardial tissue perfusion.

NURSING ACTION

1. Instruct the patient that he or she may have a light meal before the test, but nothing by mouth for 3 hours prior.
2. Advise the patient to wear clothing that allows easy access to the chest. Inform him or her that ECG electrodes will be in place during the test.
3. Secure a signed consent.
4. Instruct the patient to report fatigue, pain, or shortness of breath.
5. Immediately following the intravenous injection of dipyridamole, thallium 1.5 to 3 mCi is injected into the antecubital vein and flushed with 10 to 15 ml of normal saline solution.
6. Ask the patient to then assume a supine position under the scintillation camera. Scanning begins immediately; results are comparable to the exercise thallium perfusion study. In 4 to 6 hours thallium myocardial perfusion is evaluated again (simulating the resting state).

POSITRON EMISSION COMPUTED TOMOGRAPHY (PECT)

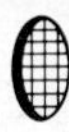

EXPLANATION OF THE TEST

Instead of using thallium, which emits photons detected by a scintillation camera, this technique uses radionuclides that decay in tissues by emitting subatomic particles (positrons). Positrons interact with electrons in tissue and produce energy in the form of photons that are detected by the PET device, which displays the radioactivity with three-dimensional techniques. Radionuclides that emit positrons (oxygen 15, carbon 11, nitrogen 13) have a very short half-life, an advantage for studying rapidly changing events such as myocardial ischemia. A disadvantage of this short half-life is the requirement that a cyclotron required for the production of the radionuclide be in close proximity to the imaging unit. The large expense and the professional expertise involved in these studies have limited their availability to a few research centers.

Further clinical validation of this technique coupled with technological development in reducing its cost and complexity may bring the test to the level of the community hospital.

VALUE OF THE TEST

Provides more accurate evaluation of myocardial perfusion and metabolism than is available with emission computed tomography.

COMPUTED TOMOGRAPHIC (CT) SCAN

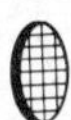

EXPLANATION OF THE TEST

The CT body scanner is sensitive to very fine variances in tissue density and thus provides detailed views of tissue and bone not possible through conventional x-ray techniques. Computerized tomography is accomplished quickly, with minimal radiation exposure. The patient is placed inside the scanner, and an x-ray tube with a diametrically opposed x-ray detector (located in a fixed position on a rotation gantry) completely encircles the body or skull at a desired cross-sectional level (Fig. 4-16, A). The tube emits a tiny stream of radiation pulses as it turns. These are collected by the detector and processed by a computer, which reconstructs the image and projects it onto a screen. The image is highly detailed, since each point within the cross-sectional field is viewed from hundreds of different angles,

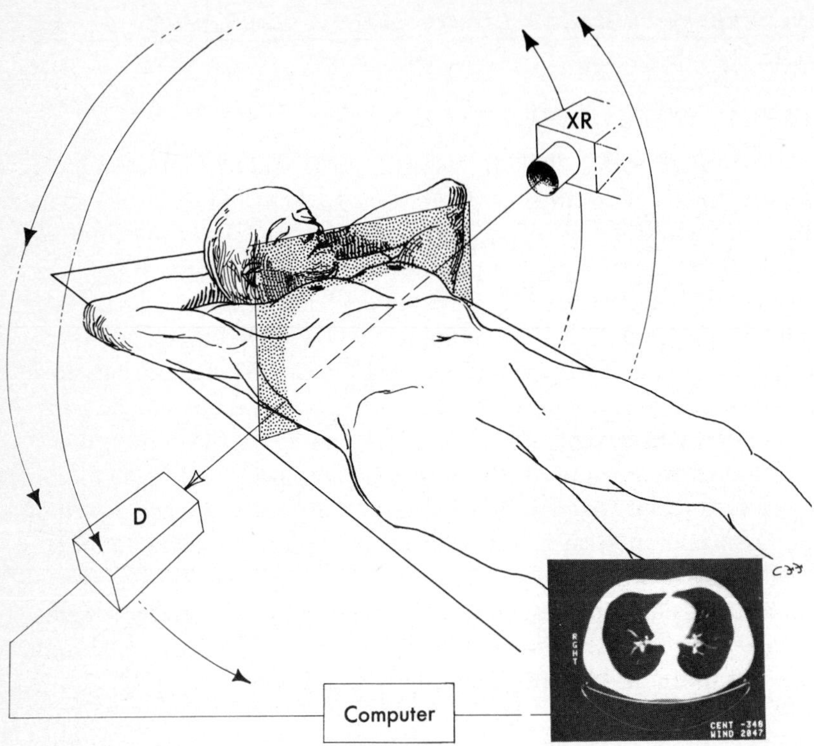

Fig. 4-16. A, *Diagrammatic representation of computerized tomography of the thorax. The image of the cathode-ray tube as projected in the lower right-hand corner is shown as though the patient were being viewed from below. This is the conventional method of viewing CT scans.* XR, *X-ray.* D, *Detectors.* ***B*** *and* **C,** *Normal 2-second CT view of the thorax.* ***B,*** *Scan is taken at the hilar level. The pulmonary vascular markings are shown throughout the lung fields* (white arrows). *The descending branch of the right pulmonary artery* (RPA) *lies slightly lateral but predominantly anterior to the intermediate bronchus, which contains air* (large white arrow). *The esophagus* (black arrow) *and azygos vein* (black arrowhead) *are evident. The descending branch of the left pulmonary artery* (LP) *is posterior to the lower lobe bronchus at this level.* DA, *Descending aorta.* **C,** *By adjusting the contrast, an examiner can look within the mediastinum at the same level as the CT scan in* ***B*** *and check for normal intrapericardial structures. The course of the right pulmonary artery can be followed to the main pulmonary artery* (MPA). *The superior vena cava* (s) *is anterior to the right pulmonary artery and behind the proximal portion of the ascending aorta* (AA). *These structures are seen because of the contrast between lower-density mediastinal fat and blood-containing vessels. (From Porgatch, R.D., and Fahling, L.J.: Computed tomography of the thorax: a status report, Chest* ***80:****618, 1981.)*

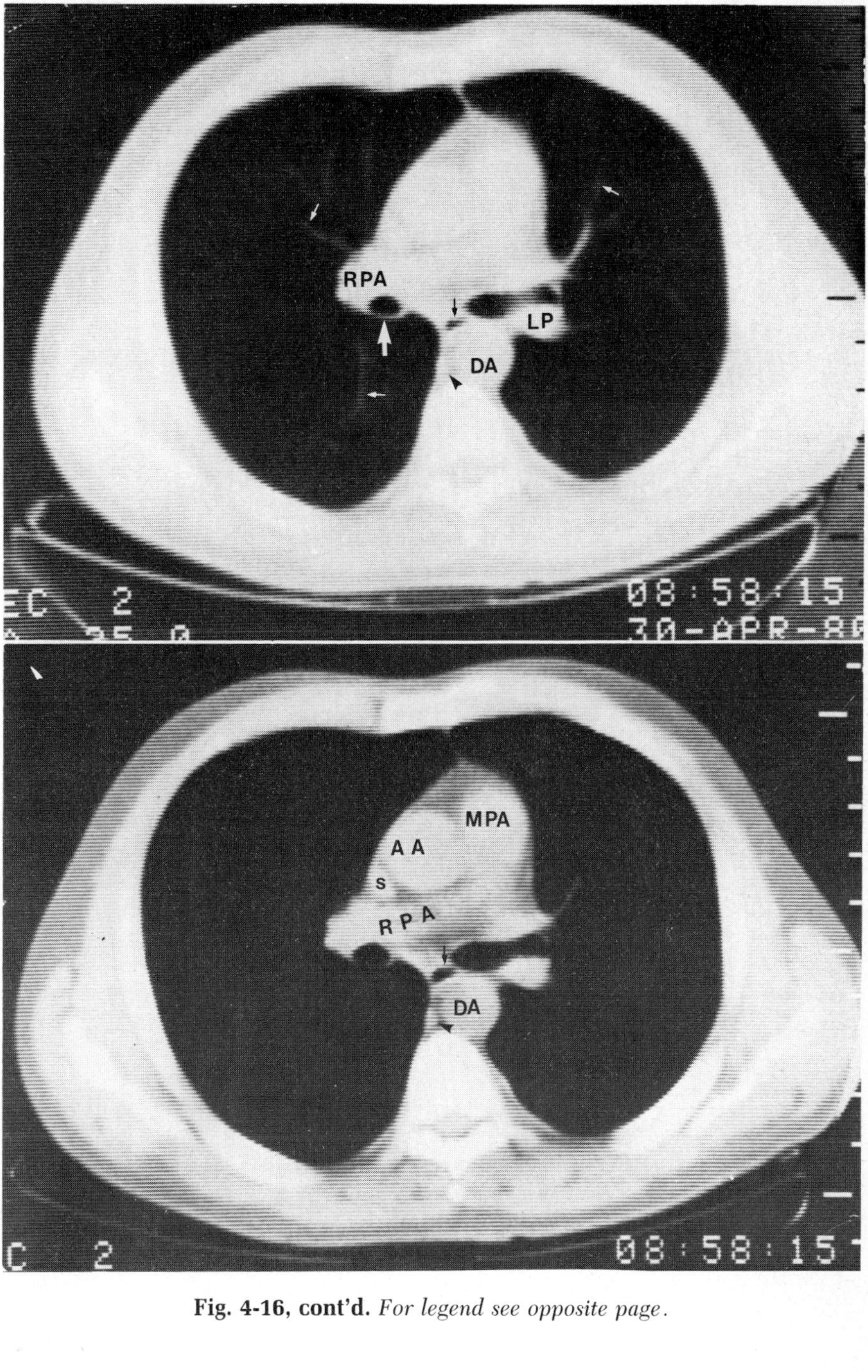

Fig. 4-16, cont'd. *For legend see opposite page.*

and the density of each point can be precisely determined, permitting the imaging of mediastinal structures that cannot be visualized with conventional x-ray procedures. Fig. 4-16, B and C, are normal CT scans of the thorax.

CT scanning of the heart uses a radiopaque contrast agent, x-ray transmission imaging, and computer reconstruction to provide tomographic images of various sections of the heart and great vessels. With currently available rapid scanners (50 msec or less, scan speed) called ultra-fast CT or cine CT, excellent resolution of cardiac structures is possible.

VALUE OF THE TEST

Used in the evaluation of left ventricular wall motion and thickness, left ventricular thrombi, and cardiac tumors.

The use of contrast permits the diagnosis of myocardial infarction and visualization of aortocoronary vein grafts.

Valuable in the determination of pericardial thickening, aortic aneurysm, and aortic dissection.

CT scanning of the heart has not achieved widespread use because of the wide availability of echocardiography, which provides an excellent alternative imaging method and is portable and less expensive. The ultimate role of CT scanning in cardiac imaging is still being evaluated.

NURSING ACTION

1. Inform the patient that, if a contrast agent is not to be used, food and drink may be taken before the procedure. If a contrast agent is to be used, instruct the patient to fast for 4 hours before the procedure.
2. Remove all jewelry and metal in the x-ray field.
3. Explain to the patient that this special x-ray test will expose him or her to only a minimal amount of radiation and that it will provide cross-sectional views of the chest that permit the physician to evaluate tissue density.
4. Tell the patient that he or she will lie upon an x-ray table and be moved into the middle of a circular piece of x-ray equipment. Instruct him or her to lie motionless and to breathe normally during the procedure.

CLINICAL IMPLICATIONS

Fig. 4-17 is an example of one of the diagnostic uses for CT scanning, detection of left ventricular thrombus.

Other possible pathological findings on CT scans of the thorax are tumors, nodules, cysts, aortic aneurysm, pleural effusion, and accumulations of blood, fluid, or fat.

NURSING ALERT

Observe the patient for adverse reactions to the radio contrast material such as anaphylactic reaction, volume overload and congestive heart failure, acute right ventricular failure, and acute renal failure.

In order to recognize a nephrotoxic response to the contrast

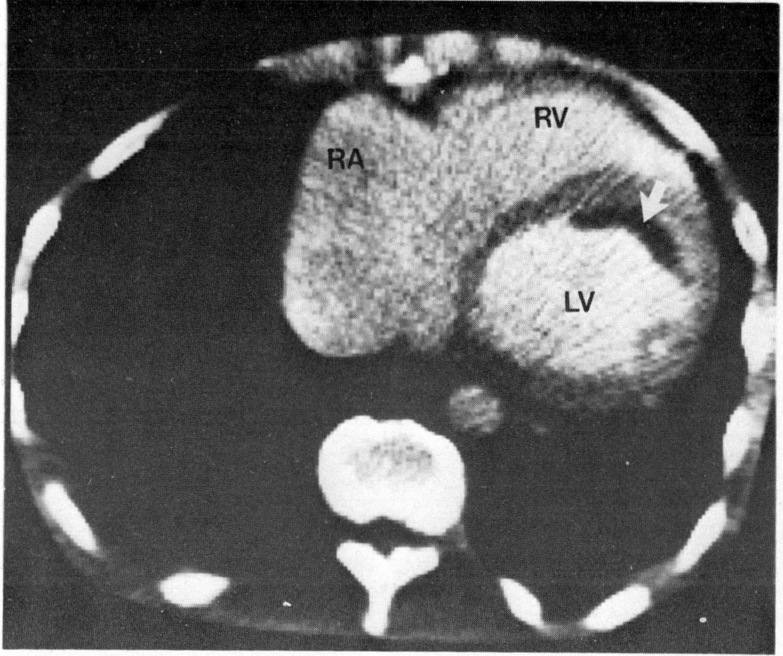

Fig. 4-17. *A contrast-enhanced CT scan. There is a large mural thrombus* (arrow) *adhering to the anterior left ventricular wall.* LV, *Left ventricle.* RV, *Right ventricle.* RA, *Right atrium. (Courtesy Bruce H. Brundage M.D., Chicago, Ill.)*

medium should it occur, closely monitor urinary output, renal function, and electrolytes 24 to 48 hours following the use of radiocontrast material.

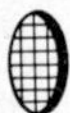

MAGNETIC RESONANCE IMAGING (MRI) OF THE HEART

EXPLANATION OF THE TEST

MRI uses static and changing magnetic fields in the body and radiofrequency pulses to generate tomographic images of the body with high contrast of soft tissue. This noninvasive technique provides excellent tissue characterization without the use of an injected contrast agent. For cardiac imaging, it is necessary to use ECG gating and acquire images over many cardiac cycles.

VALUE AND LIMITATIONS OF THE TEST

Imaging of the central nervous system, musculoskeletal system, and the cardiovascular system

Requires a metal-free environment, and therefore patients on life support equipment or with implanted metal objects such as pacemakers are not suitable candidates

CLINICAL IMPLICATIONS

MRI helps to evaluate patients with coronary artery disease (diagnosis of myocardial infarction), pericardial disease (pericardial thickening and constriction, and cysts), and cardiac masses and tumors and assists in the diagnosis of thoracic aortic aneurysm and dissection.

Fig. 4-18 illustrates its usefulness in visualizing a pericardial cyst. The exact role of MRI in the noninvasive diagnosis of cardiac disease is still being defined.

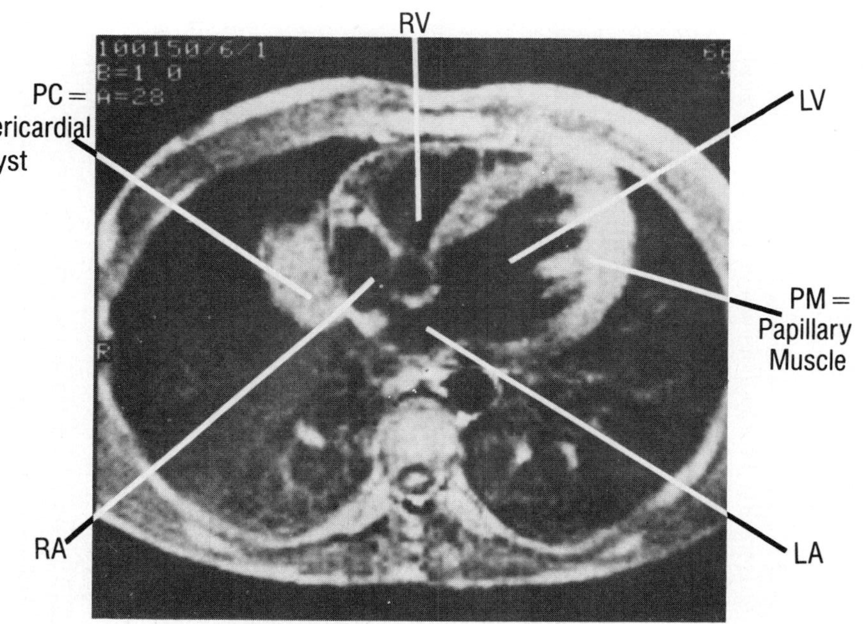

Fig. 4-18. *Gated magnetic resonance images show a right paracardiac mass and left ventricular hypertrophy. (From Higgins, C.B.: Clinical cardiovascular application of magnetic resonance imaging, Cardiac Impulse* **6**[*1*]:*1-8, 1985.)*

INVASIVE SPECIALIZED DIAGNOSTIC METHODS IN CARDIOLOGY

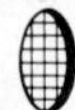

CARDIAC CATHETERIZATION

EXPLANATION OF THE TEST

Cardiac catheterization involves the passing of a catheter into the right or left side of the heart. In right-sided heart catheterization, the catheter is inserted through an arm vein (basilic or cephalic vein) or a leg vein (the femoral vein). The catheter is advanced through the vena cava, the right atrium, the right ventricle, and the pulmonary artery. Then for a brief period it is advanced further, to the distal pulmonary artery wedge position. For catheterization of the left side of the heart the catheter is introduced through an artery (either the brachial or the femoral). It is advanced through the arterial system to the ascending aorta, through the aortic valve into the left ventricle, and if necessary to the left atrium.

The cutdown technique can be used for both of these routes. In this method, the veins are usually tied at the end of the procedure while the arteries are repaired. Cardiac catheterization also can be performed percutaneously, a method in which the vessels are not surgically isolated and all catheters are introduced over guide wires or through introducer sheaths.

In the various chambers, pressures are recorded, and blood is sampled and analyzed for its oxygen content, ordinarily during rest as well as exercise. This information, coupled with measurement of the patient's rate of oxygen consumption, which is obtained by collecting gases expired by the patient, reveals (1) the patient's cardiac output (the amount of blood pumped per minute), (2) the presence and size of a right-to-left or left-to-right shunt within the cardiac chambers, and (3) the presence and severity of stenosis (narrowing of various valves). The information also makes possible the calculation of the resistance of the various vascular beds. Additional information is obtained using the indicator dilution test, angiography, and selective arteriography.

If a diagnosis from a cardiac catheterization is at variance with the clinical diagnosis, the physician will not automatically accept the catheterization diagnosis but will usually critically review it in the light of the clinical data.

Indicator dilution test. An indicator is a substance that can be harmlessly introduced into the cardiovascular system and detected with appropriate sensing apparatus. The substance commonly used for determining cardiac output is indocyanine green, which is introduced on the venous side and sampled by means of a densitometer (an instrument that is sensitive to optical changes of the blood). Curves that are thus obtained are used to calculate cardiac output, blood flow, and the size of shunts.

A slight modification of this principle involves the use of hydrogen gas that is introduced into the patient's system by inhalation. The gas is diffused into the circulation at the level of the pulmonary capillaries. Left-to-right shunts at various levels within the heart chambers can be detected by specially designed platinum-tipped electrode catheters positioned at specific sites.

Specialized catheters with thermistor (temperature-sensing) tips can be used to detect changes in temperature in various chambers after the injection of fluid at temperatures lower than the temperature of the body. This information can be used to calculate cardiac output (thermodilution techniques).

Angiography. Angiography is a modification of the basic catheterization technique. The catheter tip is positioned in a specific area of the cardiovascular system, and a contrast substance is injected to permit opacification of the area. Concomitant x-ray filming provides a permanent graphic record. Injection of contrast material into the right atrium is useful in detection of pericardial effusion and also for visualization of the tricuspid valve. Injection into the right or left ventricle gives information about the size and contraction of the respective chambers, as well as information about the tricuspid and mitral valves. Injection into the pulmonary artery makes the pulmonary arterial system visible and is the most definitive way of diagnosing a pulmonary embolus.

Selective coronary arteriography. Selective injection into the coronary arteries is performed in selective coronary arteriography. This technique was introduced in 1962 and has since served as the cornerstone for the evaluation of coronary artery disease. It has also made possible the development of surgical revascularization procedures. For selective coronary arteriography, various catheters are positioned at the coronary ostia, where contrast material is injected, and cinematographic films are taken. In selected cases in which coronary artery spasm is suspected and obstructive coronary artery disease is absent or minimal, provocative tests with intravenous ergonovine maleate are sometimes used to induce coronary artery spasm. Such spasm is promptly reversed by sublingual, intravenous, or intracoronary administration of nitroglycerine or sublingual nifedipine.

Results of vein bypass grafting are evaluated by injection of contrast agent into the graft that is interposed between the aorta and the coronary arteries.

Transluminal coronary angioplasty. This is a therapeutic extension of the technique of selective coronary arteriography. In certain cases, specifically designed balloon catheters can be introduced through a coronary catheter and positioned across the stenotic segment of a coronary artery. By means of controlled inflation of the balloon, such stenotic segments can be dilated.

Transluminal coronary recanalization. Another therapeutic extension of catheter techniques has been the introduction of thrombolytic agents into a coronary artery that has become occluded resulting in acute myocardial infarction. Clots can be lysed and occluded vessels can be recanalized. The role of such methods of treatment of coronary artery disease and myocardial infarction is under intensive evaluation.

Intracardiac electrophysiologic studies. Intracardiac electrophysiologic studies can be added to standard cardiac catheterization with the use of specially designed catheters that have recording and stimulating electrodes at their tips. When these catheters are introduced into the right and left atria and ventricles, supraventricular and ventricular arrhythmias can be induced and analyzed. The functional properties of the SA and AV nodes and accessory pathways can be evaluated. The actions of the various types of pacemakers and tachycardia-terminating devices, as well as the effects of various drugs on arrhythmias, can be assessed. Clinical intracardiac electrophysiologic studies have recently gained in popularity because of their potential for identifying patients who are prone to ventricular fibrillation, as well as for permitting a rational choice of antiarrhythmic or antitachycardia device therapy.

Digital subtraction angiography. Digital subtraction angiography is a modification of cardiac catheterization technique. Contrast is injected intravenously or within the arterial circulation. Images obtained before the injection of contrast (background) are subtracted electronically from the images obtained with contrast, providing improved contrast resolution and imaging.

The technique permits a reduction in the dose of contrast used and less need for selective vessel or cardiac chamber catheterization. It dispenses with the use of cine films. The digital format permits image manipulation and quantitative analysis. It is used in the evaluation of aortocoronary vein grafts and can be used in coronary arteriography. *Intravenous* injection of contrast can be used to visualize cardiac chambers.

VALUE AND LIMITATIONS OF THE TEST

Confirms the diagnosis and aids in the evaluation of cardiac function in congenital or acquired heart disease. Although noninvasive diagnostic methods are frequently adequate in making a diagnosis and deciding on the advisability of surgery, cardiac catheterization and angiography remain the gold standard in confirming such diagnoses and selecting proper therapy, especially in cases where surgery is considered.

Provides a diagnosis for patients with heart disease of unknown etiology in which the exact diagnosis would improve or change the mode of therapy.

Evaluates the status of prosthetic valves and of shunt procedures, the results of corrective procedures for congenital heart disease, and the adequacy and patency of grafts for coronary artery disease.

Diagnoses coronary heart disease and helps select patients for revascularization (surgery or angioplasty).

Evaluates patients with symptomatic coronary artery disease who have not responded well to medical therapy.

Associated with discomfort and a small but definite risk to the patient's life or well-being.

The test requires highly trained personnel and expensive equipment.

NURSING ACTION

1. Instruct the patient to remain fasting 6 hours before the procedure since the contrast medium may cause nausea and vomiting.
2. Ensure that a signed consent is on the patient's record. The patient should be fully informed of the intended procedure as well as the risk of complications.
3. Sedation is usually given, although some physicians avoid any medications because of the possible effect on hemodynamics.

4. ECG leads and an intravenous line will be placed before the study.
5. Adequate psychological and emotional preparation of the patient will contribute to the success and safety of the study.
6. Describe the procedure to the patient, including sensations the patient may expect to experience and the anticipated length of time of the procedure. This can help relieve the patient's fear and anxieties. Written material should be made available to the patient but should not be forced as required reading.
7. If possible, make arrangements for the patient to have a brief visit to the catheterization laboratory some time before the study. This removes some of the fear of the unknown.
8. Following the procedure:
   a. Check vital signs every 15 minutes for 2 to 4 hours and inspect the dressing for bleeding.
   b. Maintain the patient on bed rest with the limb extended for 4 to 6 hours following a procedure requiring an arterial puncture. A sandbag over the wound site is sometimes used.
   c. Check the arterial puncture site for bleeding and check pulses distal to the site.
   d. Check the venous puncture site for warmth, pain, swelling, and redness, since thrombophlebitis may be a complication.
   e. Check venous or arterial cutdown sites for signs of inflammation or infection. Sutures are usually removed 5 to 6 days following the procedure.

NURSING ALERT

Call the physician IMMEDIATELY if signs of vascular insufficiency are noted (sudden pain and cold, white blotchy skin).

Call the physician IMMEDIATELY if there is an unexplained drop in blood pressure, rise in pulse rate, or the patient becomes pale or cyanotic.

Note that there is a relative contraindication to cardiac catheterization in patients with uncontrolled hypertension, congestive heart failure, severe arrhythmias, and a history of anaphylaxis to the contrast medium.*

When the catheterization is of the right side of the heart, the morbidity is less than 1% and is limited to arrhythmias, minor bleeding, venous thromboembolism, or cardiac perforation.

When the angiography involves catheterization of the left side of the heart, be alert for signs of the development of myocardial infarction, cerebrovascular accident, arterial bleeding, and arterial thrombosis.

Watch the patient for adverse reactions to the radiocontrast material such as anaphylactic reaction, volume overload and congestive heart failure, acute right ventricular failure, and acute renal failure.

In order to recognize a nephrotoxic response to the contrast medium should it occur, closely monitor urinary output, renal function, and electrolytes 24 to 48 hours following the use of radiocontrast material.

**Recommended preparation of patients known to have had a prior anaphylactic type reaction to contrast:*

1. Prednisone or an equivalent steroid 150 mg/day is given in divided doses (24 hours before the study and 12 hours after the study).
2. Benadryl 25 to 50 mg is given slow intravenous push just before the procedure, or 50 mg orally or intramuscularly 1 hour before the procedure.

For patients who are at high risk, additional preparation may include:

1. Methylprednisolone 1 g intravenously is given 1 hour before the study.
2. Cimetidine (Tagamet) 300 mg intravenously piggyback is given over 15 minutes, 30 minutes before the study. Experience with cimetidine is limited.

PERICARDIOCENTESIS

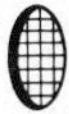

EXPLANATION OF THE TEST

Diagnostic pericardiocentesis is the removal of a small amount of fluid for laboratory examination. Therapeutic pericardiocentesis is the removal of fluid from the pericardial sac, relieving pressure on the heart when pericardial effusion is present in large quantities or has accumulated rapidly in smaller quantities.

A pericardiocentesis needle is introduced under fluoroscopic and ECG monitoring via the subxiphoid or another suitable approach into the pericardial space. Catheters can be introduced in the pericardial space for continuous drainage and introduction of medication. When echocardiography is being used in the evaluation of pericardial effusion, no air should be introduced into the pericardial space. If an x-ray examination is being used for follow-up study, a volume of air equal to the volume of fluid removed may be introduced to better define the pericardial space.

VALUE AND LIMITATIONS OF THE TEST

Detects infective pericarditis and hemopericardium.

Useful in the diagnosis of tumors or immunological disorders such as systemic lupus erythematosus or rheumatoid arthritis.

Treats or prevents life-threatening complications of pericardial tamponade.

Right atrial pressures may be monitored before and after pericardiocentesis to provide hemodynamic information diagnostic of cardiac tamponade or pericardial constriction.

The procedure may be ineffective if pericardial effusion is loculated or if it is mainly posterior without free-flowing anterior effusion. Surgical exploration may be necessary in such a situation.

NURSING ACTION AND COLLECTION OF SPECIMEN

1. Inform the patient that a local anesthetic will be used before the insertion of the aspiration needle.
2. Obtain a signed consent.
3. An intravenous line is established before the procedure.
4. The patient is usually placed in a semisitting position.
5. Send the specimen to the laboratory for determination of chemical content (protein, sugar, LDH) or the presence of malignant cells or signs of infection (bacterial, fungal, tubercular, or viral) or for other purposes as indicated.
6. Assess for abnormal ECG patterns and monitor vital signs frequently.

NURSING ALERT

If ECG monitoring is used to monitor the position of the needle tip, ensure that it is the V lead that is connected to the needle and that the electrocardiograph is properly grounded. If the needle punctures the segment, the ST segment will elevate; if the right atrium is accidentally punctured, the PR segment may elevate. This should be called to the attention of the operating physician immediately.

Strict attention to aseptic technique is essential.

Before the procedure, report to the physician any history or nursing assessment of a bleeding disorder or if the patient is undergoing anticoagulant therapy. These are contraindications to elective diagnostic pericardiocentesis, since under such circumstances accidental puncture of the cardiac chamber may precipitate cardiac tamponade.

During the procedure be alert to the development of atrial or ventricular arrhythmias.

CARDIAC BIOPSY

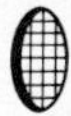

EXPLANATION OF THE TEST

Percutaneous transvenous endomyocardial biopsy is a diagnostic procedure in which a biopsy specimen is obtained from the right ventricular apex or the septum. A similar technique for the biopsy of the left ventricular endomyocardium has also been developed.

VALUE AND LIMITATIONS OF THE TEST

Diagnostic of rejection of a transplanted heart, active inflammatory carditis, or diffuse infiltrative disorders (amyloidosis or myocardial tumors).

Evaluates the effect of cardiotoxic drugs (such as Adriamycin).

Useful in the diagnosis of primary myocardial disease (cardiomyopathies), hypertrophic obstructive cardiomyopathy, hypothyroidism, some of the storage diseases (glycogen storage disease), hemochromatosis, and others.

The value is limited by the fact that the biopsy sample is very small, and sampling error may prevent an accurate diagnosis.

NURSING ACTION

1. Review the indications and possible contraindications for endomyocardial biopsy as it applies to the specific patient.

2. Explain the procedure to the patient. Emphasize the fact that this is basically a specialized form of cardiac catheterization. Avoid provoking additional anxiety.
3. Obtain consent for the procedure. This may include right-sided heart and left-sided heart catheterization and right and left endomyocardial biopsy.
4. Obtain results of studies, which may include ECG, chest x-ray study, CBC, and coagulation studies (PT, PTT).
5. Keep patient fasting for 6 hours. Small amounts of liquids may be taken by mouth. Maintain hydration intravenously, if needed.
6. Secure intravenous line and keep it open with 5% dextrose in water.
7. Shave and cleanse the appropriate area.
8. Premedication is generally not required. A mild sedative may be used.
9. Transfer patient to special procedure room or cardiac catheterization room for the procedure.

NURSING ALERT

Before the procedure. Report to the physician any history or nursing assessment of a bleeding disorder or if the patient is on anticoagulant therapy. These are among the contraindications to cardiac biopsy.

During the procedure. The patient should experience no pain. Any chest pain, especially if pleuritic or pericardial in nature, should be considered a warning of possible cardiac perforation. The procedure should be temporarily interrupted and the patient observed.

Immediately following the procedure. The patient is observed in the cardiac catheterization laboratory for 5 to 10 minutes. If the patient develops chest pain, hypotension, or dyspnea, right-heart pressures are immediately obtained, and on this basis a diagnosis of cardiac tamponade can promptly be made or excluded.

If there are no complications, sit the patient up at a 30 to 40 degree angle. The physician removes the sheath and applies gentle pressure for 5 minutes before the wound is dressed.

5

Diagnostic tests for vascular disorders

Major advances have been made during the past 10 years in the noninvasive diagnosis of peripheral vascular disease. These advances have been possible through the use of improved graphic techniques, sonography, and nuclear studies. Many patients in whom peripheral vascular disease is suspected, or who are at high risk for such disease, can now be safely screened with these studies. In addition, these tests are suitable for repeat studies to help evaluate the results of surgical treatment and to follow the progression of disease. Invasive angiographic studies can thus be reserved for patients who need surgical intervention or for situations in which noninvasive studies have yielded equivocal data.

ANATOMY AND PHYSIOLOGY

The circulation is a closed, continuous loop; the blood that is pumped by the heart must flow through each subdivision of the circuit. If blood is displaced from one segment, another segment must expand to accommodate it. Fig. 5-1 shows the principal arteries and veins.

Hemodynamics is the study of the dynamics of blood circulation. It is concerned with the physical characteristics of blood and with pressure, resistance, and flow.

Blood is composed of plasma and cells, of which more than 99% are red cells. The *hematocrit* of blood is the volume percentage of blood that consists of red cells; the hematocrit is a major determinant of the viscosity of blood. Plasma is similar to interstitial fluid, except that plasma contains more protein.

Blood pressure is the force exerted by the blood against any unit area of a vessel wall. It is usually measured in millimeters of mercury. When the heart contracts and ejects blood into the aorta, the proximal part of the aorta distends because of the pressure. A pressure wave is transmitted down the aorta, picking up speed as it reaches the less compliant vessels and finally arriving in the peripheral arteries. The pressure that exists during this rise in pressure in the arterial system after cardiac systole is called *systolic pressure;* the minimum pressure, which occurs late in diastole, is called *diastolic pressure*. The difference between the two is known as *pulse pressure*.

The rate of flow of blood through a vessel is determined by the pressure difference between the two ends of the vessel and by vascular resistance to the flow. Blood flows from the area of high pressure to the area of low pressure.

Vessels are distensible, veins more so than arteries. Veins are called the storage areas of the circulatory system, because with a given rise in pressure, 6 to 10 times more blood fills a vein than an artery of the same size. The term *compliance* refers to the ability of a vessel to increase its volume in response to a given increase in pressure. The compliance of the venous system is about 24 times greater than that of the arteries.

Resistance to blood flow is measured indirectly; it is expressed in *peripheral resistance units*. In the arteries there is little resistance to blood flow, but in the arterioles and the capillaries the resistance is considerable. In order for blood to be pumped into these small vessels, the arterial pressure must be high. The arterioles, which have strong muscular walls, are able either to close off completely or to dilate severalfold and thus to control the amount of blood going into the capillaries, which have very thin, permeable walls to permit the exchange of fluids and nutrients between the blood and the interstitial spaces. The venules gradually turn into veins, which transport the blood back to the heart.

Blood flow is the amount of blood (in milliliters or liters) passing a given point in the circulatory system each minute. *Cardiac output* represents the amount of blood pumped by the left ventricle into the aorta each minute. *Venous return* is the amount of blood flowing from the veins into the right atrium each minute.

The amount of blood that can pass through a vessel in a given time at a given pressure difference changes dramatically with slight changes in vessel diameter and resistance. Complex neural and humoral controls exist. Blood flow slows as arterial pressure falls. If arterial pressure falls to a certain point, blood flow ceases entirely. At this point (critical closing pressure) the arterioles close completely.

The blood returns very efficiently from the lower extremities, against gravity. There are valves in the veins that permit the blood to flow only toward the heart, and every time the legs are moved, muscles contract and squeeze the veins, providing a "muscle pump" to help propel venous blood back to the heart. When this muscle pump is not operating (as when a person is standing at absolute attention), venous pressure in the lower leg increases, fluid leaks into the tissue, and blood volume diminishes.

NONINVASIVE VASCULAR DIAGNOSTIC STUDIES

OPHTHALMODYNAMOMETRY (ODM)

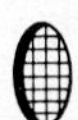

EXPLANATION OF THE TEST

Ophthalmodynamometry is a simple bedside study where calibrated strain gauges are applied to the sclera to exert increasing pressure on the eye, producing gradual obliteration of flow in the retinal arteries.

VALUE AND LIMITATIONS OF THE TEST

Aids in the detection of unilateral carotid artery obstructive disease

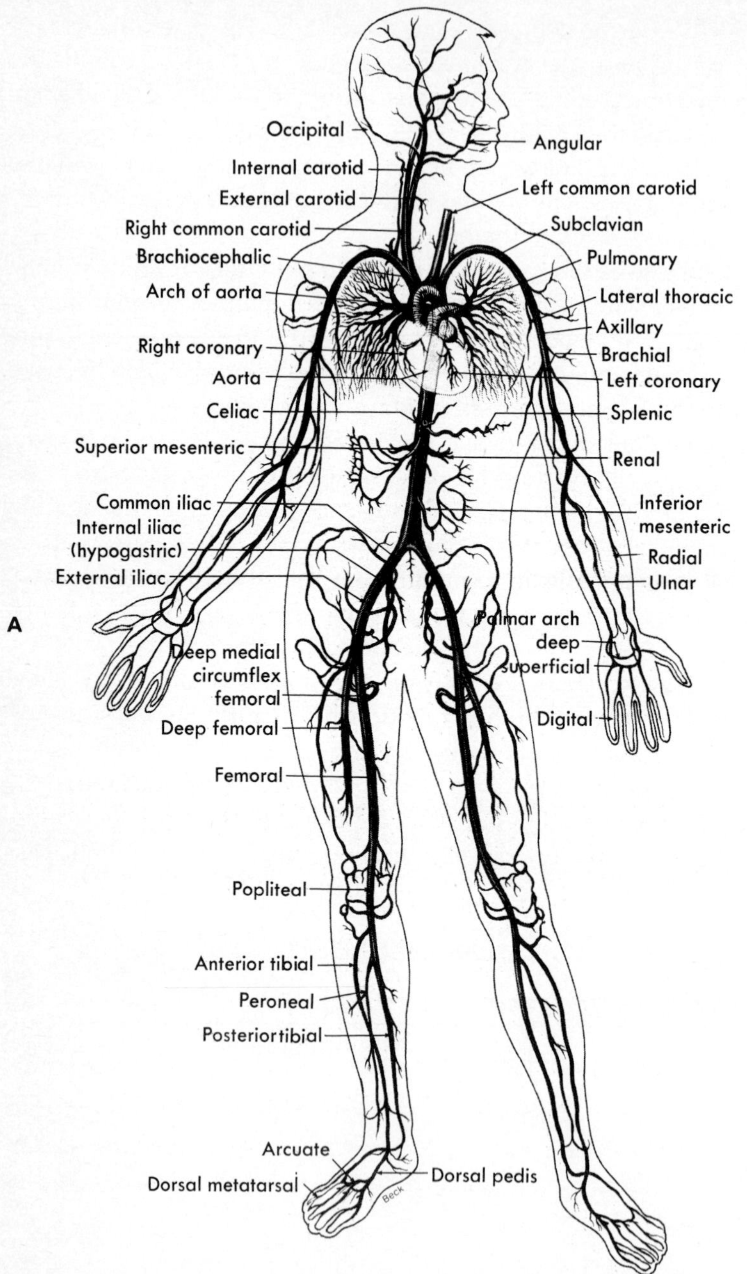

Fig. 5-1. A, *The arterial system.* ***B,*** *The venous system. (From Thibodeau, G.A.: Textbook of anatomy and physiology, ed. 12, St. Louis, 1987, Times Mirror/ Mosby College Publishing.)*

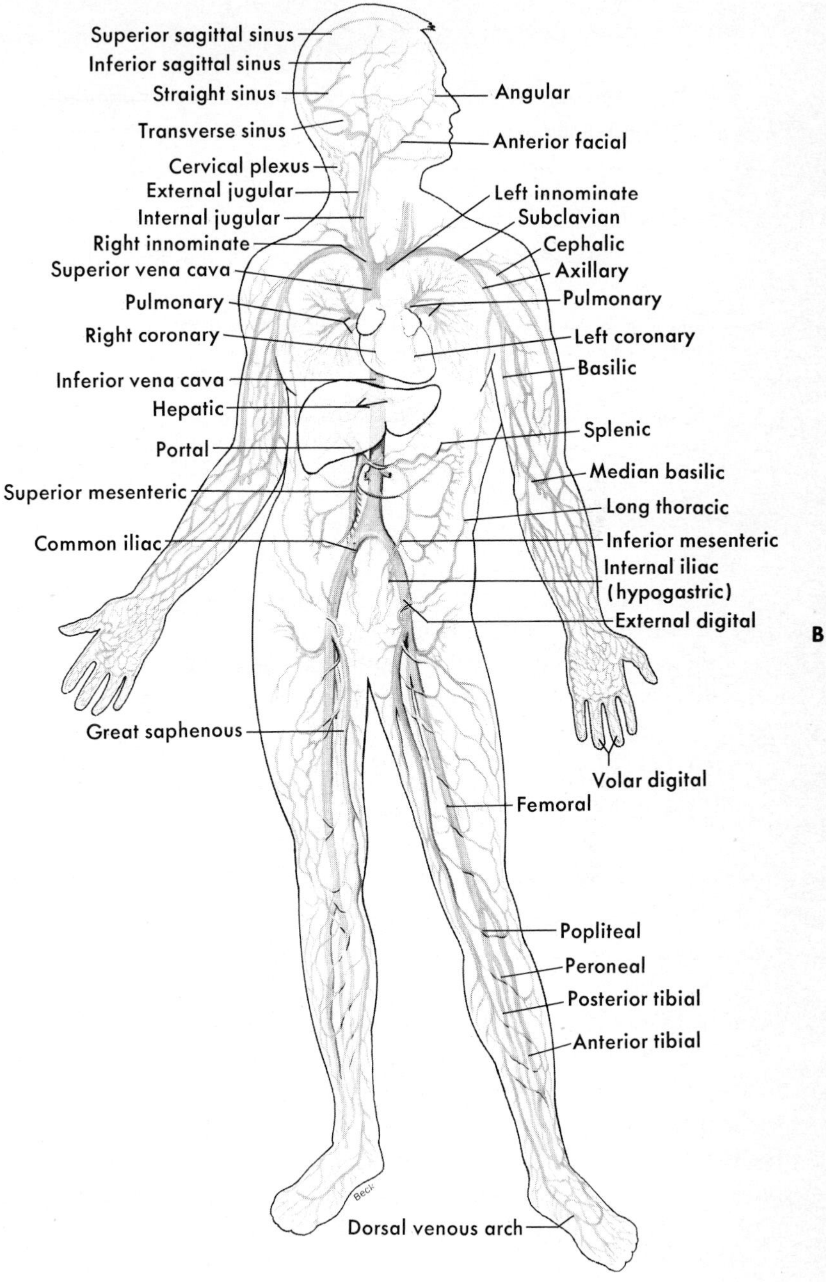

Fig. 5-1, cont'd. *For legend see opposite page.*

Bilateral carotid obstructive disease can be missed with this technique.

The test requires the skill of a physician and is rarely included in a screening test.

NURSING ACTION

1. Inform the patient that no special preparation is needed for this test.
2. Explain to the patient that an instrument will be gently applied to the eyes and that there will be slightly increasing pressure on the eye.
3. Explain to the patient that the response of the arteries in the eyes is a reflection of the pressure in the carotid arteries.

CLINICAL IMPLICATIONS

The fundus is observed with an ophthalmoscope and the pressure needed to cause intermittent collapse of the retinal artery branches (diastolic pressure) and total collapse of the retinal artery (systolic pressure) is determined. A unilateral carotid artery obstructive disease is detected by comparing one side with another.

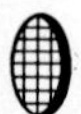

OCULOPLETHYSMOGRAPHY (OPG) AND OCULOPNEUMOPLETHYSMOGRAPHY (OPPG)

EXPLANATION OF THE TEST

In OPG, fluid-filled contact lenses or cups are applied to the eyes following administration of a local anesthetic. Cyclic changes in the volume of this fluid are recorded; these changes reflect pulsatile flow in the ophthalmic artery, the first branch of the internal carotid artery (Fig. 5-2). Narrowing of an internal carotid artery will cause a delay in the pulse wave and changes in the blood volume. The pulse wave in the ipsilateral earlobe, which reflects external carotid artery pulses, is used for reference. Twenty milliseconds or more of delay in the pulse wave in the ophthalmic artery (which reflects internal carotid pulse) is considered abnormal, signifying stenosis of that vessel.

In OPPG, air-filled transducers are applied to the lateral aspects of the sclerae; negative pressure of up to 300 mm Hg is then applied in an attempt to obliterate the ophthalmic artery pressure wave form

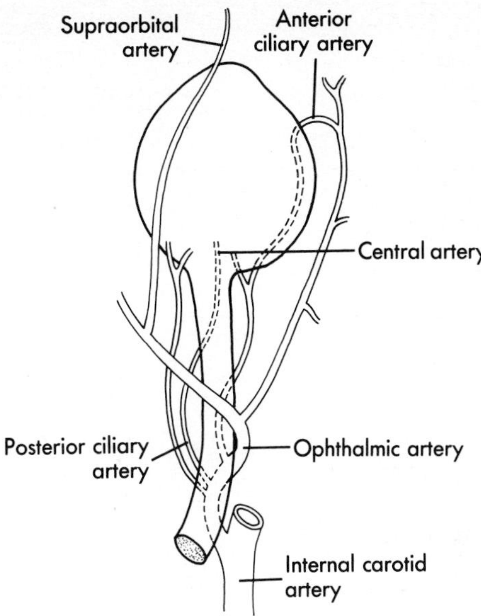

Fig. 5-2. *Ophthalmic artery and its branches.*

and thereby estimate the systolic pressure in the ophthalmic artery. This method is believed to be more accurate than OPG.

VALUE AND LIMITATIONS OF THE TEST

Provides additional graphic methods of screening for internal carotid artery stenosis or occlusion.

When combined with information from carotid phonangiography (CPA), the risk of a false-positive or false-negative result is 5%.

OPG may miss mild to moderate, bilateral, or equal narrowing of carotid arteries. OPPG is more sensitive.

NURSING ACTION

1. Inform the patient that no special preparation is needed for this test.
2. Explain to the patient that a local anesthetic will be instilled into the eyes and fluid-filled contact lenses applied so that the blood flow in the ophthalmic artery and carotid artery can be evaluated.

NURSING ALERT

When any of the following conditions are detected in the course of the nursing examination of the patient, it should be reported immediately to the physician, since they are contraindications to the procedure: conjunctivitis, uncontrolled glaucoma, history of retinal detachment, recent eye surgery (within 2 months), or allergy to topical anesthetics.

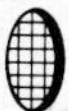

CAROTID PHONOANGIOGRAPHY (CPA)

EXPLANATION OF THE TEST

Carotid phonoangiography, also called carotid audiofrequency analysis or quantitative spectoral phonoangiography, is an extension of the technique of auscultation. Special microphones are positioned over areas of bruits, usually the carotid arteries. The sound picked up is displayed on an oscilloscope and photographed. The sound frequency pattern is analyzed with the help of computers (spectral analysis).

VALUE AND LIMITATIONS OF THE TEST

An adjunct to auscultation
Helpful in the documentation of carotid bruits and estimation of the degree and location of stenosis
Helpful in differentiating transmitted cardiac murmurs from cardiac bruits
Not reliable in the diagnosis of severe carotid stenosis, since no bruit may be recorded when the closure is greater than 90%

NURSING ACTION

1. Inform the patient that there are no dietary restrictions before taking this test.
2. Instruct the patient that the test is painless and safe and that a water-soluble conductive jelly is applied to the tip of the transducer to provide coupling between the skin and the transducer.

CLINICAL IMPLICATIONS

The longer the duration of the bruit, the greater the degree of stenosis. If the bruit extends into diastole, it usually signifies severe stenosis. The presence or absence of heart sounds and the frequency of the sounds recorded also provide diagnostic clues.

ULTRASOUND ARTERIOGRAPHY

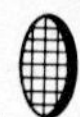

EXPLANATION OF THE TEST

The pulsed Doppler imaging instrument and the B-mode ultrasonic scanner can be used to demonstrate the anatomy of the arteries, particularly the carotid bifurcation and the internal carotid artery.

The Doppler imaging instrument uses echoes of the moving blood column to produce images of the outline of a vessel wall. It takes 10 to 20 minutes to construct these static images. Blood velocities are measured and the degree of stenosis estimated.

The B-mode ultrasonic scanner provides dynamic images of a vessel wall in real time, with a resolution of 0.5 to 1 mm. The duplex system combines the two methods.

VALUE AND LIMITATIONS OF THE TEST

Useful in the noninvasive evaluation of patients who have had strokes, transient ischemic attacks, asymptomatic bruits, or claudication.

Provides a reliable diagnosis of high-grade narrowing of an internal carotid artery.

Diagnostic for total occlusion of an internal carotid artery.

Diagnostic results require great precision and experience with ultrasound methods.

Calcification or atheromatous plaques of the artery wall will interfere with ultrasound imaging by simulating defects or "blanks" in the lumen where none may exist.

With B-mode scanning alone, the common carotid artery is seen well, but the internal carotid artery is seen less clearly. The extent of stenosis cannot be precisely gauged, and severe stenosis or total occlusion may not be clearly distinguished.

NURSING ACTION

1. There is no special patient preparation for this test.
2. Instruct the patient that the test is painless and safe and that a

water-soluble conductive jelly is applied to the tip of the transducer to provide coupling between the skin and the transducer.
3. The patient should remove all clothing over the site to be tested and assume a supine position on the examining table or bed.

CLINICAL IMPLICATIONS

The combined utilization of real-time, B-mode imaging and pulsed Doppler techniques permits visualization of plaque and analysis of the flow disturbance it creates. Improved signal processing methods and the use of computerized pattern recognition systems should make such studies even more reliable than they are now.

In Fig. 5-3 internal carotid artery obstruction is demonstrated by carotid phonoangiography and ultrasonic arteriography and is confirmed by contrast arteriography. Fig. 5-4 shows how a duplex scanner visualizes and analyzes blood flow at a carotid bifurcation.

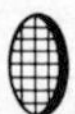

IMPEDANCE PLETHYSMOGRAPHY

EXPLANATION OF THE TEST

In impedance plethysmography a pneumatic cuff is applied to a limb for the purpose of occluding the venous return. As the blood volume in the limb increases, so does the electrical resistance; by measuring the electrical resistance, one can obtain information about blood flow. Two electrodes are applied to the limb, and a very weak electrical current is passed through it. The resistance of the limb to this current is then recorded on graph paper.

VALUE AND LIMITATIONS OF THE TEST

Helpful in the diagnosis of proximal deep-vein thrombosis and other types of obstruction

Particularly helpful in the diagnosis of recurrent venous thrombosis. When combined with fibrinogen leg scanning (discussed later in the chapter), its accuracy is improved.

Insensitive to obstruction in distal extremity veins.

NURSING ACTION

1. Inform the patient that there is no special dietary patient preparation for this test.

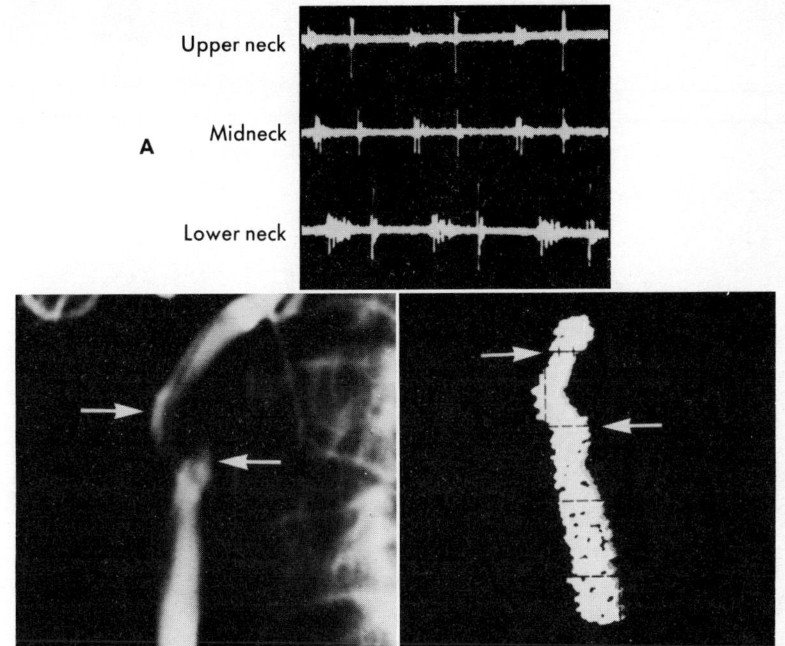

Fig. 5-3. *Noninvasive studies of an occluded internal carotid artery yielded varying amounts of information, but in combination were as conclusive as contrast arteriography.* ***A,*** *Microphone recordings along the neck revealed a bruit only in the lower neck.* ***B,*** *Contrast arteriogram showed total occlusion of proximal internal carotid artery* (right arrow) *and a patent external carotid artery* (left arrow). ***C,*** *Ultrasonic arteriogram gave corresponding image* (arrows *mark same arteries*). *(From Strandness, D.E.: Noninvasive evaluation of carotid artery disease, J. Cardiovasc. Med., September 1980, p. 841.)*

2. Before the test instruct the patient to void and put on a hospital gown.
3. Help the patient assume a supine position on the examining table or bed with the leg elevated 30 to 35 degrees to promote venous drainage.
4. Ask the patient to flex the knee slightly and shift the weight to the same side as the leg being tested.
5. Attach electrodes loosely to the calf about 4 inches apart and wrap the pressure cuff around the thigh 2 inches above the knee.

CLINICAL IMPLICATIONS

In patients with venous thrombosis the resting blood volume in the leg is greater than normal. Therefore, when venous return is

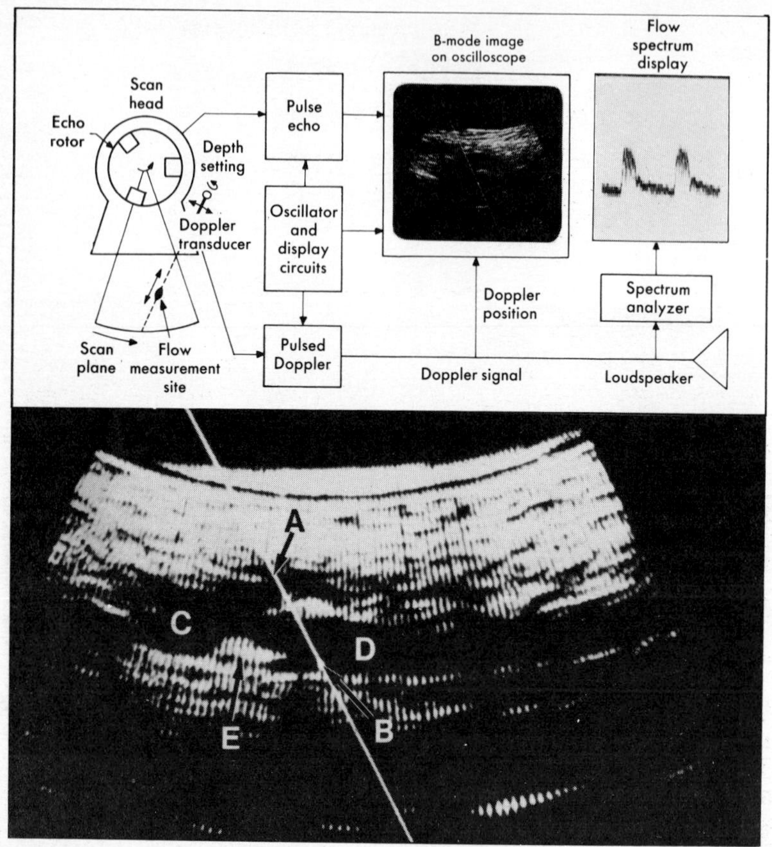

Fig. 5-4. Top, *Electronic-component diagram showing an ultrasonic duplex scanner processing pulse echo information to provide a real-time B-mode image of the carotid bifurcation. In addition, pulsed Doppler signals are used to measure flow velocity at specific sites, providing both an audible output via a loudspeaker and a display of the analyzed flow spectrum.* Bottom, *In this enlarged B-mode image, the diagonal line* (A) *indicates the path of the Doppler beam along which flow at point* B *is being analyzed. In the imaged view of the bifurcation, a plaque* (E) *is seen at the midportion of the bulb, between the common carotid* (C) *and the internal carotid* (D) *arteries. (From Strandness, D.E.: Noninvasive evaluation of carotid artery disease, J. Cardiovasc. Med., September 1980, p. 841.)*

occluded by the cuff, the increase in blood volume and the increase in electrical resistance are smaller than normal; after the cuff is deflated, the decrease in blood volume and the decrease in electrical resistance are smaller than normal. Fig. 5-5 illustrates this procedure and compares the results from a normal leg with those from a leg with venous thrombosis.

INVASIVE DIAGNOSTIC STUDIES

RADIONUCLIDE PHLEBOGRAPHY (VENOGRAPHY)

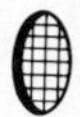

EXPLANATION OF THE TEST

Technetium Tc 99m microaggregated albumin is injected into the dorsal veins of the feet and is directed into the deep veins by tourniquets above the ankles. An anterior scintigram enables one to view the veins as the circulation carries the isotope through the field of view. Overlapping views of the thighs and pelvis are also obtained by repeating the procedure. After injection, the albumin is trapped in the pulmonary capillaries; thus a perfusion lung scan can also be obtained at the end of the study.

VALUE AND LIMITATIONS OF THE TEST

Aids in the diagnosis of deep vein thrombosis.

There is the possibility of false-positive results because of valve incompetence. Tagged human albumin microspheres can be used to try to improve the yield.

NURSING ACTION

1. Inform the patient that there is no dietary preparation for this test.
2. Instruct the patient that there will be an injection into the feet veins and then the legs and pelvis will be imaged. Tell him or her that this test permits the evaluation of blood flow in the deep veins.
3. Make sure that the patient understands that this is a painless and safe procedure.

CLINICAL IMPLICATIONS

Deep vein thrombosis can be visualized by this procedure.

VALUE OF THE TEST

Iodine 125 leg scanning is most helpful in the diagnosis of thrombi in the calf veins and in the distal half of the thigh. Thus, its great utility is when used in conjunction with impedance plethysmography.

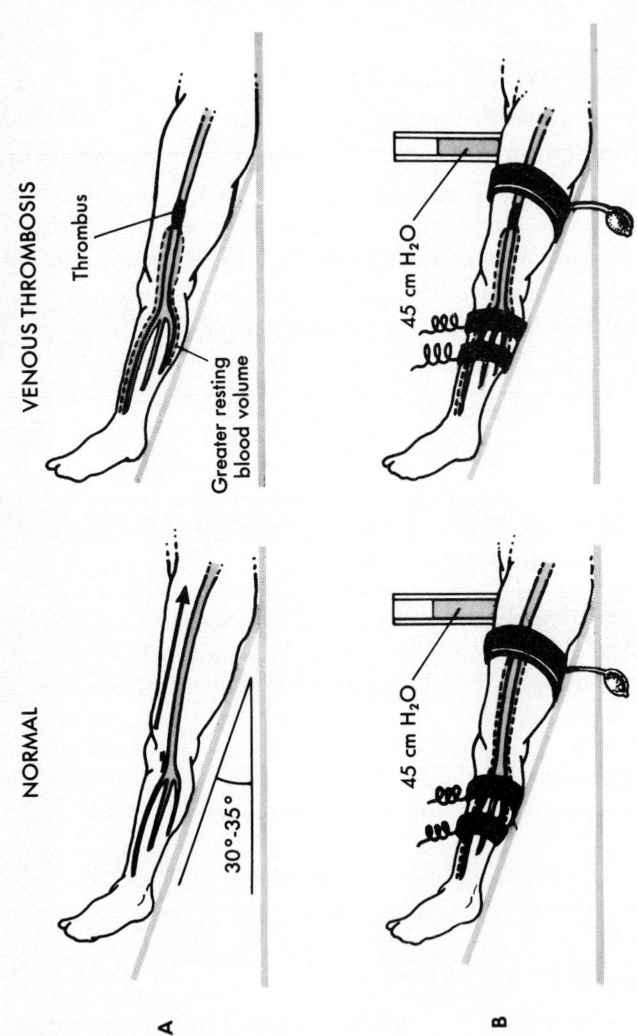
A
NORMAL
30°-35°
VENOUS THROMBOSIS
Thrombus
Greater resting blood volume
B
45 cm H_2O
45 cm H_2O

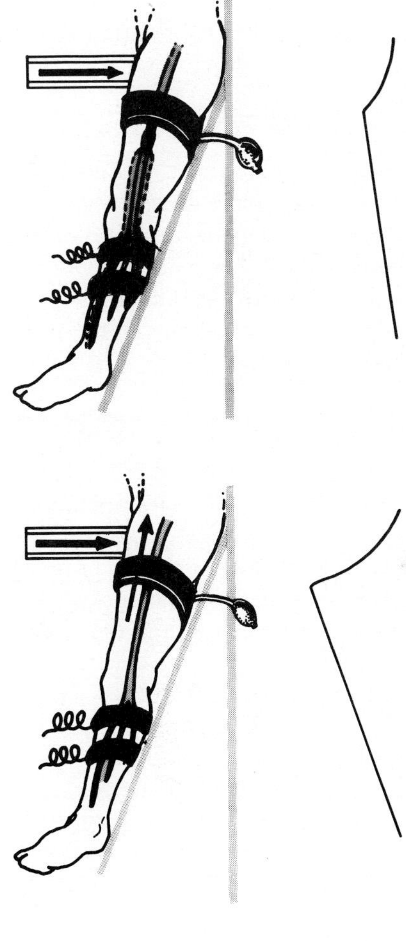

Fig. 5-5. *Impedance plethysmography.* **A,** *The resting blood volume is greater in the leg with venous thrombosis than in the normal leg.* **B,** *Two electrodes are applied, to deliver a weak electrical current, and the cuff is inflated to 45 cm* H_2O *to occlude venous return. In the leg with venous thrombosis, there is a smaller increase in blood volume and less resistance to the current. Thus the tracing (***D***) does not rise as high as for the normal leg.* **C,** *When the cuff is deflated, the decrease in electrical resistance, recorded in* **D,** *is smaller in the leg with venous thrombosis than in the normal leg.*

FIBRINOGEN I 125 UPTAKE TEST (FIBRINOGEN LEG SCANNING)

EXPLANATION OF THE TEST

Fibrinogen I 125 is a radiopharmaceutical used in the detection of deep vein thrombosis of the legs. The iodine 125-tagged fibrinogen is injected intravenously and is incorporated into the blood clots. The patient's legs are then scanned with scintillation detectors to identify sites of increased radioactivity (clots).

VALUE AND LIMITATIONS OF THE TEST

Iodine 125 leg scanning is most helpful in the diagnosis of thrombi in the calf veins and the distal half of the thigh. Its greatest utility is when used in conjunction with impedance plethysmography.

Limitations include delays of 24 to 72 hours in the performance of the test, the possibility of false-positive results in the presence of inflammation and hematoma, and the inability of the test to evaluate the high femoral and iliac veins.

NURSING ACTION

1. Inform the patient that there is no dietary preparation for this test.
2. Instruct the patient that there will be an injection into the feet veins and then the legs and pelvis will be photographed. Tell him or her that this test permits the evaluation of blood flow in the deep veins.
3. Make sure that the patient understands that this is a painless and safe procedure.
4. Following the test do not wash the markings from the patient's legs, since the procedure may be repeated later.
5. Before lowering the patient's legs, be certain that the procedure has been completed.

CLINICAL IMPLICATIONS

Fig. 5-6 shows the procedure for the diagnosis of venous thrombosis by leg scanning. Increased radioactivity can be detected in the region overlying a thrombus as a result of the incorporation of the radioactive fibrinogen into the thrombus.

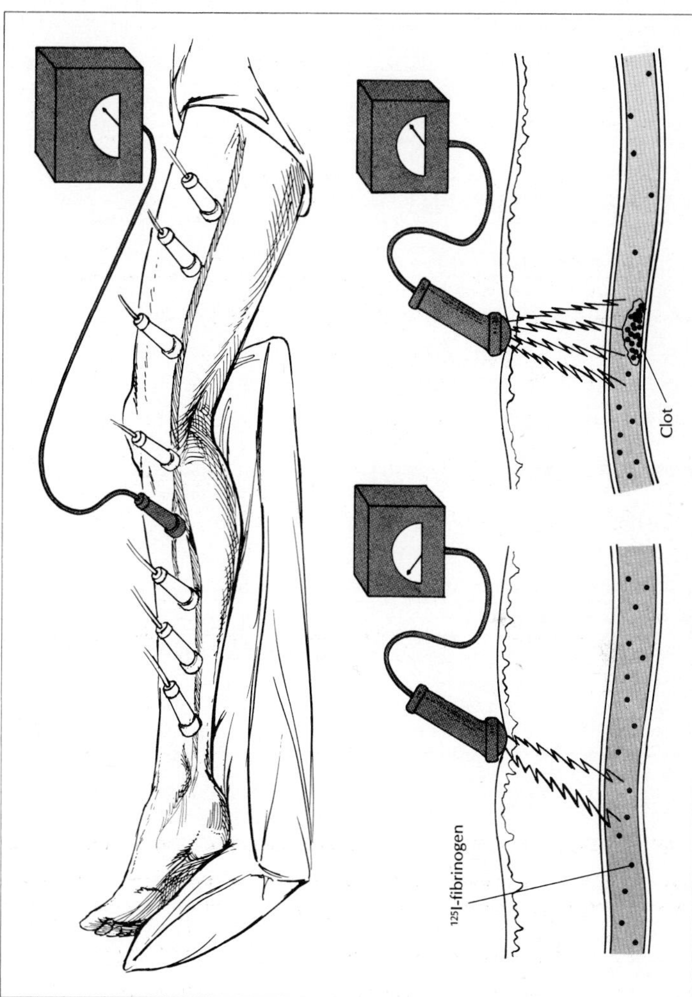

Fig. 5-6. *Leg scanning. A single intravenous injection of fibrinogen I 125 is incorporated into the blood clots and is scanned with a scintillation detector. The sites of increased radioactivity are identified.* (From Hirsh, J.: Noninvasive tests for thromboembolic disease, Hosp. Prac., September 1982, p. 82.)

NURSING ALERT

In taking the nursing history, ask the patient whether he or she has used heparin in the last 24 to 48 hours and report this to the physician; this may render the results of the test unreliable.

CONTRAST VENOGRAPHY

EXPLANATION OF THE TEST

Contrast medium is injected into a superficial vein of the foot or ankle, and sequential radiological visualization of the veins is done by means of rapid serial radiography. The technique may also be applied to a vein in an upper extremity.

VALUE AND LIMITATIONS OF THE TEST

The definitive way of diagnosing venous thrombosis; it is done when noninvasive studies yield equivocal results.

Careful attention to technique is necessary to prevent extravasation and secondary inflammation.

Insufficient injection of contrast medium may give false-positive results.

The procedure can be painful.

NURSING ACTION

1. Inform the patient that there is no dietary preparation for this test.
2. Instruct the patient that there will be an injection into the feet veins and then x-ray films will be taken of the legs. Tell the patient that this test permits the evaluation of blood flow in the deep veins.

CLINICAL IMPLICATIONS

Venous thrombosis can be visualized.

CONTRAST ARTERIOGRAPHY

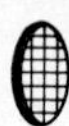

EXPLANATION OF THE TEST

Contrast arteriography remains the gold standard in vascular diagnostic imaging. The techniques are similar to those of cardiac catheterization and angiography (see Chapter 4).

VALUE OF THE TEST

Permits diagnostic visualization of the arterial system.

NURSING ACTION

Prepare the patient as for cardiac catheterization and obtain an informed consent.

DIGITAL SUBTRACTION INTRAVENOUS ANGIOGRAPHY

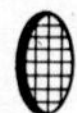

EXPLANATION OF THE TEST

This computerized fluoroscopic method permits adequate visualization of extracranial and intracranial vessels and systemic arteries after the intravenous injection of contrast material.

VALUE OF THE TEST

Useful for screening patients who have carotid or cerebrovascular disease, or abnormalities of the renal or peripheral arteries.

NURSING ACTION

1. Inform the patient that there is no dietary preparation for this test.
2. Instruct the patient that there will be an injection of contrast material followed by fluoroscopic examination for the purpose of visualizing the veins of the body.
3. Secure informed consent.
4. Determine if there is history of reaction to contrast agents.

6

Diagnostic tests for bronchopulmonary disease

ANATOMY AND PHYSIOLOGY

The lung is an organ dedicated to the exchange of gases, primarily oxygen and carbon dioxide. This exchange occurs at the level of the alveolus where the distance between red blood cells and outside or ambient air is minimal but the surface area for this gas exchange maximal.

Ventilation

The movement of air into and out of the alveoli is generally dependent on the integrity of the respiratory muscles, the resistance to air flow within the airways, and the elasticity of the lung. The lung, being an elastic organ, would tend to contract into a small ball if it were removed from the chest. The chest wall can be thought of as a container made up of muscle and bone that may also change its volume but is more rigid than the elastic lung and requires muscle activity to significantly change its size. Normally at the end of expiration, when there is no air movement into or out of the lung, the tendency for the elastic lung to contract is exactly balanced by the negative pressure that exists in the pleural space between the lung and the chest wall. During inspiration, the inspiratory muscles enlarge the chest wall, reducing the pleural pressure surrounding the lung, thereby reducing the pressure actually within the alveolar air spaces. With the glottis open, ambient air, which at sea level is at one atmosphere of pressure (1 atm), will then flow into the lung, which contains air at this reduced pressure. At the end of inspiration, the lung is at a larger volume and, like a stretched spring, exerts a greater tendency to collapse. This greater elastic pressure is exactly balanced by a more negative pressure within the pleural space. During normal relaxed breathing, exhalation occurs simply by relaxing the expiratory muscles. It follows, then, that without the muscular effort of the inspiratory muscles to hold the chest wall out, the very same negative pressure that caused the elastic lung to expand will now pull the chest wall inward, reducing the pleural pressure and allowing the elastic lung to rebound toward its original shape, until once again the tendency of the lung to collapse is exactly balanced by the relative rigidity of the chest wall and once again a minimal negative pressure is formed within this pleural space (approximately 5 cm H_2O less than atmospheric pressure). Thus, during relaxed breathing expiration is passive. It is only during exercise, talking, singing, or coughing that expiratory muscles are used to more forcefully push air out of the lungs.

Respiratory muscles

The diaphragm, the external intercostals, and the parasternal intercartilaginous muscles are the chief muscles of respiration, with the diaphragm accounting for more than two thirds of the air entering the lung during quiet breathing. The primary muscles of expiration are the internal intercostal muscles, the external and internal oblique abdominal muscles, and the transversus and rectus abdominis muscles, the contraction of which depresses the ribs.

Gas exchange

Atmospheric air is composed primarily of nitrogen and oxygen with small amounts of water vapor, carbon dioxide, and other gases. At sea level the pressure of all the gases is equal to 760 mm Hg (1 atm, one atmosphere). However, the actual pressure exerted by each gas is proportional to its concentration. In the lung, gases are fully humidified. Since the pressure of water vapor is 47 mm Hg, the total pressure exerted by all the gases must be 713 mm Hg. Since the concentration of oxygen is approximately 21% in atmospheric air, then the total pressure of oxygen is 150 or 21% of 713. Obviously, at altitude, as the atmospheric pressure decreases, so does the pressure of oxygen contained within the lung. The actual pressure of oxygen (Po_2) in the venous end of the pulmonary capillary is only 40. One can see the very obvious pressure gradient between the two, which influences the movement of oxygen from inspired air moving into the pulmonary capillary blood.

The actual volume of the gas that is in solution in a fluid is dependent on the pressure of that gas. Thus, if the pressure of oxygen were raised (e.g., in a hyperbaric chamber), the actual amount dissolved in solution would also be greater. At ordinary atmospheric pressures, however, the actual amount of oxygen dissolved in blood is very small and without another mechanism to increase the amount of oxygen taken up and carried by the blood, human life could not be sustained.

Hemoglobin

Hemoglobin is a protein found in red blood cells. Each hemoglobin molecule can carry four molecules of oxygen by means of a reversible chemical combination. It is only through hemoglobin that sufficient oxygen can be taken up from the alveolar air and carried within the blood to sustain life. The actual volume of oxygen carried in the blood is related in a nonlinear fashion to the oxygen pressure or tension. Ordinarily, oxygen pressures above 60 mm Hg are associated with 90% or more of the maximal amount of oxygen that can be carried by hemoglobin. Below an oxygen pressure of 60 mm Hg, there is rapid loading or unloading of oxygen, whereas in atmospheric air carbon dioxide pressure is less than 1 mm Hg. Within the alveolus the levels are much higher depending on the degree of ventilation. Ordinarily, the carbon dioxide pressure is 46 mm Hg and the oxygen pressure is reduced accordingly to approximately 100 mm Hg. This 100 mm Hg oxygen pressure equilibrates with blood as it traverses the pulmonary capillaries and is responsible for a small volume of oxygen carried in physical solution and for a much larger volume of oxygen that is carried in reversible chemical combination with hemoglobin. Any lung disease that reduces the amount of air, and hence oxygen, at the alveolar level will cause a reduction in oxygen tensions and, if the tensions are less than 60 mm Hg, will result in a significant reduction in the volume of oxygen carried by hemoglobin.

Carbon dioxide transport

The movement of carbon dioxide can be thought of as being the reverse of oxygen flow. Since oxygen is taken up by tissues, blood returning to the lung contains less oxygen and hence the gradient favors the uptake of oxygen within the lung. On the other hand, as oxygen is taken up by body tissues carbon dioxide is produced and the concentration in venous blood is higher than that in arterial blood, roughly 46 and 40 mm Hg respectively. Within blood, carbon dioxide is carried in three forms: physically dissolved, 10%; chemically combined with amino groups on the hemoglobin molecule, 25% to 30%; and converted to bicarbonate, 60%. When blood reaches the alveolar capillaries, a rapid conversion of the bicarbonate, as well as of the bound carbon dioxide, occurs to the carbon dioxide molecule. Although the gradient between pulmonary capillary blood carbon dioxide tensions and alveolar tensions is much smaller than with oxygen, the carbon dioxide diffusibility is much greater, and the major determinant to the carbon dioxide tension of the blood is ventilation. That is, the more rapidly air can be moved into and out of the lung, the lower will be the carbon dioxide tensions. Thus, an individual breathing twice the normal rate will have a carbon dioxide tension of only 20 (normal being 40 mm Hg). Similarly, in a patient who is hypoventilating with an overall ventilation of only one-half normal, the carbon dioxide tension will be greater (80 mm Hg).

PATHOPHYSIOLOGY AND CLINICAL IMPLICATIONS OF LABORATORY TESTS

Pulmonary embolism

Pulmonary embolism is commonly diagnosed under the dramatic circumstances of pulmonary infarction with pleuritic chest pain and hemoptysis, or in the setting of acute dyspnea, tachypnea, and tachycardia in a patient who has an obvious predisposition to this disorder (postoperative state, obesity, heart failure). Frequently, pulmonary embolism occurs without such a classic presentation. Occasionally, patients who have had dyspnea for a long time—even many months—are ultimately diagnosed as having chronic multiple pulmonary emboli.

Chest x-ray studies and *resting ECG data* are frequently normal (in the absence of cor pulmonale). *Pulmonary function studies* reveal normal spirograms or flow-volume loops and normal lung volumes. However, the *carbon monoxide diffusing capacity* is reduced and the *resting arterial oxygen pressure* ($Pa{O_2}$) is often decreased, although it may be normal.

With exercise there are frequently characteristic changes, depending on the degree of pulmonary vascular obstruction. These include

Decreased arterial oxygen tension
Decreased maximal oxygen consumption
Unusually high pulse rate for actual oxygen consumed
The generation of an unusually high base deficit (metabolic acidosis) presumably resulting from poor cardiac output, tissue hypoxia, and anaerobic metabolism with lactic acid production

In the absence of cardiac disease, which can explain these abnormalities, pulmonary vascular disease must be carefully ruled out. *Ventilation-perfusion scanning,* and even catheterization of the right side of the heart, with pulmonary angiography, should be considered.

Perfusion lung scanning is helpful if used correctly. A normal scan with rare exceptions excludes a clinically significant pulmonary embolus. On the other hand, an abnormal scan should not be equated with a pulmonary embolus. Numerous other disorders that may alter pulmonary blood flow and be confused with the clinical picture of pulmonary embolism may produce an abnormal or "positive" perfusion lung scan. *Ventilation lung scanning* in conjunction with perfusion lung scanning may help exclude some of these other causes.

Pulmonary angiography is the most specific diagnostic test for pulmonary embolism. It is used when the less specific tests have not yielded a clear picture or when surgical intervention (e.g., inferior vena cava ligation or pulmonary embolectomy) is being considered. Pressures on the right side of the heart may be obtained during angiography to provide a hemodynamic assessment. In major vascular occlusion there is increased pulmonary artery pressure and possibly secondary tricuspid regurgitation.

Pulmonary edema

Pulmonary edema may be caused by elevated pulmonary venous pressure secondary to cardiac disease, as in left ventricular failure or mitral stenosis, or it may be secondary to increased permeability of the pulmonary capillaries, as seen in the adult respiratory distress syndrome (ARDS), frequently related to shock, trauma, and most commonly sepsis. Uncommonly, it may mimic bronchial asthma or interstitial lung disease.

The differential diagnosis is made by means of clinical history, cardiac examination, hemodynamic assessment, and response to therapy. Pulmonary function tests are generally not used.

Pneumonias

The diagnosis is suspected clinically because of the history and physical examination. The most useful test is the *chest radiograph,* in which a parenchymal infiltrate is seen. When cavities are observed, lung necrosis is likely and the clinician should consider such infections as tuberculosis, fungal infections, and staphylococcal, anaerobic, and gram-negative pneumonias. The *sputum examination* is very helpful, a Gram stain of which determines the gram positivity or gram negativity and the morphology of the predominant organism and helps in guiding initial antibiotic treatment. The sputum is cultured to isolate the organism.

Pleural disease

Pleural disease may be secondary to inflammation, infection, or neoplasm. The diagnosis is suspected on clinical examination and confirmed by the *x-ray examination of the chest,* sometimes including *CT scanning*. In the presence of pleural fluid, thoracentesis may be performed to help in the differential diagnosis and when indicated a *pleural biopsy* may be obtained by a specially modified needle under local anesthesia.

RADIOGRAPHIC EVALUATION OF LUNG DISEASE

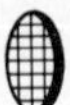

ROUTINE CHEST RADIOGRAPHY

EXPLANATION OF THE TEST

The basic chest x-ray study consists of two views of the chest, posterior to anterior (PA) and left lateral (LL). Supplementary views can also be taken as needed, for example, decubitus views to determine if pleural fluid is present and if it is mobile or loculated.

Fluoroscopy augments routine radiography by permitting visualization of the lungs and diaphragm during respiratory motion and thus one can better evaluate diaphragmatic function and visualize subtle nodular or parenchymal calcifications and the extent of inflation and deflation of the lungs. Fluoroscopy exposes the patient to more radiation than standard chest radiography and should be used selectively. It is used most commonly in conjunction with biopsy of the lung by needle or bronchoscopic means.

Whenever possible, these studies should be done with the patient in the upright position. When pneumothorax is considered, x-ray views should be taken in the upright position because small degrees of pneumothorax may be readily missed in supine views. For further details of routine radiographic examination of the chest relating to the cardiovascular system see Chapter 4.

VALUE AND LIMITATIONS OF THE TEST

Oblique views (15 or 45 degrees) permit visualization of lung periphery without interference from breast or pectoral shadows, and help localize pulmonary abnormalities.

Lateral decubitus views permit the detection of small amounts of pleural fluid or a small pneumothorax when upright films cannot be obtained and help distinguish infrapulmonary effusion from high diaphragmatic effusion.

Expiratory films help detect a small pneumothorax, may demonstrate air trapping, and may be used to evaluate the extent of diaphragmatic excursion.

Apical lordotic views are sometimes used to visualize abnormalities that are superimposed on the head of the clavicle or on the first rib, for example, reactivation tuberculosis.

Portable chest radiographic equipment generally produces radiographs of inferior quality; thus its use should be limited to patients who cannot safely be transferred to a radiology department.

NURSING ACTION

1. Inform the patient that there are no food or fluid restrictions before the test.
2. Instruct the patient to remove all jewelry in the x-ray field.
3. Assure that the patient understands the nature of the procedure and that the routine chest film causes minimal radiation exposure.

TOMOGRAPHY

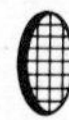

EXPLANATION OF THE TEST

Tomography is an extension of the technique of plain chest radiography. A series of x-ray films is exposed, with each film visualizing a "slice" of the lung at a different depth. Radiographic shadows outside of the selected plane are blurred.

VALUE OF THE TEST

Identifies features not clearly seen on routine chest radiography, including hilar masses, calcium or a cavity in a lesion, and tracheobronchial abnormalities.

Emphysema may be better evaluated.

NURSING ACTION

1. Inform the patient that there are no food or fluid restrictions before the test.
2. Instruct the patient to remove all jewelry in the x-ray field.
3. Instruct the patient that he or she will assume a supine position and remain immobile during the test.

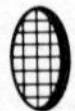

ESOPHAGOGRAM (BARIUM SWALLOW)

EXPLANATION OF THE TEST

Esophagogram is the procedure where radiopaque material is swallowed while x-ray films of the chest are taken. Aspiration may be documented during this test and displacement or abnormal impression of the esophagus may indicate the presence of mediastinal lymphadenopathy or metastatic disease involving the esophagus. This test has been discussed more completely in Chapter 8.

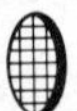

BRONCHOGRAPHY

EXPLANATION OF THE TEST

Bronchography is the procedure by which a radiopaque material is instilled into the tracheobronchial tree through a catheter introduced through the mouth, nose, or cricothyroid membrane. Regions of interest may be filled with radiopaque material selectively. Multiple views are obtained, including oblique views.

VALUE OF THE TEST

This test is rarely done but remains the definitive test for diagnosing and establishing the extent of bronchiectasis.

NURSING ACTION

1. Instruct the patient to perform thorough oral hygiene the evening before and the morning of the test.
2. Assess for loose teeth, capped teeth, bridges, or dentures before the test.

3. Inspect and report any oral inflammation of the mucosa.
4. Obtain informed consent.
5. Assess for allergies to iodine or seafood.
6. Instruct the patient to fast for 12 hours before the test.
7. Explain to the patient that this test helps the physician detect bronchial abnormalities.
8. Instruct the patient regarding the procedure. Have the patient practice relaxation techniques to assist with intubation and try different breathing techniques before the procedure (mouth versus nose breathing). Inform the patient that he or she may be tilted into various positions during the procedure.
9. Inform the patient that the procedure may cause or exacerbate coughing and may worsen underlying lung function.
10. A local anesthetic is sprayed on the patient's throat before the procedure.
11. Instruct the patient that nothing should be taken by mouth after the procedure until a gag reflex returns. Show the patient how this will be checked.

NURSING ALERT

Following the procedure, encourage the patient to take deep breaths and cough to expectorate the contrast agent.

Be alert to the development of laryngeal spasm in asthma patients. This may be secondary to the instillation of the contrast agent.

Be alert to the development of insidious respiratory failure (airway occlusion) in the patient with chronic obstructive pulmonary disease.

Be alert to the development of complications, which include atelectasis, chemical and bacterial pneumonias, and bronchospasm.

Bronchography is contraindicated during pregnancy and in patients who are hypersensitive to iodine or contrast material or have respiratory insufficiency.

Observe the patient for adverse reactions to the radiocontrast material, such as anaphylactic reaction or exacerbation of respiratory failure.

COMPUTERIZED TOMOGRAPHY (CT)

Normal

See Fig. 6-1, B and C.

EXPLANATION OF THE TEST FOR THE EVALUATION OF LUNG DISEASE

In the radiographical evaluation of lung disease, CT scanning can detect small peripheral nodules, evaluate coin lesions (solid versus cystic versus calcified), and distinguish the chest wall from areas of pleural or parenchymal disease. Also well seen are loculated and subpulmonic effusion, mediastinal and hilar masses, and the tracheobronchial tree. When contrast material is used, vascular structures can also be identified and a diagnosis of aortic dissection or aneurysm can be made. CT scanning is further described on p. 161.

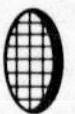

SPUTUM EXAMINATION

EXPLANATION OF THE TEST

Sputum is material raised from lung parenchyma and bronchi by coughing. A sputum specimen may be obtained for microbiological and/or cytological examination and is helpful in the evaluation of pneumonias and suspected malignancies.

VALUE OF THE TEST

Cytologic evaluation of the sputum is a relatively simple method of detecting malignant disease of the lung.

May reveal eosinophilia in allergic disorders.

NURSING ACTION

1. If the specimen will be collected by expectoration, the patient should have an adequate fluid intake the night before collection of the specimen to help in sputum production. Sputum specimens are most easily obtained and should be obtained when the patient first awakens in the morning, since secretions pool during sleep. Give the patient a specimen cup the night before so that mucus from the first expectorate on awakening may be obtained.
2. Instruct the patient on the proper method of expectorating—to take three deep breaths and then force a deep cough, expectorating into the specimen container.

Make sure that the patient understands the difference between sputum and saliva. No useful information is gained in microscopic or bacteriologic evaluation of saliva.

3. For nonproductive coughs, chest physiotherapy, heated aerosol spray, or intermittent positive pressure breathing with prescribed sputum-inducing aerosol may be used by an inhalation therapist to promote a deep and productive cough. In rare instances one may resort to transtracheal aspiration to obtain a satisfactory sputum specimen.
4. The patient should not brush the teeth or use a mouthwash before specimen collection. He or she may rinse the mouth with water.

CLINICAL IMPLICATIONS

In bronchiectasis, chronic bronchitis, and pneumonia the volume of sputum is increased.

In bacterial infections of the lung, purulent sputum is seen and Gram-stained smears and cultures are often very helpful in defining a specific causative organism. Tuberculosis and fungal lung infections may similarly be diagnosed if the organisms can be seen with special stains of sputa (e.g., acid-fast stain for tuberculosis) or can be cultured on special media.

NURSING ALERT

Examine the specimen to make sure it is sputum; it is futile to perform the test on saliva.

If the patient has underlying asthma or chronic bronchitis, bronchospasm may occur following inhalation of acetylcysteine, high concentration of sodium chloride, and with the inhalation of sterile water.

If tracheal suctioning is needed, suction for only 5 to 10 seconds at a time. Always provide oxygen before and during suctioning, particularly if the patient has an underlying pulmonary condition associated with reduced oxygen tensions. Stop suctioning promptly if the patient becomes cyanotic.

Wearing a mask to protect yourself from respiratory pathogens during patient coughing may be helpful, but it is more important to cover the patient's mouth to prevent generation of infectious aerosol.

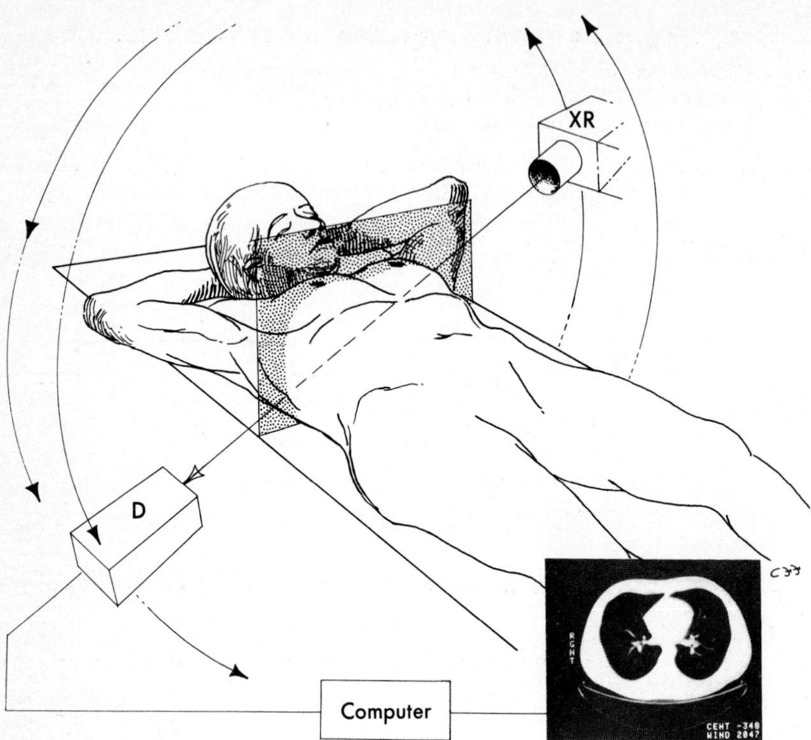

Fig. 6-1. A, *Diagrammatic representation of computerized tomography of the thorax. The image of the cathode-ray tube as projected in the lower right-hand corner is shown as though the patient were being viewed from below. This is the conventional method of viewing CT scans.* XR, *X-ray.* D, *Detectors.* ***B*** *and* ***C****, Normal 2-second CT of the thorax.* ***B****, Scan is taken at the hilar level. The pulmonary vascular markings are shown throughout the lung fields* (white arrows). *The descending branch of the right pulmonary artery* (RPA) *lies slightly lateral but predominantly anterior to the intermediate bronchus, which contains air* (large white arrow). *The esophagus* (black arrow) *and azygos vein* (black arrowhead) *are evident. The descending branch of the left pulmonary artery* (LP) *is posterior to the lower lobe bronchus at this level.* DA, *Descending aorta.* ***C****, By adjusting the contrast, an examiner can look within the mediastinum at the same level as the CT scan in* ***B*** *and check for normal intrapericardial structures. The course of the right pulmonary artery can be followed to the main pulmonary artery* (MPA). *The superior vena cava* (s) *is anterior to the right pulmonary artery and behind the proximal portion of the ascending aorta* (AA). *These structures are seen because of the contrast between lower-density mediastinal fat and blood-containing vessels. (From Porgatch, R.D., and Fahling, L.J.: Computed tomography of the thorax: a status report, Chest* ***80:*** *618, 1981.)*

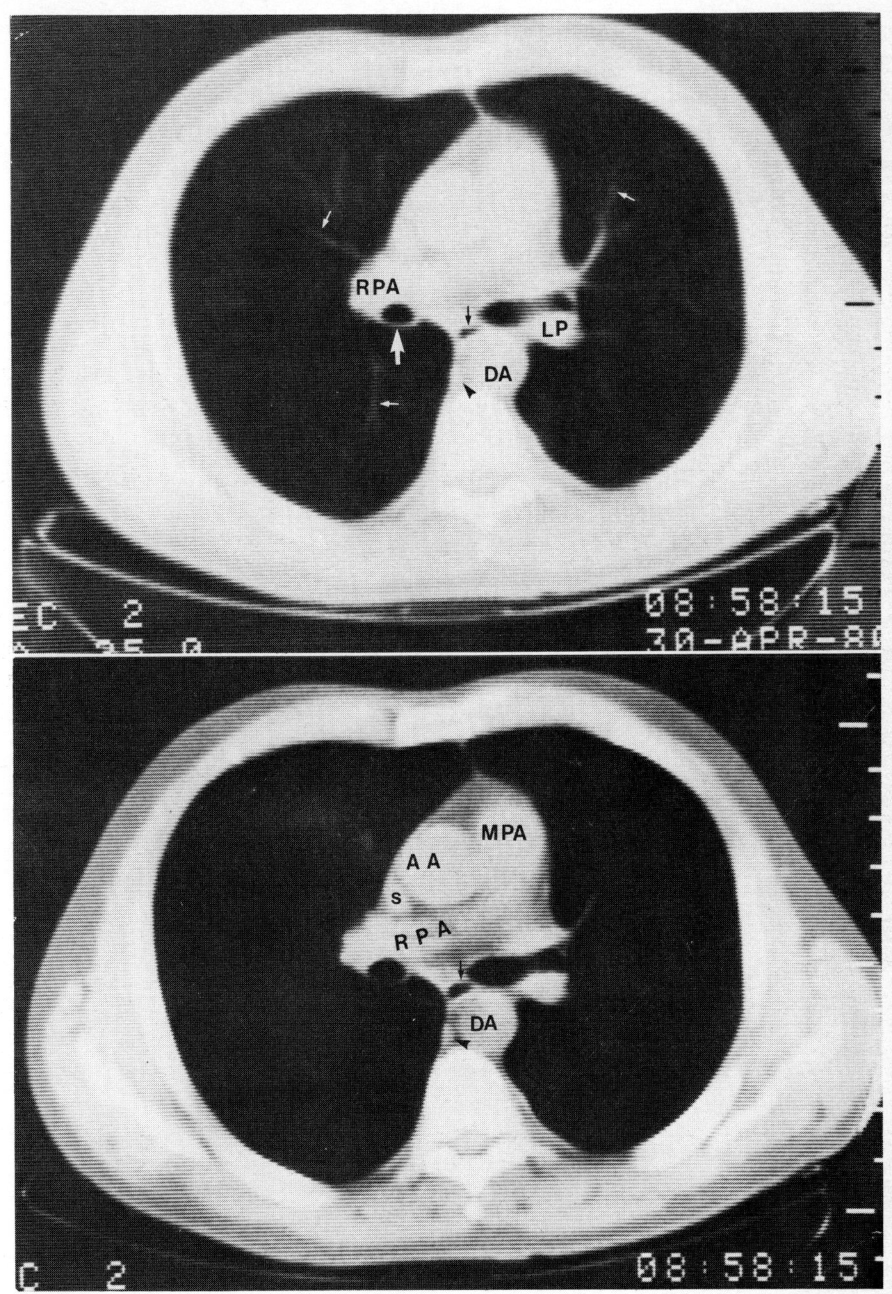

Fig. 6-1, cont'd. *For legend see opposite page.*

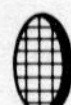

ALPHA$_1$-ANTITRYPSIN ASSAY (SERUM)

Normal for the trypsin inhibitory capability (TIC) assay

MM genotype: 2.1-3.8 U/ml
MZ phenotype: 1.05-2.1 U/ml
ZZ phenotype: 0.5-0.7 U/ml

EXPLANATION OF THE TEST

Alpha$_1$-antitrypsin is a plasma protein that is synthesized in the liver. It is a major inhibitor of trypsin in the serum and of enzymatic proteolysis. A deficiency of this protein leads to severe pulmonary disease in adults or hepatic disease in infants and children. Assays are ordered when there is family history of emphysema, or when emphysema develops at an unusually early age or without associated cigarette smoking. The test can be done by routine serum protein electrophoresis, trypsin inhibitory capability (TIC) assay, radial immunodiffusion, or electroimmunodiffusion using an antiserum specific for alpha$_1$-antitrypsin.

VALUE OF THE TEST

Identifies patients with a genetic abnormality that leads to emphysema.

NURSING ACTION

1. Inform the patient that there are no dietary restrictions for this test.
2. Withdraw venous blood into a 7 ml collection tube. Handle the specimen gently to prevent hemolysis and send it immediately to the laboratory.

CLINICAL IMPLICATIONS

Two results are significant: (1) intermediate deficiency associated with a heterozygous genotype, and (2) severe deficiency associated with a homozygous genotype. The heterozygous state is suspected of being a risk factor for the development of emphysema, while the homozygous state is definitely associated with the early development of severe emphysema. It is imperative that patients with the homozygous state give up cigarette smoking immediately. Therapy with infusion of alpha$_1$-antitrypsin is being studied in hope of preventing further emphysematous lung destruction.

RADIOISOTOPE TECHNIQUES

PULMONARY PERFUSION SCANNING (Q SCAN)

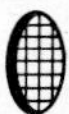

EXPLANATION OF THE TEST

A pulmonary perfusion scan is a technique that utilizes radioactive particles and a scintillation camera to visualize the lungs. Macroaggregates of albumin labeled with technetium or radioactive iodine are injected into a peripheral vein. The macroaggregates are trapped in the pulmonary capillaries, blocking 0.1% of the pulmonary capillary bed and providing an indirect measure of blood flow to the lungs. In 8 hours the albumin microspheres disintegrate and clear from the circulation. A scintillation camera obtains images in multiple views, and computers process the data and quantitate the perfusion.

VALUE AND LIMITATIONS OF THE TEST

Aids in the assessment of pulmonary arterial perfusion.

Aids in the detection of pulmonary embolism.

In a patient with marginal pulmonary reserve, aids in quantitating the effect of removal of a lung or part of a lung on overall postoperative (residual) lung function.

The test is nonspecific, since numerous lung disorders can also compromise pulmonary blood flow.

NURSING ACTION

1. Inform the patient that there are no food or fluid restrictions.
2. Explain to the patient that the trace radioactive agent will be injected into an arm vein and that the amount of radioactivity is minimal. Make sure that the patient understands that neither the camera nor the uptake probe emits any radiation.
3. Explain to the patient that the radioactive agent will be injected while he or she is supine and that the gamma camera then takes a series of single stationary images in the anterior, posterior, and lateral views. The distribution of radioactive particles is then projected on an oscilloscope screen.

INTERFERING FACTORS

Injection of the radionuclide agent while the patient is sitting.
Another radionuclide test having been performed that day.

CLINICAL IMPLICATIONS

An abnormal result is rarely in itself diagnostic of pulmonary embolism; such a result must be interpreted in the context of the clinical problem, the chest x-ray film, and the ventilation scan.

Pulmonary embolism. In the clinical setting suggestive of pulmonary embolism, if the chest x-ray film is normal and no abnormalities are seen on ventilation scanning, a perfusion defect would indicate pulmonary embolism with a high degree of probability. In the presence of pulmonary infiltrates or a ventilation scan that shows abnormalities, a perfusion defect has little diagnostic value and cannot be used for the diagnosis of pulmonary embolism. When a pulmonary perfusion scan is normal, clinically significant pulmonary embolism is very unlikely.

Arteriovenous fistula. If, during pulmonary perfusion scanning, other organs are visualized (e.g., the kidneys or spleen), one would then search for a pulmonary arteriovenous fistula, which has allowed the passage of the macroaggregates to the arterial side.

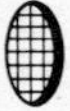

PULMONARY VENTILATION SCANNING (V SCANNING)

EXPLANATION OF THE TEST

The pulmonary ventilation scan is a scintillation camera scan of the lungs. The patient inhales a mixture of air, oxygen, and radioactive gas, usually xenon (xenon 133 or xenon 137). An initial breath is taken to total lung capacity, and a scan is done (a single-breath scan). Next, the patient breathes tidally while the distribution of the radioactive gas is recorded (wash-in phase). After equilibrium has been achieved, the patient resumes breathing room air (washout phase).

VALUE OF THE TEST

Used in the diagnosis of various obstructive lung diseases and in the evaluation of abnormal perfusion scans of the lung.
Useful in the evaluation of pulmonary function prior to surgery.

NURSING ACTION

1. Inform the patient that there are no food or fluid restrictions.
2. Instruct the patient regarding the procedure and tell him or her that the test involves minimal radiation.

CLINICAL IMPLICATIONS

Pulmonary embolism and airway obstruction. In an otherwise normal lung, if a perfusion defect is the result of pulmonary embolism the ventilation scan will be normal. If the pulmonary defect is due to airway obstruction and decreased ventilation (obstructive lung disease, pneumonia, atelectasis), the ventilation scan may be abnormal, showing ventilation defects. However, emboli may occur in lungs so deranged by underlying emphysema or neoplasm (among other conditions) that the resulting ventilation and perfusion scans are both abnormal. In this case, when the clinical suspicion is high enough, a *pulmonary angiogram* must be done to rule out the suspected additional disorder of pulmonary embolism.

BLOOD GASES AND ACID-BASE HOMEOSTASIS

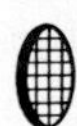

Normal

	Arterial blood	*Mixed venous blood*
pH	7.40 (7.37-7.43)	7.36 (7.32-7.40)
PaO_2	80-100 mm Hg	35-40 mm Hg
O_2 saturation	95%	65%-75%
HCO_3	22-26 mEq/L	23-27 mEq/L
Base excess	−2 to +2	−2 to +2

EXPLANATION OF THE TEST

Arterial blood gas analysis evaluates gas exchange in the lungs by measuring (1) arterial oxygen tension (PaO_2), (2) saturation, (3) carboxyhemoglobin, (4) carbon dioxide tension ($PaCO_2$), and (5) pH. The proper interpretation of blood gas data requires knowledge of the clinical state of the patient, types of therapy being applied (i.e., oxygen), hemoglobin content, cardiac output, and other clinical information.

A "mixed venous" blood gas analysis is one obtained from the pulmonary artery, where there is complete mixing of venous blood. Mixed venous blood samples are frequently obtained in the critical care setting in patients being monitored with Swan-Ganz catheters. The difference between arterial oxygen content and mixed venous oxygen content (arteriovenous oxygen difference) is inversely related to the cardiac output. Thus, cardiac output can be estimated by concurrent measurements of arterial and mixed venous oxygen content, with an estimated value being used for oxygen consumption.

Arterial oxygen tension. Arterial oxygen tension (Pao_2) is a measurement of the partial pressure of oxygen dissolved in blood. The concentration of oxygen generally increases in blood with increasing oxygen partial pressures, the actual amount being primarily a function of the oxygen dissociation curve at oxygen tensions of less than 100. In a person with normal pulmonary function, who is breathing air at sea level, the Pao_2 is usually 80 to 100 mm Hg, and decreases with age, pulmonary disease, reduced oxygen pressures in inspired air (altitude), and is dependent on body position. Normally, the Pao_2 is less in the supine position than it is when the individual is sitting or standing, but in the presence of disease (primarily in the lower lobes) this relationship may be reversed. A Pao_2 of less than 70 mm Hg is abnormal at any age or in any position (Table 6-1).

Table 6-1 Predicted Pao_2 at various ages and body positions

Age	Seated	Supine
15	100	97
20	99	95
25	97	93
30	96	91
35	95	89
40	93	87
45	92	85
50	91	83
55	89	80
60	88	78
65	87	76
70	85	74
75	84	72
80	83	70
85	81	68

Oxygen saturation of the blood. Oxygen taken up in the lungs is delivered to the tissues through the circulatory system. A small amount is carried dissolved in the blood, while the bulk of oxygen is transported in chemical combination with hemoglobin as oxyhemoglobin. Oxygen taken up in the lungs combines reversibly with hemoglobin in the blood and forms oxyhemoglobin. The ratio of total oxyhemoglobin (Hbg combined with oxygen) to total hemoglobin in the blood is referred to as the *oxygen saturation of blood*. Normally, arterial blood is almost fully saturated, with an O_2 saturation of 95% to 99%, while mixed venous (pulmonary artery) blood is 65% to 75% saturated with O_2.

Oxyhemoglobin dissociation curve. Oxygen is transported bound to hemoglobin, each gram of which, when fully saturated, can carry 1.34 ml of oxygen. The amount of oxygen dissolved in plasma is very small and is generally disregarded in clinical evaluation. The oxyhemoglobin dissociation curve (Fig. 6-2) represents the relationship between the PaO_2 and the amount of hemoglobin bound with oxygen.

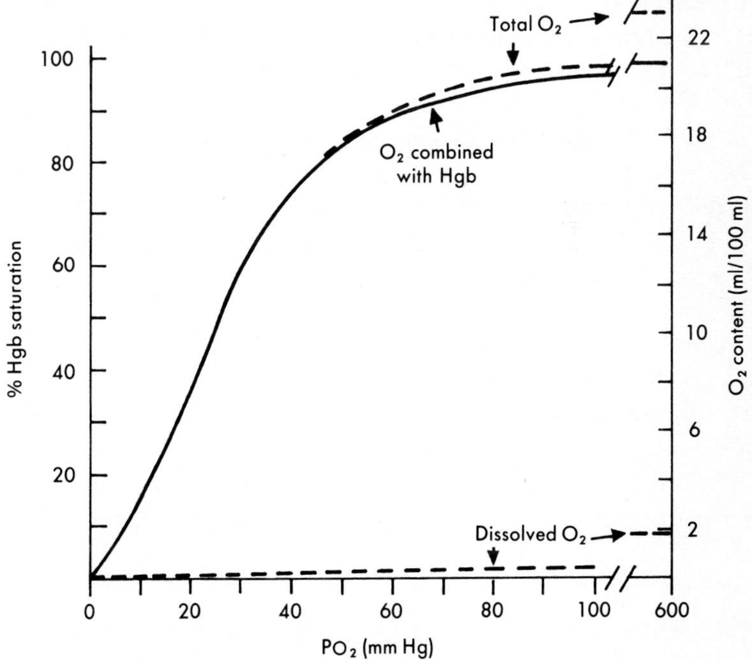

Fig. 6-2. *Oxyhemoglobin dissociation curve. The* solid line *is the oxygen dissociation curve at pH 7.4,* $PaCO_2$ *40 mm Hg, and 37° C. The total blood oxygen content is also shown for a hemoglobin concentration of 15 g/dl of blood.*

Note the progressive increase in the percentage of hemoglobin that is bound with oxygen (percent saturation of the hemoglobin) as the PaO_2 increases.

In general, hemoglobin saturation is at least 90% as long as the PaO_2 is greater than 60 mm Hg. As arterial oxygen tension drops below 60 mm Hg, oxygen saturation falls steeply, with the drops in saturation being relatively larger than the changes in oxygen tension. Temperature changes and the acid-base state will also affect the degree of oxygen saturation of hemoglobin for a given PaO_2. The amount of oxygen that is actually delivered to the cellular level depends on the oxygen saturation of the hemoglobin, as well as on the hemoglobin concentration and the cardiac output. Thus, in cases of severe anemia or markedly decreased cardiac output, even if the PaO_2 and the oxygen saturation of the hemoglobin are normal, delivery of oxygen to the tissue level may be inadequate.

Carboxyhemoglobin. Carboxyhemoglobin is formed when hemoglobin is exposed to carbon monoxide, as in cigarette smoking. This carbon monoxide–bound hemoglobin is unable to carry oxygen. Also, the remaining hemoglobin binds oxygen more tightly and gives off less oxygen to tissue cells. Hence, even though carbon monoxide may be bound only to a certain percentage of hemoglobin, the overall consequences are more serious than the same degree of anemia. Therefore, PaO_2 should be interpreted in the context of (1) the hemoglobin concentration and whether there is abnormal hemoglobin present, such as carboxyhemoglobin or methemoglobin, (2) the status of cardiac output, and (3) other factors that affect oxygen-hemoglobin binding (temperature, pH, and drugs).

Carbon dioxide tension ($PaCO_2$). CO_2 tension in arterial blood reflects the balance between CO_2 production (metabolic) and excretion through ventilation. Thus, alveolar hypoventilation would cause an elevated $PaCO_2$ (hypercapnia), while hyperventilation would cause a decreased $PaCO_2$ (hypocapnia). The normal range for $PaCO_2$ is 35 to 44 mm Hg. An arbitrary classification of severity of changes in $PaCO_2$ follows:

	Mild	*Moderate*	*Severe*
Hypocapnia	30-33	20-29	<20
Hypercapnia	45-55	55-65	>65

Hypocapnia and hypercapnia reflect underlying hyperventilation or hypoventilation, respectively, which may be primary or compensatory to a metabolic or other condition. In the absence of other metabolic forces (acids or alkalies) hypoventilation would lead to respiratory acidosis, while hyperventilation would cause respiratory alkalosis.

As a working rule, the sum of PaO_2 and $PaCO_2$ should be less than 140 mm Hg, if a person is breathing air at sea level. A sum greater than 140 mm Hg indicates a laboratory error or the fact that a person is receiving supplemental oxygen.

Blood pH. Since the pH is the negative logarithm of the hydrogen ion concentration, it is an expression of the degree of acidity or alkalinity. Normal values for arterial blood range from 7.37 to 7.43.

Acidemia. A low pH indicates acidemia. The source of excess acid can be respiratory, metabolic, or both. In respiratory acidemia an increased $PaCO_2$ (hypoventilation) causes an increase in the amount of carbonic acid. In metabolic acidemia accumulation of various metabolic acids causes the increase in hydrogen ion concentration.

Alkalemia. A high pH reflects alkalemia. In respiratory alkalemia (hyperventilation) too much carbon dioxide is lost, resulting in a decrease in the amount of carbonic acid. In metabolic alkalemia excessive amounts of various body acids are lost (e.g., hydrochloric acid as a result of vomiting or gastric suction).

Metabolic acidosis and alkalosis. The kidneys are also intimately involved in acid-base balance. Daily they excrete 50 to 100 mEq of hydrogen ions, which are formed as a result of carbohydrate and protein metabolism.

In metabolic alkalosis the kidneys respond by excreting bicarbonate. Respiratory compensation consists of hypoventilation with an increase in $PaCO_2$ and carbonic acid. In metabolic acidosis the kidneys reabsorb bicarbonate ions and secrete hydrogen ions. This renal process occurs gradually over several days, whereas the respiratory compensation of increased ventilation and hypocapnia occurs within minutes.

The term *base excess* refers to an excess of bicarbonate as well as other bases in the blood. An elevation in the bicarbonate level indicates metabolic alkalosis, while a decrease in the bicarbonate level indicates metabolic acidosis.

It is now apparent that a complete assessment of acid-base balance should include determinations of $PaCO_2$, pH, and bicarbonate concentration, as well as the levels of the other serum electrolytes. Diagnostic possibilities include pure metabolic or respiratory acidosis, or a combination of the two, and pure respiratory or metabolic alkalosis, or a combination of the two. Respiratory and metabolic compensatory mechanisms are frequently involved, and acid-base disturbances in clinical circumstances frequently are of a mixed variety.

VALUE OF THE TEST

Provides the single best assessment of the adequacy of pulmonary gas exchange and the presence and severity of acid-base disturbances.

NURSING ACTION

1. Inform the patient that there are no dietary restrictions before this test.
2. Explain to the patient that this test evaluates the ability of the lungs to deliver oxygen to the blood and clear carbon dioxide.
3. Use a 22-gauge or smaller needle to minimize trauma to the artery and precoat the syringe with a small amount of heparin.
4. Radial or brachial arteries are frequently used, although the femoral artery may also be used.
5. Indwelling catheters may be used if multiple samples are needed.
6. All bubbles should be expelled, exposure to air avoided, and samples placed on ice.
7. The patient's rectal temperature should be taken as measurements of arterial blood gases are corrected to body temperature.
8. Delay the test for 20 minutes if any breathing treatment has been done.
9. Ascertain whether the measurement of blood gases is to be made with the patient breathing room air or oxygen, and note the liter flow or inspired oxygen concentration on the laboratory slip.
10. Apply firm pressure for 2 to 3 minutes after the puncture. Longer periods of pressure are needed if the patient is taking anticoagulants.

INTERFERING FACTORS

Exposure of the blood specimen to air (interferes with PaO_2 and $PaCO_2$ levels).

Failure to heparinize the syringe, ice the specimen, or send it promptly to the laboratory.

Venous blood mixed in the arterial sample (lowers PaO_2 and elevates $PaCO_2$ levels).

A recent breathing treatment may alter blood gas values.

CLINICAL IMPLICATIONS

The oxygen saturation (and therefore the content) in pulmonary arterial blood is an excellent indicator of the adequacy of oxygen delivery to the tissues.

Normal PaO_2 in pulmonary arterial sample is 35 to 40 mm Hg. Inadequate cardiac output, unable to meet the O_2 demands of the body, is reflected by reduced O_2 tension; and with PaO_2 of less than 27, lactic acidosis generally is present.

NURSING ALERT

Watch for bleeding from the puncture site.

Observe closely for signs of circulatory impairment (swelling, discoloration, numbness, tingling, pain) in the arm with the puncture site.

If the patient is receiving anticoagulants exercise caution and apply prolonged pressure to the puncture site.

If thrombolytic agents are in use, arterial puncture is generally contraindicated.

PULMONARY FUNCTION TESTS

SPIROMETRY

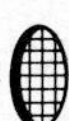

NORMAL VALUES

These are predicted for individual patients relative to age, height, weight, and sex. They are compared with standard measurements and expressed as a percentage. Abnormal results are less than 80% of the predicted value. The commonly obtained lung volumes and capacities as seen on a spirogram are shown in Fig. 6-3.

EXPLANATION OF THE TEST

Spirometry involves the use of an instrument, a spirometer, to measure and record the changes in the gas volume in the lungs with time and thus ventilatory capacity and flow rate. The commonly

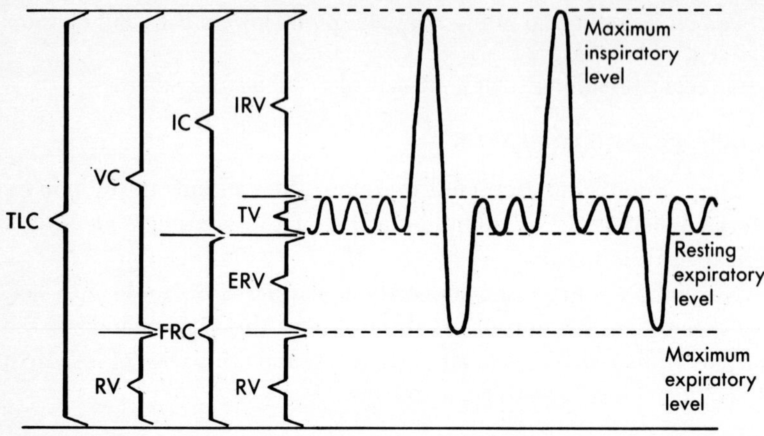

Fig. 6-3. *Spirogram.* TLC, *Total lung capacity.* VC, *Vital capacity.* IC, *Inspiratory capacity.* IRV, *Inspiratory reserve volume.* TV, *Tidal volume.* ERV, *Expiratory reserve volume.* FRC, *Functional reserve capacity.* RV, *Residual volume.*

obtained lung volumes and capacities as seen on a spirogram are shown in Fig. 6-3. They include total lung capacity (TLC), vital capacity (VC), residual volume (RV), inspiratory capacity (IC), and tidal volume (TV). Table 6-2 lists some normal spirometric values adjusted for age and sex.

Procedures

Lung volumes. There are four standard lung volumes. Three are measured by the spirometer: tidal volume, inspiratory reserve volume, and expiratory reserve volume. The fourth, residual volume, is ascertained by subtracting expiratory reserve volume (ERV) from the functional residual capacity (FRC). The functional residual capacity cannot be measured by simple spirometry. It is routinely measured by means of a nitrogen washout test, helium dilution test, or by means of body plethysmography. Most pulmonary function laboratories do at least one of these tests to quantitate the FRC and hence the RV.

The sum of the four volumes is the maximal volume to which the lungs can be expanded, that is, the total lung capacity (TLC = RV + TV + FRC + ERV). All figures for lung volumes and capacities given in this chapter are those of a normal young male

Table 6-2 Normal spirometric values

Test	Age 20-39	Age 40-59	Age 60+
VC (liters)			
Men	3.35-5.90	2.72-5.30	2.42-4.70
Women	2.45-4.38	2.09-4.02	1.91-3.66
FEV_1 (liters)			
Men	3.11-4.64	2.45-3.98	2.09-3.32
Women	2.16-3.65	1.60-3.09	1.30-2.53
FEV% (FEV_1/VC%)			
Men	77	70	60
Women	82	77	74
RV (liters)			
Men	1.13-2.32	1.45-2.62	1.77-2.77
Women	1.00-2.00	1.16-2.20	1.32-2.40
TLC (liters)			
Men	4.80-7.92	4.50-7.62	4.35-7.32
Women	3.61-6.18	3.41-6.02	3.31-5.86

adult; the figures for a female adult are about 20% to 25% lower.

Tidal volume (TV) is the volume of air inspired or expired with each normal breath (about 500 ml).

Inspiratory reserve volume (IRV) is the maximal volume of air that can still be inspired after the end of a normal tidal inspiration (approximately 3000 ml).

Expiratory reserve volume (ERV) is the maximal amount of air that can still be expired, by forceful expiration, after the end of normal tidal expiration (about 1100 ml).

Residual volume (RV) is the volume of air that remains in the lung after a forced maximal expiration (about 1200 ml). This volume provides oxygen for the blood between breaths and prevents the concentrations of oxygen and carbon dioxide in the blood from rising and falling markedly with each breath.

Lung capacities. A lung capacity comprises two or more lung volumes.

Inspiratory capacity (IC) is the *tidal volume* plus the *inspiratory reserve volume* (about 3500 ml). This is the amount of air that can be inspired during a maximal inspiratory effort that starts at the normal resting expiratory level.

Functional residual capacity (FRC) is the *expiratory reserve volume* plus the *residual volume*. This is the amount of air remaining in the lungs at the end of normal expiration (about 2300 ml).

Vital capacity (VC) is the *inspiratory reserve volume* plus the *tidal volume* plus the *expiratory reserve volume*. This is the maximum amount of air that can be expelled from the lungs after maximal inspiration. It is sometimes called expiratory vital capacity. The major factors affecting the measurement of vital capacity are the patient's position during the test, the strength of the muscles of respiration, and pulmonary compliance (distensibility of lungs and chest cage).

Total lung capacity (TLC) is the total volume to which the lungs can be expanded with the greatest inspiratory effort (about 5800 ml).

Flow rates. Simple spirometry can usually differentiate obstructive from restrictive pulmonary disorders simply on the basis of lung volume measurements combined with expiratory flow rates. Fig. 6-4 compares a normal spirogram with those of obstructive and restrictive lung disease.

In obstructive pulmonary disorders (chronic bronchitis, emphysema, and asthma), the resistance to air flow increases and flow rates decrease. As obstruction to air flow increases, hyperinflation occurs and both residual volume and, to a lesser extent, total lung capacity increase. With the increase in residual volume, vital capacity decreases. In restrictive pulmonary disorders (pulmonary fibrosis) the lungs shrink and flow rates decrease in proportion to the decrease in lung size.

Forced expiratory volume during the first second of expiration after full inspiration (FEV_1) is the most reproducible flow rate and one of the most useful measurements of airway obstruction. It is used often in monitoring response to therapy. FEV_1 decreases linearly with time, both in normal persons and in persons with chronic obstructive lung disease (more rapidly in the latter). Thus the rate of decline in FEV_1 with time is a very useful prognostic factor.

Maximal mid-expiratory flow (MMEF) is a more sensitive indicator of expired air flow than is FEV_1; it is obtained from the mid-portion of the spirogram.

Maximal breathing capacity or maximal voluntary ventilation (MVV) is another useful index of overall lung mechanics. The patient breathes as deeply and as rapidly as possible for 15 seconds. The

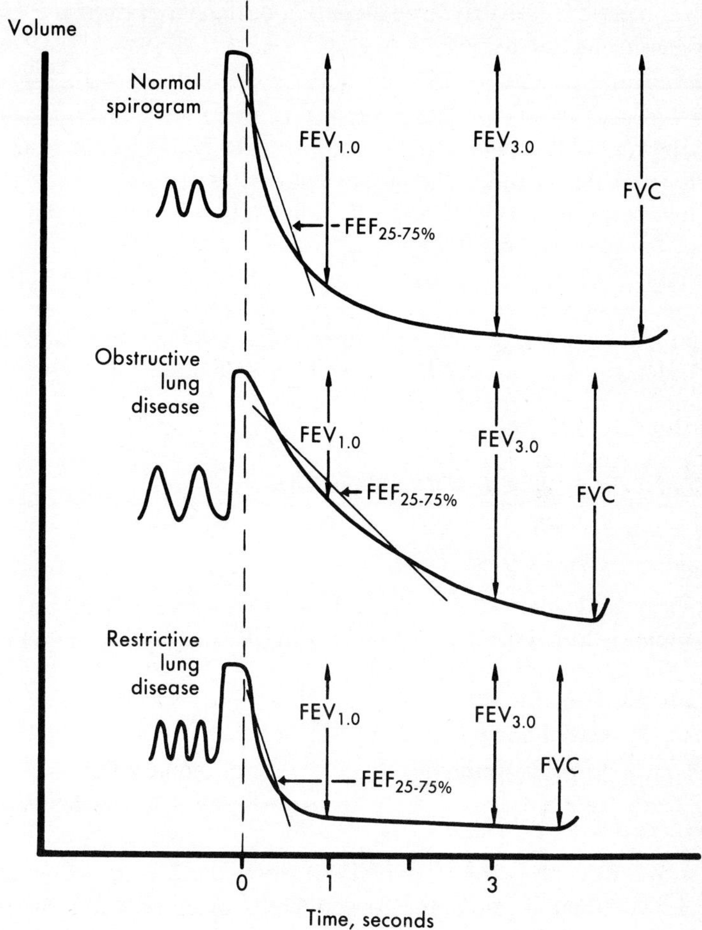

Fig. 6-4. *Simple spirometry usually allows differentiation between obstructive and restrictive patterns. Note that in both, the forced vital capacity* (FVC) *is reduced; however, flows are reduced in obstruction and normal or "supernormal" in restriction. (From Slonim, N.B., and Hamilton, L.H.: Respiratory physiology, ed. 4, St. Louis, 1981, The C.V. Mosby Co.)*

volume of exhaled air is multiplied by 4, yielding an estimate of 1 minute of MVV. A normal value is 80% or more of the predicted value.

The results and success of this test are very effort dependent.

Thus if the patient is overly tired, sedated, or uncooperative, a useful result cannot be achieved.

VALUE OF THE TEST

Useful in the documentation of the presence, type, and degree of functional impairment in various pulmonary disease states.

When performed serially, helps to evaluate the response to therapy or the progression of disease.

Helpful in differentiating dyspnea of cardiac origin from that of pulmonary origin.

Spirometry, determination of lung volumes and flow rates, and diffusion capacity are used in the differentiation of obstructive pulmonary disease from restrictive pulmonary disease.

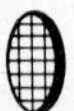

FLOW-VOLUME LOOP ANALYSIS

EXPLANATION OF THE TEST

This analysis relates the instantaneous expiratory air flow reached during a forced vital capacity maneuver to the lung volume at which the particular flow occurs.

VALUE OF THE TEST

More useful than the conventional spirogram.

CLINICAL IMPLICATIONS

Fig. 6-5 illustrates the characteristic flow-volume loops from the normal individual as compared to patients with chronic obstructive airway disease (COPD), fixed large airway obstruction, variable intrathoracic large airway obstruction, variable extrathoracic large airway obstruction, variable effort, and restrictive defect.

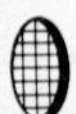

DETERMINATION OF DIFFUSING CAPACITY

EXPLANATION OF THE TEST

Diffusing capacity of the lungs refers to the ability of gases to diffuse across the alveolar-capillary membrane. This is determined in a special pulmonary test where carbon monoxide is inhaled in a single breath and its concentration in the blood is measured.

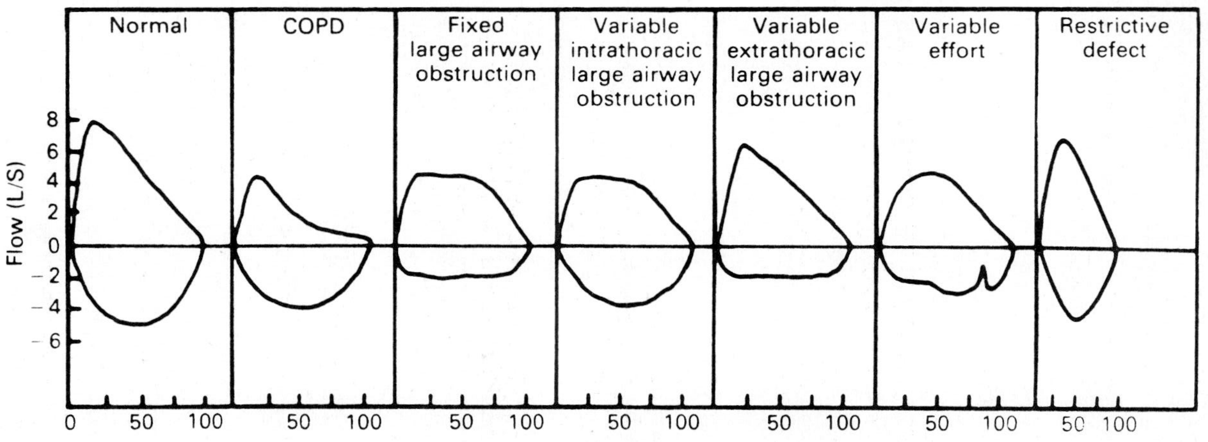

Fig. 6-5. *Characteristic flow-volume loops from various lesions. The TLC is to the left of each panel. (From Burton, G.G., and Hopkins, J.E., editors: Respiratory care, a guide to clinical practice, ed. 2, Philadelphia, 1985, J.B. Lippincott Co., p. 246.*

VALUE OF THE TEST

Helps in the detection of interstitial lung disease
Helps in the evaluation of pulmonary vascular disease, vasculitis, and embolism
A sensitive, noninvasive test for following the effects of therapeutic interventions or for following the progression of pulmonary disease

CLINICAL IMPLICATIONS

Interstitial lung disease. The ability of carbon monoxide to diffuse from the alveolar to the capillary space is reduced in the presence of interstitial lung disease. Factors including alveolar-capillary membrane surface area, alveolar ventilation, lung perfusion, matching of ventilation and perfusion, red cell mass, and hemoglobin all can affect the diffusing capacity. Nevertheless, clinically this is a very useful test in the detection of interstitial lung disease.

Emphysema. The combination of a reduced diffusing capacity and an abnormal flow-volume loop is of value in facilitating the early diagnosis of emphysema even before x-ray and spirometric abnormalities appear or symptoms may be recognized.

Pulmonary embolism. In the presence of normal lung mechanics, a reduced diffusing capacity in a dyspneic patient may be an important clue to pulmonary embolism, in which condition the uptake of carbon monoxide is reduced by a partially blocked pulmonary vascular bed.

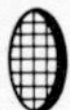

MAXIMAL INSPIRATORY PRESSURE (MIP)

EXPLANATION OF THE TEST

MIP is the pressure generated on maximal inspiratory effort, starting at residual volume, against a closed system. This is a direct test of inspiratory muscle strength.

VALUE AND LIMITATION OF THE TEST

Helpful in the evaluation of neuromuscular diseases
Assessment of patient motivation and performance is crucial to the proper interpretation of results

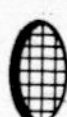

PULMONARY FUNCTION TESTING DURING INTERVENTIONS

EXPLANATION OF THE TEST

Pulmonary function testing may be performed during various interventions. Some of the commonly used interventions include bronchodilators, bronchial provocation, and exercise.

If abnormal flow rates or volumes are recorded, bronchodilators may be given and the pulmonary function test repeated to determine if improvement has occurred.

Bronchial provocative testing may be used when resting flow rates and volumes are normal and the clinical presentation suggests episodic bronchospasm. Bronchospasm can be induced in the pulmonary laboratory by inhalation of a suspected agent (smog, cold air, atmospheric pollutants, or specific drugs or antigens). Whether the response is positive or negative is determined from spirograms produced before and after the provocative test.

Exercise during pulmonary function testing is valuable in patients who complain of effort dyspnea or fatigue or who have cardiopulmonary disease or exercise-induced bronchospasm. During graded levels of exercise, heart rate, blood pressure, respiratory rate and volume, and volumes of expired gases are measured, electrocardiographic data are recorded, and samples are taken for arterial blood gas determinations.

VALUE OF THE TESTS

Use of bronchodilators helps to identify reversible bronchial obstruction.

Provocative testing helps to identify the agent that triggers episodic bronchospasm when resting pulmonary function tests are normal.

Exercise testing helps to determine the extent of exercise limitation and the cause of that limitation, and the functional capacity of the oxygen transport system may be evaluated by measuring maximal oxygen consumption.

During exercise, hypoxemia or hypercapnia that is not apparent from the resting data may be recognized, limitations to exercise assessed, need for supplemental oxygen evaluated, and the degree of improvement achieved through treatment or rehabilitative efforts measured.

CLINICAL IMPLICATIONS

Bronchospasm. A significant improvement in abnormal flow rates and volumes following the administration of a bronchodilator indicates reversible bronchial obstruction (bronchospasm). Note that bronchodilators should be used with caution in patients with coronary artery disease, angina pectoris, or arrhythmias.

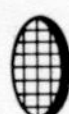

PLEURAL FLUID EXAMINATION AND BIOPSY

EXPLANATION OF THE TEST

Normally the pleural cavity is only a potential space; it has moist membranes and contains only a few milliliters of fluid, which acts as a lubricant between the visceral and parietal portions of the pleura. Pleural effusion is an abnormal accumulation of fluid within this pleural space.

Numerous systemic and intrathoracic diseases can cause pleural effusion, a sample of which may be obtained by means of thoracentesis. In this technique fluid is removed by means of a needle or catheter that has been introduced into the pleural space at the appropriate intercostal level. The fluid is sent to the laboratory for chemical, cytological, and bacteriological evaluation.

VALUE OF THE TEST

Pleural effusion may be removed to improve respiratory status.

Cultures may be obtained.

Distinguishes exudate from transudate as an aid to the differential diagnosis.

May confirm the diagnosis of malignancy.

Aids in the diagnosis of acute pancreatitis, ruptured esophagus, emphysema, and tuberculosis.

NURSING ACTION

1. Inform the patient that there are no food or fluid restrictions before this test.
2. Instruct the patient regarding the procedure and secure a signed consent. Remind the patient that during the procedure he or she should not cough, breathe deeply, or move suddenly.

3. Reassure the patient that a local anesthetic is to be used and the procedure is not usually painful.
4. Record baseline vital signs.
5. It is rarely if ever necessary to shave the site intended for needle entry.
6. The patient should be positioned so that the intercostal spaces are as wide as possible, that is, (a) sitting on the edge of the bed, feet on a chair, and arms on a pillow on the overbed table; (b) sitting up in bed with legs on the bed and arms on two to three pillows on the overbed table; or (c) lying on the unaffected side with arms over the head and a rolled-up towel under the thoracic cage.

CLINICAL IMPLICATIONS

Up to 2 L of pleural effusion may be removed to improve a patient's respiratory status. When volumes much larger than this are rapidly removed, hypotension and pulmonary edema may occur.

A complete bacteriological evaluation of the fluid is done, including evaluations for tuberculosis and fungal diseases.

A cell count and a differential count help in the diagnosis of emphysema.

Protein analysis distinguishes exudate (high in protein) from transudate (low in protein).

Malignant effusions are diagnosed by means of cytological and cell-block evaluations.

If acute pancreatitis is the cause of pleural effusion, elevated amylase levels in the pleural effusion will be noted.

Meigs' syndrome is associated with tumors on the ovaries and pleural effusion that disappears when the tumor is removed.

Pleural fluid collected in an arterial blood gas syringe and promptly analyzed in a blood gas machine provides an accurate pH measurement, which may be of diagnostic help, for example:

<6: A very low pH is most likely caused by a ruptured esophagus.

6 to 7: pH within this range may be an indication of infection (e.g., emphysema). This diagnosis should be carefully pursued, even in the absence of positive pleural fluid cultures. Such cultures are frequently negative, especially if the patient was given a course of antibiotics before hospitalization.

A pH of less than *7.20* usually characterizes tuberculous effusions.

NURSING ALERT

Following thoracentesis or pleural biopsy, a chest x-ray study should be obtained to check for the possibility of pneumothorax.

Thoracentesis is relatively contraindicated in patients with bleeding disorders.

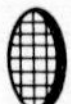

BRONCHOSCOPY AND BRONCHIAL BIOPSY

EXPLANATION OF THE TEST

A flexible fiberoptic bronchoscope is introduced into the tracheobronchial tree via the nose, mouth, tracheotomy tube, or endotracheal tube, permitting inspection of the trachea, carina, and all segmental branches and orifices. The nasopharynx and the oropharynx-larynx may be similarly examined at the same time. Abnormal masses or lesions are brushed or biopsied, and all specimens are sent for complete bacteriologic, cytologic, and histologic evaluation.

A lung biopsy may also be obtained through the fiberoptic bronchoscope. In cases of diffuse involvement of the lung, a biopsy may yield satisfactory results.

VALUE AND LIMITATIONS OF THE TEST

Evaluates cases of hemoptysis of unknown cause and suspected neoplasm
Aids in the localization of airway obstruction
Aids in the removal of tenacious secretions and mucous plugs
Helpful in the treatment of atelectasis
Valuable in the removal of foreign bodies
Useful for lung lavage

NURSING ACTION

1. Instruct the patient to take nothing by mouth for 6 to 8 hours before the procedure and until cough and gag reflexes have returned following the procedure.
2. Explain to the patient that this test helps to evaluate abnormalities of bronchial structure.
3. Obtain informed consent.
4. Explain to the patient that he or she will be given medications

to help control coughing and to decrease secretions, and that the physician may order light sedation.

5. Make sure that the patient understands that the airway will not be blocked during the procedure.
6. The patient is sedated as ordered and assumes a supine position on a table or bed.
7. Instruct the patient to remain relaxed with arms at the sides and to breathe through the nose.
8. The bronchoscope is introduced following an anesthetic throat spray.
9. Lidocaine 2% to 4% (3 to 4 ml) is flushed through the inner channel of the scope to the vocal cords.
10. If distal lesions are to be visualized or transbronchial biopsy to be taken, fluoroscopic guidance is required.
11. Place biopsy specimens in properly labeled containers.

NURSING ALERT

Following the procedure be alert to the complications associated with premedication (respiratory depression, hypotension or syncope, hyperexcitement), local anesthesia (laryngospasm, bronchospasm, seizures, cardiorespiratory arrest), the procedure itself (bronchospasm and laryngospasm, hypoxemia, arrhythmias, fever, pneumonia), and the use of biopsy (pneumothorax, hemorrhage, pneumonia).

Fiberoptic bronchoscopy is relatively contraindicated in asthma, severe hypoxemia, uncontrolled arrhythmia, unstable angina pectoris, recent myocardial infarction, and uncooperative patient.

Biopsy procedures are contraindicated in uncorrected bleeding diatheses, uremia, pulmonary hypertension, mechanical ventilation or positive end-expiratory pressure (PEEP), and severe anemia.

MEDIASTINOSCOPY

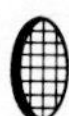

EXPLANATION OF THE TEST

Mediastinoscopy is an operative procedure in which a 3 to 5 cm incision is made in the suprasternal notch. Blunt dissection is done with the finger anterior to the trachea. A mediastinoscope is introduced through the incision, and the lymph nodes around the trachea and the right main stem bronchus are evaluated.

VALUE OF THE TEST

Diagnosis of primary and secondary mediastinal disease.

Usually performed preoperatively to determine whether a primary lung carcinoma has metastasized to mediastinal nodes and whether resection is contraindicated.

Permits visualization and biopsy of paratracheal and subcarinal lymph nodes.

NURSING ACTION

1. Instruct the patient to fast from midnight prior to the test.
2. Obtain informed consent.
3. Transported the patient to surgery for the procedure.

NURSING ALERT

Be alert to signs of complications such as hemorrhage, pneumothorax, damage to the left recurrent laryngeal nerve, and infection. Death of a patient as a result of this procedure is very rare and is almost always secondary to biopsy of a major intrathoracic vessel.

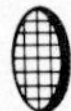

PULMONARY ANGIOGRAPHY

EXPLANATION OF THE TEST

Selective pulmonary angiography is the procedure whereby radiocontrast material is injected into the main pulmonary artery or its branches with visualization of the vessels on radiographic film. Pulmonary angiography, by visualizing the pulmonary artery and its branches, is useful in the diagnosis of numerous types of congenital or acquired disease of the pulmonary vessels. By far the most common indication for this procedure is its application in the diagnosis of pulmonary thromboembolic disease.

A catheter is introduced into the pulmonary artery from a peripheral vein. Pressures are recorded in the right atrium, right ventricle, and pulmonary artery, and blood samples are obtained for analysis of gases. Contrast material is injected while radiographic films are exposed in rapid sequence. Various projections may be used. Selective injection into a branch of the pulmonary artery may be done, permitting detailed visualization of the pulmonary artery and veins.

VALUE OF THE TEST

Provides definitive diagnosis of suspected pulmonary embolism that cannot be excluded or confirmed by other studies.

Helps with quantification of the extent of vascular obstruction, and evaluation of hemodynamic effects of pulmonary embolism.

Test is helpful before surgical intervention for treatment of pulmonary embolism.

Test is diagnostic of peripheral pulmonary artery stenosis, anomalous pulmonary venous drainage, and pulmonary arteriovenous fistulae.

Hemodynamic measurements obtained during the procedure can aid in the diagnosis of pulmonary hypertension and cor pulmonale.

Selective pulmonary angiography is useful in situations in which clinical, radiological, and isotope studies have failed to produce a specific diagnosis, or when surgical procedures (inferior vena cava interruption or embolectomy) are being considered.

NURSING ACTION

Patient preparation for selective pulmonary angiography is similar to that for any cardiac catheterization with angiography.

1. Inform the patient regarding procedure, risks, and what to expect, and obtain informed consent.
2. Ensure that the patient takes nothing by mouth for 4 to 6 hours except for sips of water.
3. Ensure that the patient has adequate hydration and intravenous fluids if necessary.
4. Review recent ECG, electrolytes, blood urea nitrogen (BUN), creatinine, and arterial blood gases. Correct any abnormalities if possible.
5. Shave and prepare anticipated venous entry site.

NURSING ALERT

Ensure that a signed consent is on the patient's record.

Check vital signs every 15 minutes for 2 to 4 hours and inspect the dressing for bleeding. The patient is at bed rest 2 to 4 hours following the procedure.

A venous puncture site should be checked for warmth, pain, swelling, and redness, since thrombophlebitis may be a complication.

Venous sites should be checked for signs of inflammation or infection. Sutures are usually removed 4 to 5 days following the procedure.

Watch the patient for adverse reactions to the radiocontrast material such as anaphylactic reaction, volume overload and congestive heart failure, acute right ventricular failure, and acute renal failure.

In order to recognize a nephrotoxic response to the contrast media should it occur, closely monitor urinary output, renal function, and electrolytes 24 to 48 hours following the use of radiocontrast material.

For patients known to be allergic to contrast material, the following preparation is usually used before any angiography procedure.

Routine

Prednisone or an equivalent steroid 150 mg/day is given in divided doses (24 hours before the study and 12 hours after the study).

Benadryl 25 to 50 mg is given by slow intravenous push just before the procedure, or 50 mg orally or intramuscularly 1 hour before the procedure.

For patients at especially high risk for reaction to contrast media

Methylprednisolone 1 g intravenously is given 1 hour before the study to patients who are at high risk of a major reaction.

Cimetidine (Tagamet) 300 mg intravenously piggyback may be given over 15 minutes, 30 minutes before the study. Experience with this drug is limited.

7

Diagnostic tests for renal disorders

ANATOMY AND PHYSIOLOGY

Each kidney contains over 1 million nephrons, the functioning units of the kidney, each being capable of forming urine. Two of the major functions of the nephrons are:

1. Excretion of some of the waste products of metabolism (urea, creatinine, uric acid) by means of glomerular filtration and tubular secretion.
2. Maintenance of water and electrolyte balance by means of changes in tubular reabsorption or secretion, which is in turn mediated by hormones, such as changes in antidiuretic hormone (ADH), renin, aldosterone, parathyroid hormone.

There are two major units in the nephron: the glomerulus, through which the blood is filtered, and the tubule, where the filtered blood is modified by the processes of reabsorption and secretion and converted into urine. The tubule has a blind end that begins in the cortex of the kidney (Fig. 7-1) to follow a tortuous path (the proximal convoluted tubule) and then to straighten and plunge down into the medulla, bending back to form a loop (loop of Henle) and return to the cortex. Within the cortex again, the tubule twists and turns (distal convoluted tubule). Its path and blood supply are illustrated in Fig. 7-2. It finally joins the collecting tubule, which ends in the pyramid and empties into the calyx.

The glomerulus is a tuft of up to 50 capillaries that begins with an afferent and terminates with an efferent arteriole. The capillary walls of the glomerulus have three layers, endothelial and epithelial cells with glomerular basement membrane between them. The glomerulus is invaginated into the blind end of the tubule. The little sac thus formed is Bowman's space, the inside surface of which is the outermost layer of capillary wall (epithelial cells). The plasma is filtered from the blood, across the capillary walls of the glomerulus, into Bowman's space. The amount of ultrafiltrate formed depends on (1) the hydrostatic pressure difference between the capillary lumen and Bowman's space, (2) the permeability of the capillary wall, and (3) the difference of the colloid osmotic pressure between Bowman's space and the capillary lumen. As the ultrafiltrate passes down

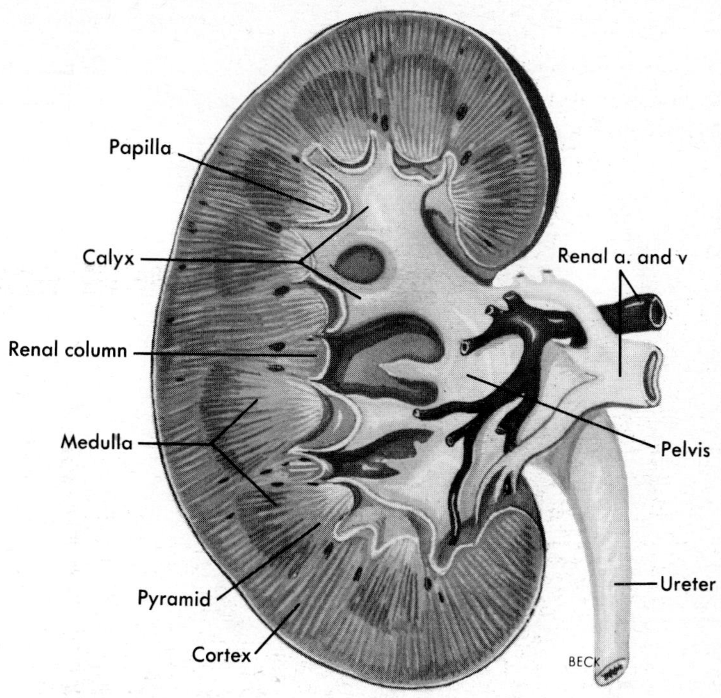

Fig. 7-1. *Coronal section of the right kidney. (From Thibodeau, G.A.: Textbook of anatomy and physiology, ed. 12, St. Louis, 1987, Times Mirror/Mosby College Publishing.)*

through the tubules, substances are modified by reabsorption and secretion, processes that change in response to the need of keeping the internal milieu of the body within a narrow, safe range.

Because of their size and electrical charge, red blood cells and protein do not normally pass through the glomerular filter. Thus the fluid in Bowman's capsule is a protein-free filtrate of blood plasma; the rate of its formation is called the *glomerular filtration rate*. Normally this averages about 125 ml/min, but may be as high as 200 ml/min. Usually over 99% of the glomerular filtrate is reabsorbed in the tubules, the remainder passing into the urinary bladder as the final urine.

The glomerulus is not the only capillary bed supplying the nephron. The efferent arteriole leaving Bowman's capsule goes on to form

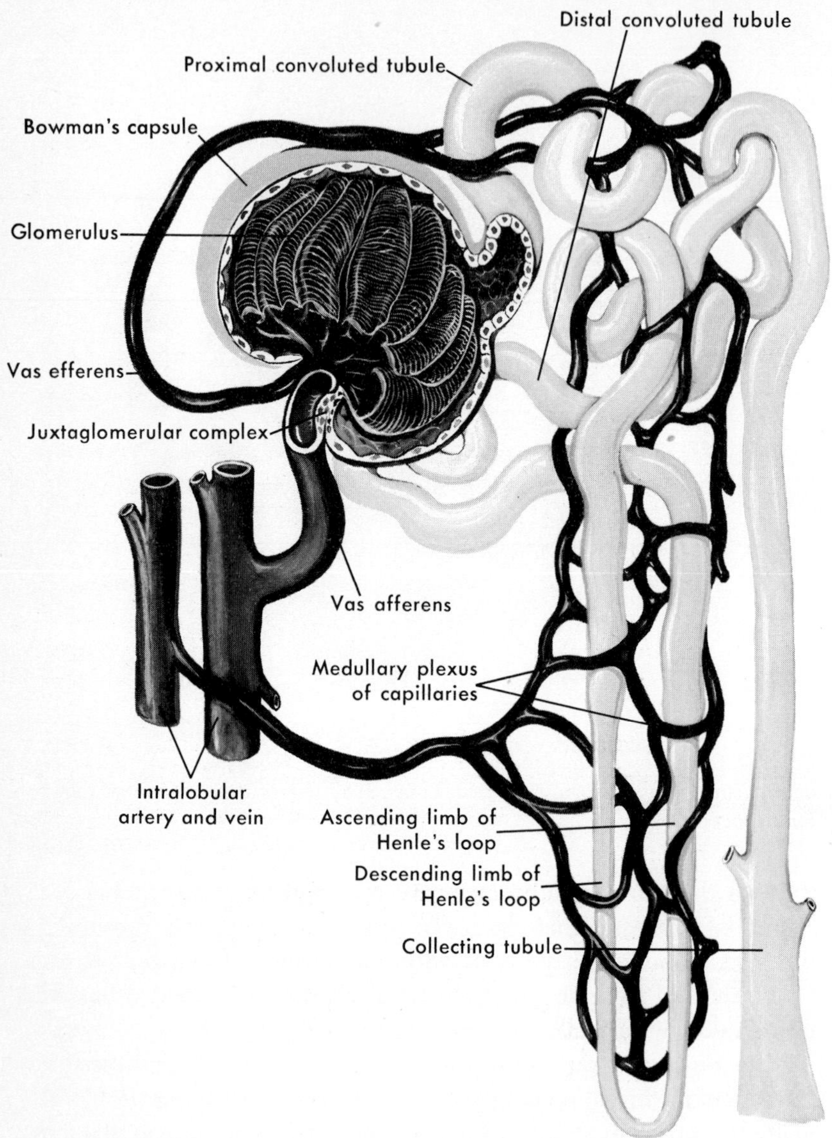

Fig. 7-2. *The nephron and its blood supply. The wall of Bowman's capsule has been cut away to reveal the detail of the glomerulus. (From Schottelius, B.A., and Schottelius, D.D.: Textbook of physiology, ed. 17, St. Louis, 1973, The C.V. Mosby Co.)*

another capillary bed, this time a low-pressure bed that supplies the tubules (Fig. 7-2). Changes in hydrostatic and oncotic pressures in these peritubular capillaries change the rate of sodium and water reabsorption from the tubular fluid and the concentrating ability of the kidney.

PATHOPHYSIOLOGY

Diseases of the kidney have different manifestations depending on the preferential area involved in the nephron—glomerular or tubular.

Glomerular disease may present with some of these abnormalities:

1. Microscopic or gross hematuria such as in glomerulonephritis of various types
2. Proteinuria, which in excessive amounts (nephrotic syndrome) will present with hypoalbuminemia and edema such as in diabetic nephropathy and childhood minimal lesion disease
3. Hypertension because of salt and water retention.
4. Acute or chronic renal failure, causing elevation in blood urea nitrogen (BUN) and creatinine and other toxic metabolites. The renal failure is due to destruction of glomerular capillary surface area secondary to the disease. In acute renal failure, there may be decreased urine flow.

Tubular disease may present with some of these abnormalities:

1. Urinary volume changes, such as oliguria (<400 ml/24h); most commonly seen with acute tubular necrosis or polyuria, which may occur in interstitial diseases owing to loss of concentrating ability.
2. Diminution in urinary acidification, which causes systemic metabolic acidosis. This condition is usually associated with hypokalemia, presenting with generalized muscular weakness, urinary calculi, or nephrocalcinosis. In some cases, hyperkalemia may be present, especially in diabetes mellitus associated with renal failure.
3. Rise in BUN and creatinine (with severe damage).

Recent animal studies show that after any renal disease with residual damage, the remaining normal nephrons receive a higher blood flow and are thus hyperperfused. If unchecked, this hyperperfusion leads to progressive sclerosis of the glomeruli and end-stage renal disease. It has also been demonstrated that dietary protein restriction, if started very early in the course of the disease, will decrease the hyperperfusion and slow down the rapid progression of renal failure.

CLINICAL APPLICATION OF LABORATORY TESTS

In many renal glomerular diseases there is loss of the integrity of the capillary wall with resultant proteinuria, hematuria, or both. Thus the most useful major noninvasive laboratory test for the evaluation of kidney disease is a careful *examination of the urine* correlated with the clinical signs and symptoms. Some form of renal disease is clearly present when the urinalysis is abnormal and the *glomerular filtration rate* reduced.

Measurement of the glomerular filtration rate (GFR) is used to estimate the severity and follow the course of known renal disease. It is evaluated through clearance tests, the gold standard of which is *inulin clearance*. *Creatinine clearance* and clearance using *radionuclides* are used in clinical practice. The *urea clearance* test is not frequently used in clinical medicine because it is not very reliable. The severity and rate of progression of glomerular nephritis and other renal disorders can be assessed through serial GFR measurements.

Tubular function is best measured by a test that determines the ability of the tubules to concentrate and dilute urine *(urine and serum osmolality)*. The first function to be lost in renal disease is the ability of the kidney to concentrate urine. Since the concentration of urine occurs in the renal medulla where the loop of Henle and collecting tubules are, it is the disease processes that affect the medulla that produce early signs of impairment of concentration of urine. Such disorders are acute interstitial nephritis, obstructive uropathy, pyelonephritis, papillary necrosis, medullary cysts, hypokalemic and hypercalcemic nephropathy, and sickle cell disease. *Urinary sodium concentration* is another tubular function test that is helpful in the diagnosis and differentiation of dehydration and decreased urine output versus acute tubular necrosis.

Other helpful tests include *antinuclear antibody titer*, *anti-DNA*, *anti-ribonucleoprotein (RNP)*, *anti-GBM titers*, *circulating immune complexes*, *cryoglobulins*, *serum complement levels*, *hepatic B antigen and antibody*, *ASO titers*, and *VDRL* levels, which may help differentiate collagen vascular diseases from other glomerulonephritides. These are discussed in Chapter 12. Renal plasma flow is measured only in research situations *(para-aminohippurate [PAH] clearance test)*.

KIDNEY FUNCTION TESTS

Laboratory tests for renal function are related to the three main functions of the nephron—glomerular filtration, tubular reabsorption, and tubular secretion. It is through these three mechanisms that the kidney clears the blood of unwanted substances. The routine urinalysis is completely covered in Chapter 3. Urine osmolality and sodium are discussed later in this chapter.

TESTS OF GLOMERULAR FILTRATION RATE

CREATININE CLEARANCE

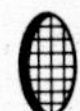

Reference range

Adult males: 120 (82-160) ml/min
Adult females: 95 (74-130) ml/min

EXPLANATION OF THE TEST

For a true picture of glomerular filtration rate, which is 105 to 135 ml/min, the tested substance must be freely filtered and neither reabsorbed nor secreted by the tubules. Such a substance is inulin, a polysaccharide that is completely cleared by the kidney. However, its use involves both an intravenous infusion of, and an assay for, inulin that is not widely available. In clinical nephrology, although creatinine is modified slightly by the tubules through reabsorption and secretion, its final clearance comes quite close to inulin clearance, making creatinine clearance the most widely used test to evaluate glomerular filtration rate in clinical medicine.

Creatinine is an endogenous waste product originating from the creatine and phosphocreatine of skeletal muscle. The serum creatinine level, therefore, rises and the creatinine clearance rate falls when the GFR is impaired. Urine and plasma concentrations of creatinine are measured, and a urine specimen is collected and measured for volume at 2, 12, or 24 hours. Thus:

$$\text{Creatinine clearance} = \frac{\text{Urine creatinine concentration (mg\%)} \times \text{Urine volume (ml/min)}}{\text{Plasma creatinine concentration (mg\%)}}$$

VALUE OF THE TEST

Essential in the evaluation of any kidney dysfunction.
Assesses renal function (GFR).
Serial measurements help in the decision of whether to start protein restriction, vitamin D supplementation, and later on, as renal function deteriorates to levels of glomerular filtration of 10% of normal, in the initiation of renal replacement therapy, such as hemodialysis, peritoneal dialysis, or transplantation.

NURSING ACTION

1. Inform the patient that there are no fluid restrictions but that an excessive amount of meat should not be eaten before the test.
2. Explain to the patient that this test helps to evaluate kidney function, and that it involves a timed urine specimen collection and at least one blood sample.
3. Instruct the patient to avoid strenuous physical exercise during the collection period.
4. Instruct the patient to empty bladder and then collect a urine specimen at either 2, 6, 12, or 24 hours in a bottle containing a preservative.

INTERFERING FACTORS

Incomplete urine collection
A high-protein diet before the test
Strenuous exercise during the collection period

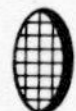

USE OF RADIOISOTOPES FOR RENAL CLEARANCE

EXPLANATION OF THE TEST

The glomerular filtration rate can also be measured by means of radioisotopes, which enter the tubules by proximal tubular secretion and, to a lesser degree, by glomerular filtration. They may also be used for outlining the kidneys by also using a scintillation camera. Iothalamate labeled with *iodine 125* is injected subcutaneously or intravenously. There is no protein binding, and the renal clearance of the iodine 125 remains independent of variations in the plasma level. By measuring the iodine 125 levels in the urine and the plasma, iodine 125 clearance can be calculated, reflecting GFR.

More recently, *technetium pyrophosphate* is being used for the determination of glomerular filtration rate with the distinct advantage that the difficulties and errors involved in timed urine collections are eliminated. The infusion rate of the technetium pyrophosphate is kept at a steady state. The amount infused in a given time is then divided by the plasma level, giving a glomerular clearance rate that is very close in accuracy to that of inulin clearance.

VALUE OF THE TEST

Essential in the evaluation of any kidney dysfunction.
Assesses renal function (GFR).
Serial measurements help in the decision of whether to start protein restriction and vitamin D supplementation and, later on, as renal function deteriorates to levels of glomerular filtration of 10% of normal, in the initiation of renal replacement therapy, such as hemodialysis, peritoneal dialysis, or transplant.

NURSING ACTION

1. Inform the patient that there are no dietary restrictions before this test.
2. Inform him or her that the radiation received will be minimal.
3. Inform the patient that this test helps the physician evaluate kidney function.

UREA CLEARANCE AND BLOOD UREA NITROGEN (BUN)

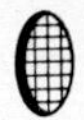

Reference range

8-25 mg/dl (SI units: 0.18-0.42 mmol/L)

EXPLANATION OF THE TEST

Urea is the end product of protein metabolism and is excreted primarily by glomerular filtration. Thus the BUN tends to vary inversely with the glomerular filtration rate. Two factors make the BUN and urea clearance tests less reliable than the creatinine clearance test: (1) urea, after being filtered, tends to diffuse back into the renal tubular cells and thus its clearance is dependent on the rate of urine formation, and (2) urea production varies according to the state of liver function and protein intake and breakdown.

LIMITATIONS OF THE TEST

The creatinine clearance is the preferred clinical method for measuring glomerular filtration rate because of the variability in urea production and reabsorption.

NURSING ACTION

1. Inform the patient that there are no food or fluid restrictions before this test.
2. Inform him or her that this test helps to evaluate kidney function.
3. Collect venous blood in a 10-ml to 15-ml red-top tube. Handle the sample gently to prevent hemolysis.

INTERFERING FACTORS

Chloramphenicol may depress BUN.

CLINICAL IMPLICATIONS

Urea clearance is less than inulin clearance when there is decrease in urine flow and therefore is not very useful. However, the ratio of BUN to serum creatinine may be helpful in certain conditions. A ratio greater than 10:1 may be suggestive of dehydration, gastrointestinal bleeding, increased protein intakes, decreased cardiac output, increased catabolism causing increased protein breakdown, or intake of tetracycline (an antianabolic agent).

TUBULAR FUNCTION TESTS

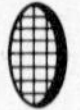

URINE AND SERUM OSMOLALITY

Reference range, urine osmolality

50-1400 mOsm/L (range)

500-800 mOsm/L (random specimen)

Note: Normal urine osmolality can be as much as 1400 mOsm/L with maximal ADH stimulation and as little as 50 mOsm/kg with maximal ADH suppression. Thus, urine osmolality should be interpreted in the light of what is known about the patient's hydration status and plasma osmolality.

Reference range, serum osmolality

280-295 mOsm/L (range)

EXPLANATION OF THE TEST

Osmolality is an expression of the total number of particles in a solution. Plasma osmolality is the main regulator of the release of antidiuretic hormone (ADH). When sufficient water is not being taken in, the osmolality of the plasma rises, ADH is released from the pituitary gland, and the kidneys respond by reabsorbing water from the distal and collecting tubules and producing a more concentrated urine. The converse occurs with excessive water ingestion. With the decrease in plasma osmolality, ADH is not released, more water is lost, and the urine becomes more dilute. A change in plasma osmolality of as little as 1% will either suppress or stimulate thirst and ADH secretion.

In normal kidney function there is tremendous flexibility in the volume of water that can be ingested (as little as 500 ml or as much as 25 L/24 h). Abnormalities in urine diluting or concentrating capacity markedly reduce this flexibility and since sodium is the most abundant plasma electrolyte, such an abnormality is reflected in changes in plasma sodium concentration, which can vary in extremes from 100 to 180 mEq/L, normal being 136 to 145 mEq/L.

VALUE OF THE TEST

Helps in the differential diagnosis of polyuric and oliguric states; and hyponatremic and hypernatremic states.

NURSING ACTION

See also p. 441. This test requires an osmometer; thus it is not a bedside procedure. If an osmometer is not available, the concentration of the urine can be estimated from the specific gravity, which is measured with a hydrometer. Such a measurement would reflect only major deviations from normal, but can be done at the bedside and helps in the treatment of diabetes insipidus following head injuries. However, the measurement of urine osmolality is a more accurate method than specific gravity for determining the diluting and concentrating ability of the kidneys.

INTERFERING FACTORS

Other stimuli besides changes in plasma osmolality can increase the secretion of ADH. Some of these are:

Hypovolemia

Angiotensin II

Drugs such as chlorpropamide (Diabinese), vincristine (Oncovin), clofibrate (Atromid-S), carbamazepine (Tegretol), and thiazides (Hydrodiuril).

Disease states such as cancer of the lung, cerebrovascular accidents, or brain tumors can also increase ADH secretion by themselves and thus lead to hyponatremia if fluid intake is not restricted (in the absence of any intrinsic renal tubular disease).

CLINICAL IMPLICATIONS

Inadequate ADH secretion or decreased responsiveness of the distal tubules to circulating ADH

Simultaneous determination of serum and urine osmolality is often valuable in assessing the distal and collecting tubular response to circulating ADH. There may be inadequate ADH secretion (central diabetes insipidus) or decreased responsiveness of the distal tubules to circulating ADH (nephrogenic diabetes insipidus). A hyperosmolar serum with a much lower concurrent urine osmolality suggests central diabetes insipidus (low or absent ADH secretion). In nephrogenic diabetes insipidus owing to unresponsiveness of diseased tubules to normal or even high circulatory ADH levels, the urine osmolarity is usually equal to serum osmolarity (isosthenuria).

Urinary hyperosmolalities

In oliguric states secondary to hypovolemia, ADH secretion is stimulated and therefore urine osmolarity will be high as long as the tubules have not sustained ischemic damage. However, if damage has occurred, the tubules are unresponsive to ADH and therefore urine will be isosthenuric, the result of acute tubular necrosis.

Increased urinary osmolarity can also occur when there is excretion of solutes in the urine that are osmotically active, such as glucose in hyperglycemic situations when the tubular threshold is surpassed or in patients who are receiving mannitol infusion.

SODIUM (URINE)

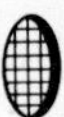

Reference range

80-180 mEq/24 hr

Note: In hypovolemic patients with normal kidney function the normal sodium concentration in the urine is less than 10 mEq/L and may be as low as 1 mEq/L.

EXPLANATION OF THE TEST

The excretion of sodium is very sensitive to extracellular fluid volume. This is because sodium is an extracellular ion and acts to hold water in the extracellular compartment and keep it at a constant level by varying water and sodium excretion in the urine. If sodium is taken in, volume expansion occurs and sodium is excreted in the urine to maintain homeostasis. If sodium is lost (e.g., vomiting or diarrhea), volume depletion results and the amount of sodium excreted in the urine is reduced, in an attempt to prevent further dehydration.

VALUE OF THE TEST

Helps differentiate between the two most common causes of renal failure in hospitalized patients—prerenal failure (secondary to dehydration or hemorrhage) and acute tubular necrosis (secondary to hypotension and ischemic tubular necrosis).

Helps in the decision of when rehydration has been accomplished in a hypovolemic patient who requires fluid repletion.

NURSING ACTION

1. Inform the patient that there are no dietary restrictions before the test.
2. The test is done on a random urine sample.

CLINICAL IMPLICATIONS

Renal disease. The urinary sodium level usually is more than 40 mEq/L in most forms of renal disease. This is because the kidney is unable to conserve sodium.

Prerenal failure. In prerenal failure there is decreased blood volume secondary to dehydration from vomiting, diarrhea, and so on.

In hemorrhage with hypovolemia there is decreased renal perfusion and therefore a urine sodium concentration of less than 10 to 20 mEq/L. If the hypovolemia is not reversed, further ischemia to the kidney will ensue resulting in acute tubular necrosis. This will manifest with a urine sodium concentration of greater than 40 mEq/L. In some situations, such as vomiting and severe hypochloremic alkalosis, the urine sodium may be high in spite of the fact that the patient may be in prerenal failure. Chloride in this situation may be low and thus support the diagnosis of prerenal failure. Usually, however, the urine sodium and chloride will be simultaneously elevated or simultaneously depressed. Occasionally the sodium will be low and the chloride high. If the urine potassium concentration is elevated in oliguric states it indicates that the tubules are responding normally to the aldosterone levels and that the patient may not have acute tubular necrosis.

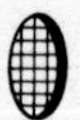

PLASMA RENIN ACTIVITY

Reference range

Conventional	*SI Units*
Normal diet	
Supine 1.1 ± 0.8 ng/ml/hr	0.9 ± 0.6 nmol/L/hr
Upright 1.9 ± 1.7 ng/ml/hr	1.5 ± 1.3 nmol/L/hr
Low sodium diet	
Supine 2.7 ± 1.8 ng/ml/hr	2.1 ± 1.4 nmol/L/hr
Upright 6.6 ± 2.5 ng/ml/hr	5.1 ± 1.9 nmol/L/hr

EXPLANATION OF THE TEST

Renin is an enzyme secreted into the renal veins by the juxtaglomerular cells of the afferent arteriole of the glomerulus. Renin catalyzes the conversion of angiotensinogen to angiotensin I, which is converted into angiotensin II by a converting enzyme. Angiotensin II is a potent vasoconstrictor and stimulates aldosterone production by the adrenal cortex. Excessive amounts of angiotensin II, when not caused by hypovolemia, result in renal hypertension.

The release of renin is determined by many factors including plasma levels of potassium, ADH, catecholamines, ACTH, prostaglandins, blood volume, various drugs, and age. The most important protective mechanism when there is hypovolemia is elevated renin and elevated angiotensin, which keep the blood pressure from falling, and the elevated aldosterone and increased sodium reabsorption help to bring the blood volume back to normal.

Radioimmunoassay techniques are used in the determination of plasma renin activity. A peripheral or renal venous blood sample is used, and the results are expressed as the rate of angiotensin I formation per unit of time.

VALUE AND LIMITATIONS OF THE TEST

Important in the diagnosis of primary aldosteronism.

Selective renal vein sampling is important in the confirmation of unilateral renal artery stenosis in the causation of hypertension.

Patient dietary preparation is crucial to the accuracy of the test.

NURSING ACTION

1. Instruct the patient to maintain a normal sodium diet (3 g/day) for 4 weeks before the test and to follow the physician's orders regarding abstention from medications. Dietary instructions should be in writing and should emphasize the importance of preparing all foods without salt and of eating only the foods listed on the teaching aid provided by the physician.
2. Instruct the patient to remain in bed until the blood sample is obtained, if it is to be a recumbent sample (used in renovascular disease such as renal artery stenosis). Otherwise he or she should be upright, walking or standing for 2 to 4 hours after taking the baseline supine sample to rule out primary aldosteronism (both samples will be low in this situation).
3. An informed consent should be obtained for renal vein catheterization.
4. For a peripheral vein sample, withdraw venous blood in a 7-ml lavender-top tube, completely filling it and gently inverting it several times to mix the anticoagulant. The syringe and collection tube should be chilled. Place it on ice and send it to the laboratory immediately. For a renal vein sample, the patient is taken to the radiology department, a local anesthetic used, and a catheter advanced to the renal vein through the femoral vein under fluoroscopic control.

CLINICAL IMPLICATIONS
Elevated levels

Malignant and accelerated hypertension
Renal artery stenosis
Contraceptive-induced hypertension
Renin-producing renal tumors (hemangiopericytoma)
Hypokalemia
Adrenal hypofunction (Addison's disease)
Chronic renal failure with parenchymal disease
Bartter's syndrome
Transplantation rejection
Cirrhosis of the liver
Congestive heart failure
Nephrotic syndrome
Hypovolemia due to hemorrhage or other causes
Drugs: hydralazine, sodium nitroprusside, converting enzyme inhibition, and diuretics

Decreased levels

Primary aldosteronism
Cushing's syndrome
Salt-retaining steroids
Licorice ingestion or chewing tobacco
Essential hypertension (20%)
Hypervolemia due to a high-sodium diet
Drugs: beta blockers, methyldopa (Aldomet), clonidine hydrochloride (Catapres)

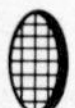

ALDOSTERONE ASSAY (PLASMA AND URINE)

Reference ranges

	Conventional	*SI Units*
Excretion:	5-19 μg/24 hr	14-53 nmol/day
Supine:	48 ± 29 pg/ml	133 ± 80 pmol/L
Upright (2 hr):	65 ± 23 pg/ml	180 ± 64 pmol/L

EXPLANATION OF THE TEST

Aldosterone is the major electrolyte-regulating steroid of the adrenal cortex. It is instrumental in sodium and potassium homeostasis and in maintenance of blood pressure. Renin-angiotensin system and circulating potassium primarily stimulate aldosterone production and secretion (although the production of aldosterone is stimulated by adrenocorticotropic hormone [ACTH], it is not dependent on this). Aldosterone levels are also influenced by sodium, potassium, and magnesium. Aldosterone production is decreased in (1) adrenal insufficiency, (2) high sodium intake, (3) hypokalemia, and (4) other excess mineralocorticoids such as found in licorice ingestion and chewing tobacco. It is increased by low sodium intake and hyperkalemia. Its function is to promote tubular reabsorption of sodium and chloride in exchange for potassium and hydrogen ions, thus maintaining blood pressure and blood volume and regulating fluid and electrolyte balance.

VALUE AND LIMITATIONS OF THE TEST

Aids in the diagnosis of aldosteronism.

Along with plasma renin levels, distinguishes between primary and secondary aldosteronism.

Aids in the diagnosis of adrenal adenoma and adrenal hyperplasia.

Its interpretation has to be done by accurately collected 24-hour urine specimen for sodium.

NURSING ACTION

1. Before the patient arises in the morning, withdraw venous blood in a 7-ml red-top collection tube. Draw another sample 4 hours later after the patient has been up and around and while the patient is standing.
2. Advise the patient regarding controlled sodium intake.
3. Note that the physician will order tests for plasma renin activity and plasma aldosterone levels, and a 24-hour urine sample for sodium and aldosterone.
4. Collect a 24-hour urine specimen; refrigerate it during collection.

INTERFERING FACTORS

Increased aldosterone secretion results from any medications or disease states that raise the plasma renin activity.

Decreased aldosterone secretion results from heparin, licorice, chewing tobacco.

CLINICAL IMPLICATIONS
Elevated levels

Adenoma (increased secretion; primary aldosteronism; low renin). This is associated with hypertension and hypokalemia.

Increased levels of aldosterone with increased angiotensin II (high renin), such as renovascular disease. Aldosterone levels are also increased in congestive heart failure, liver cirrhosis with ascites, nephrotic syndrome, or hypovolemia (sodium excretion is decreased with resultant sodium and fluid retention). This may or may not be associated with hypertension and/or hypokalemia. However, in primary or secondary aldosteronism associated with hypertension there is wastage of potassium, and thus presence of hypokalemia. The reverse can occur in conditions of low aldosterone secretion, that is, hypotension and hyperkalemia. Table 7-1 lists typical renin-aldosterone patterns in various clinical conditions.

Table 7-1 Typical renin-aldosterone patterns in various clinical conditions

	Plasma renin	Aldosterone
Primary aldosteronism	Low	High
Low-renin essential hypertension	Low	Normal
Cushing's syndrome	Low	Low/normal
Licorice ingestion syndrome	Low	Low
High-salt diet	Low	Low
Oral contraceptives	High	Normal
Cirrhosis	High	High
Malignant hypertension	High	High
Unilateral renal disease	High	High
High-renin essential hypertension	High	High
Pregnancy	High	High
Diuretic overuse	High	High
Juxtaglomerular tumor	High	High
Bartter's syndrome	High	High
Low-salt diet	High	High
Addison's disease	High	Low
Hypokalemia	High	Low

Adapted from Ravel, R.: Clinical laboratory medicine, Chicago, 1984, Year Book Medical Publishers.

LABORATORY DETECTION OF URINARY TRACT INFECTIONS

URINE CULTURE

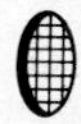

EXPLANATION OF THE TEST

Urine is cultured in order to identify urinary tract infections. A test of antimicrobial sensitivity of any organism detected should be ordered in cases of suspected genitourinary infection. New methods of detecting infection and identifying the organism sometimes eliminate the need for lengthy culture and sensitivity testing (e.g., dipstik, the nitride test).

VALUE OF THE TEST

Aids in the diagnosis of pyelonephritis as well as urinary tract infection.

NURSING ACTION

1. Inform the patient that there are no dietary restrictions before this test.
2. Instruct the patient regarding the collection of a clean-voided midstream specimen. The first-voided specimen in the morning is best.
3. Check the patient's history for current antibiotic therapy and report this on the laboratory slip.
4. The amount of urine collected should be at least 3 ml and not more than half a specimen cup. Seal the cup with a sterile lid and send to the laboratory immediately. If transport to the laboratory will be delayed more than a half hour, refrigerate the specimen.

CLINICAL IMPLICATIONS

Colony count

In a urine culture the colony count is important. The presence of fewer than 10,000 viable bacterial units per milliliter of urine is probably of no significance. If 10,000 to 100,000 colonies are cultured, no positive conclusion can be drawn. There should be over 100,000 colonies before an infection is considered significant. However, samples of urine from the ureters and renal pelvis might contain fewer bacteria and still indicate infection because bacteria multiply while urine is being held in the bladder.

A positive culture without symptoms

In the absence of symptoms, a positive urine culture should elicit an inquiry into how the specimen was collected. Unless a catheter was used or the sample is a midstream-voided specimen obtained after proper cleansing of the genitalia, contamination will occur. It should also be remembered that a negative urine culture does not necessarily rule out chronic low-grade pyelonephritis. Asymptomatic bacteruria is quite common in elderly women and especially in patients with indwelling catheters and may not require treatment.

A positive culture with symptoms

A positive urine culture, flank pain, and elevated temperature help differentiate pyelonephritis from lower urinary tract infection. Pyelonephritis represents active infection of the pelvis and medulla of the kidney. A positive culture and symptoms of dysuria, frequency, and urgency suggest cystitis.

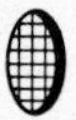

NEW TESTS

The *urine culture* remains the gold standard for the diagnosis of urinary tract infections. However, because the standard culture time is 24 hours there has been intense research to develop more rapid tests for determining urinary tract infections. The result has been the development of biochemical methods such as the Griess test (nitrate reduction test), which is highly specific but lacks sensitivity, and automated methods (photometry and bioluminescence) that eliminate negative specimens and identify potential positive specimens rapidly and accurately.

Photometry detects significant bacterial growth by changes in turbidity or light transmission through inoculated media. There are three systems at the present time, Autobac (General Diagnostics), Automicrobic (Vitek Systems), and MS-2 (Abbott Laboratories).

Bioluminescence (the Lumac system [3M] detects significant bacteriuria because it detects bacterial adenosine triphosphate. Other rapid automated methods in development include a Bactometer microbial monitoring system (Bactomatic) that monitors the electrical impedance of broth inoculated with a urine specimen; a filtering and staining technique (Baca-T-Screen [Marion Laboratories]); carbon 14 labeling; microcalorimetry, which measures heat generated by bacterial growth; and particle size distribution analysis (Coulter counter).

METHODS OF IMAGING THE KIDNEY

INTRAVENOUS PYELOGRAM (IVP)

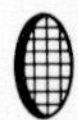

EXPLANATION OF THE TEST

An IVP is obtained by the intravenous injection of contrast media that is cleared from the blood by glomerular filtration and thus permits visualization of the renal parenchyma and collecting system on multiple x-ray films.

Before ordering a contrast study of the kidney, it is helpful to check the serum creatinine. If it is more than 2 mg/dl there is a distinct possibility of precipitating contrast nephrotoxicity and acute renal failure. Other risk factors are diabetes mellitus, dehydration, hypertension, old age, congestive heart failure, and multiple myeloma. Using nonionic contrast media or contrast with low osmolality may cause fewer problems with nephrotoxicity. The use of computerized digital subtration angiogram where smaller volumes of contrast media are utilized with good visualization has also contributed to a decrease in incidence of nephrotoxicity.

Timed-sequence IVP is a modification of the standard IVP. Films are made every minute for 5 minutes after injection of the contrast media. A difference between the times of excretion of the dye from the two kidneys indicates unilateral kidney disease. In such a case, the normal kidney shows some concentration of the dye before the abnormal one does. Note that a negative timed sequence IVP does not rule out renal artery stenosis (it is positive in only 70% of proven cases). Thus if the clinical suspicion is high for this condition, the physician will use arterial digital subtraction angiography, where the diagnostic yield approaches 100%.

VALUE AND LIMITATIONS OF THE TEST

Provides visualization of the entire urinary tract.

Helpful in the diagnosis of renal masses and cysts, ureteral obstruction, retroperitoneal tumors, renal trauma, bladder abnormalities, and so on.

Provides an estimate of renal function based on the appearance time and concentration of the contrast media in each kidney.

Visualization may be poor in the presence of moderate to severe renal disease with a compromised glomerular filtration rate.

The timed sequence IVP does not differentiate between renal artery disease, intrinsic renal disease, or renal venous thrombosis.

In patients with hypertension, the timed sequence IVP does not differentiate between hypertension resulting from renal parenchymal disease or diffuse small-vessel disease and that caused by obstruction of a major renal artery.

NURSING ACTION

1. Instruct the patient to remain fasting after midnight prior to the test. Explain to the patient that this helps to produce a moderate dehydration and better concentration of the contrast medium.
2. Explain the procedure to the patient and tell him or her that it will allow the physician to visualize the renal system.
3. Secure an informed consent.
4. Check the patient's history for hypersensitivity to iodine, iodine-containing foods, or contrast media containing iodine.
5. The patient should take a strong cathartic the afternoon before the test so that films will not be obscured by the intestinal contents.
6. Have the patient void immediately before the test.

NURSING ALERT

Watch the patient for adverse reactions to the radiocontrast material such as anaphylactic reaction, volume overload and congestive heart failure, and acute renal failure.

In order to recognize a nephrotoxic response to the contrast media should it occur, closely monitor urinary output, renal function (BUN and serum creatinine), and electrolytes 24 to 48 hours following the use of radiocontrast material.

RENAL ANGIOGRAPHY

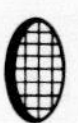

EXPLANATION OF THE TEST

Renal angiography provides visualization of the entire renal arterial, capillary, and venous system. This test is performed by introducing a catheter into the renal artery or the renal vein (selective angiography), or into the aorta proximal to the origin of the renal arteries (aortorenal angiography), and injecting contrast material while rapid x-ray filming is performed. In digital subtraction angiography, smaller amounts of contrast media are used.

VALUE OF THE TEST

Helpful in the diagnosis of renal artery stenosis (renal vascular hypertension), renal masses, trauma, and venous thrombosis.

NURSING ACTION

1. Instruct the patient to remain fasting after midnight prior to the test.
2. Explain the procedure to the patient and tell him or her that it will allow the physician to visualize the renal vasculature.
3. Secure an informed consent.
4. Check the patient's history for hypersensitivity to iodine, iodine-containing foods, or contrast media. Review the Nursing Alert box in this section relative to the administration of contrast media.
5. Establish baseline values for vital signs and peripheral pulses.
6. Have the patient void immediately before the test to avoid an overdistended bladder, since the contrast medium is an osmotic diuretic.
7. While taking the patient's history, ascertain if he or she has been taking crystalline warfarin sodium (Coumadin) or heparin; the physician may order vitamin K or protamine sulfate if such is the case.
8. Instruct the patient to remain on bed rest for 4 to 10 hours following the procedure.
9. Check vital signs and peripheral pulses frequently and compare them with the baseline values that were established before the procedure.

NURSING ALERT

Note that for patients with multiple myeloma or diabetes melitis with dehydration the physician may limit the volume of contrast medium injected and hydrate the patient before the study is done in order to avoid renal shutdown.

Watch the patient for adverse reactions to the radiocontrast material such as anaphylactic reaction, volume overload and congestive heart failure, and acute renal failure.

In order to recognize a nephrotoxic response to the contrast media should it occur, closely monitor urinary output, renal function (BUN and serum creatinine), and electrolytes 24 to 48 hours following the use of radiocontrast material.

Following the procedure observe the puncture site closely for swelling and bleeding (hematoma formation). Apply manual pressure and notify the physician immediately if this occurs.

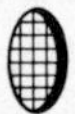

RETROGRADE PYELOGRAPHY

EXPLANATION OF THE TEST

Retrograde pyelography is performed by passing a catheter from the urethra to the urinary bladder, then to the right or left ureter, and injecting a contrast medium. This test is more involved than regular IVP. If the obstruction is so severe that the catheter cannot be passed across it (Fig. 7-3), an antegrade pyelogram may be indicated (p. 260).

VALUE OF THE TEST

Provides detailed visualization of the urinary collecting system independent of the status of renal function
Helpful in the diagnosis of ureteral obstruction
Fewer allergic reactions

NURSING ACTION

1. If a general anesthetic is ordered, instruct the patient to fast for 8 hours before the test.

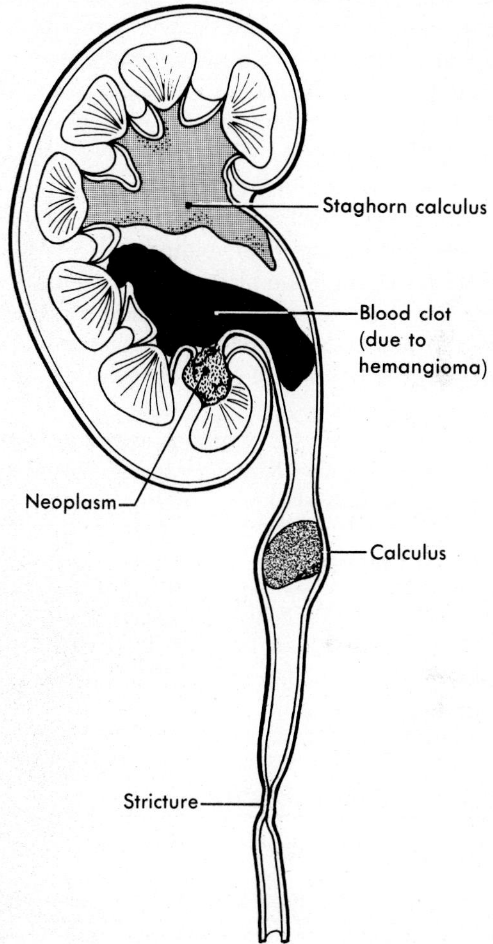

Fig. 7-3. *Types of obstruction that may be seen with pyelography. It is possible to determine the site and type of obstruction to the flow of urine in the calices, pelvis, or ureter.*

2. Inform the patient that this test allows the physician to visualize the urinary collecting system.
3. Obtain a signed informed consent.
4. Explain to the patient that the legs will be placed in stirrups and that the physician will first examine the bladder with a cystoscope followed by catheterization of the ureters and injection of a small amount of contrast media.
5. Following the procedure, check vital signs every 15 minutes for the first 4 hours, every hour for the next 4 hours, and every 4 hours for 24 hours.
6. Record intake and output for 24 hours.
7. Check for signs of hematuria in the urine; it should not be gross or continue beyond the third voiding.
8. Notify the physician if the bladder is distended.
9. If ureteral catheters are in place, be alert to inadequate output since the catheters may need to be irrigated by the physician.
10. Be alert to the symptoms of sepsis (pain, chills, fever, hypotension).
11. Be alert to the nursing precautions associated with the use of contrast media (see the Nursing Alert in the discussion of the intravenous pyelogram).

CLINICAL IMPLICATIONS

Fig. 7-3 illustrates the types and exact sites of obstructions in the renal collecting system that can be visualized with retrograde and antegrade pyelography. Note that blood clots, calculi, neoplasm, and stricture can be diagnosed.

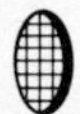

ANTEGRADE PYELOGRAPHY

EXPLANATION OF THE TEST

Percutaneous catheterization of the kidney pelvis, antegrade injection of contrast media, and insertion of a catheter past the obstruction may be used if it is not possible to relieve it by retrograde catheterization. Such a maneuver may help to localize the area and clarify the nature of the obstruction; the obstruction may also be relieved by leaving the catheter in place.

VALUE OF THE TEST

Provides detailed visualization of the urinary collecting system independent of the status of renal function.

Is helpful in the diagnosis of obstruction in the upper collecting system.
Evaluates hydronephrosis and allows the placement of a percutaneous nephrostomy tube and stints.

NURSING ACTION

1. Instruct the patient to fast for 4 hours before the procedure, but to drink fluids.
2. Inform the patient that this test allows the physician to visualize the urinary collecting system and that he or she will be given a sedative and a local anesthetic before the contrast medium is injected into the kidney.
3. Be alert to the nursing precautions associated with the use of contrast media (p. 234).

ULTRASOUND

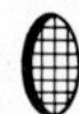

EXPLANATION OF THE TEST

Ultrasonic examination of the kidney is part of an abdominal ultrasonic examination. For a full discussion of the test and nursing action see p. 234.

VALUE OF THE TEST

Detects renal or perirenal masses.
Aids in the differential diagnosis of renal cysts versus solid masses.
Very valuable in the evaluation of ureteral obstruction with hydronephrosis.
Very valuable in the workup of renal failure where small kidneys with decreased cortex are diagnostic of chronic renal failure and large kidneys with thick cortex suggest infiltrative diseases.

COMPUTERIZED TOMOGRAPHY (CT) FOR EVALUATION OF THE KIDNEYS

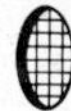

EXPLANATION OF THE TEST

CT scanning with nursing action has already been discussed in Chapter 4.

VALUE OF THE TEST IN RENAL DISORDERS

Provides excellent visualization of the kidneys.
Kidney size can be evaluated.
Kidney tumors and suprarenal masses (adrenal tumors, pheochromocytoma) can be detected.
Hydronephrosis can easily be seen.
Benign cysts can be differentiated from malignant cysts and intrarenal abscesses.
Retroperitoneal bleeding from the kidney or fluid collection (as with an abcess) is noted.
The injection of contrast material further improves image quality.
Loss of kidney cortex and small size suggests chronic renal failure.

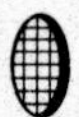

RENAL SCANS (RADIONUCLIDE RENAL IMAGING)

EXPLANATION OF THE TEST

Radioactive material is injected intravenously and its distribution in the kidney mapped by scintiphotography. The amount of radioactivity over each kidney, as measured with a gamma camera or a probe, rises rapidly (within minutes) and then declines as the radioactive tracer leaves the kidney via the ureters. The curve describing these changes as a function of time is called a renogram (Fig. 7-4). It makes possible a composite evaluation of renal plasma flow, glomerular filtration, and tubular secretion, as well as excretory function. Any process that interferes with these functions will produce an abnormal renogram. The data are usually evaluated in a qualitative manner. Computer processing of the data permits semiquantitation of renal function. Various patterns in abnormal renograms can be recognized and equated with specific conditions, such as renal vascular hypertension, tubular disease, urinary obstruction, or absence of kidney function. Initially, this test was important in the diagnosis of hypertension, particularly unilateral renal vascular hypertension. However the diagnostic yield is only 70%, whereas the diagnostic yield of digital subtraction angiography is close to 100%.

VALUE OF THE TEST

Reveals the location, size, and shape of the kidneys
Assesses renal blood perfusion and the ability of the kidney to secrete urine

Differentiates tumors, which are usually vascular, from cysts
Evaluates transplant rejection and indicates obstruction of vascular grafts
Detects abnormalities of the collecting system and extravasation of the urine
Defines the level of ureteral obstruction

NURSING ACTION

1. Instruct the patient to fast from midnight prior to the test.
2. Explain to the patient that this test allows the physician to evaluate kidney function. Make sure that he or she understands that the amount of radioactivity is minimal and that the radionuclide is excreted within 24 hours.
3. Obtain a signed informed consent.

CLINICAL IMPLICATIONS

In Fig. 7-4 the normal renal scan is compared to that of renal artery obstruction and polycystic kidneys. Note in Fig. 7-4, *B*, there is obvious failure of the left kidney to perfuse. The right kidney is perfusing well with diffuse uptake of the radionuclide; however, because of a thrombus and partial obstruction of the left renal artery, only slight perfusion of the lower part of the left kidney is apparent. Before this renal scan, the patient had had complete obstruction of the renal artery; this is the renal scan taken following administration of a thrombolytic agent (Streptokinase). Fig. 7-4, *C* shows the blotchy appearance of the kidneys, the typical appearance of the renal scan in patients with polycystic kidneys.

Other conditions visualized on a renal scan include:

Abscesses, emboli, and tumors: May appear as "cold spots" because of the presence of nonfunctioning tissue.
Markedly decreased tubular function: Radionuclide activity in the collecting system is reduced.
Outflow obstruction: Radionuclide activity in the tubules is reduced and that of the collecting system increased.
Lesions, congenital abnormalities, traumatic injury, space-occupying lesions within or around the kidney (tumors, abscesses, infarcts): Demonstrated by static images.

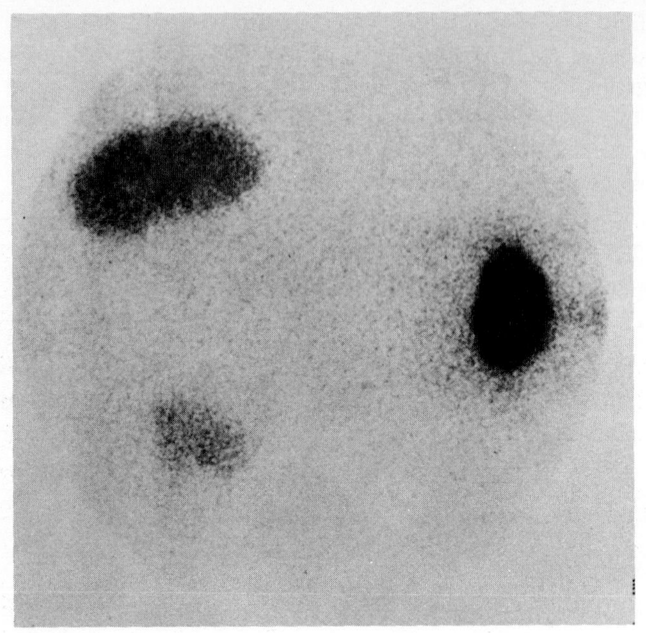

B

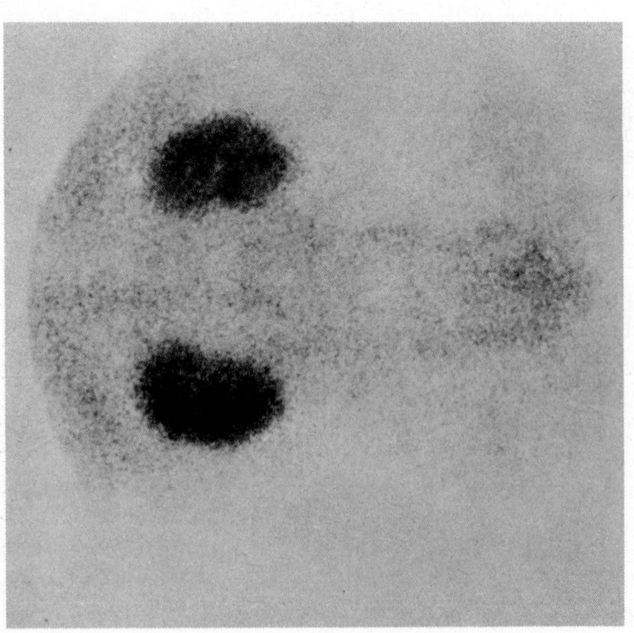

A

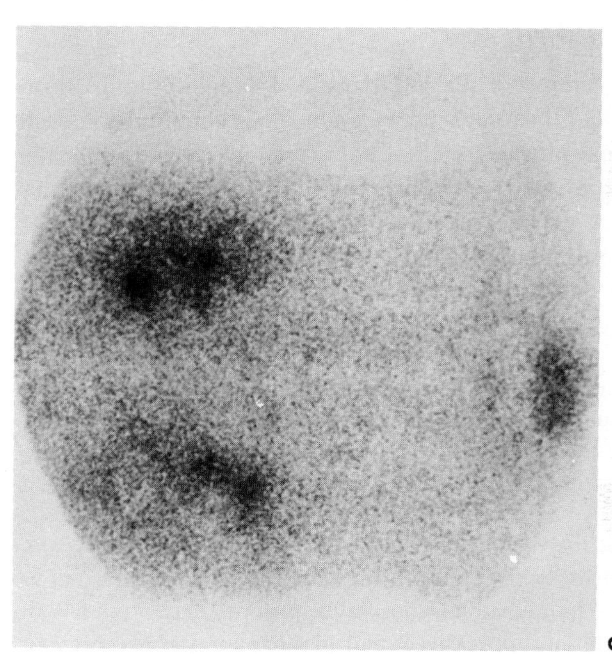

Fig. 7-4. *Renal scans.* **A,** *Normal.* **B,** *Renal artery thrombus partially blocking perfusion of the left kidney.* **C,** *Polycystic kidney disease. (Courtesy Mike Balabanian M.D., Mission Hills, Calif.)*

Diffuse renal disorder (acute tubular necrosis, severe infection, ischemia): Lower than normal total concentration of the radionuclide, but also delayed excretion in contrast to organ rejection with decreased radionuclide uptake.

Congenital ectopia or aplasia: Failure to visualize. Definitive diagnosis usually requires the combination of static images, perfusion studies, and function studies.

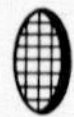

RENAL BIOPSY

EXPLANATION OF THE TEST

Percutaneous biopsy of the kidney under fluoroscopic or ultrasonic guidance yields histologic information about both the glomeruli and the tubules and thus is the most important definitive test for the final diagnosis of intrinsic renal disease. The tissue is processed for light and electron microscopy as well as immunofluorescent studies and cultures when indicated.

VALUE OF THE TEST

Helpful in establishing the diagnosis of the underlying renal disease, prognosis, and choice of therapy.

Most useful in the differential diagnosis of nephrotic syndrome, classification of lupus nephritis, and transplant rejection from other renal diseases in the posttransplant period.

Most useful in the differential diagnosis of rapidly progressive glomerulonephritis where it has very important therapeutic implications, since immediate diagnosis and appropriate treatment with steroids, immunosuppressives, and plasmapheresis may prevent the inflammatory disease from proceeding into end-stage renal failure (e.g., Goodpasture's syndrome).

NURSING ACTION

1. Instruct the patient to restrict food and fluids for 8 hours before the test.
2. Tell the patient that the test helps the physician diagnose kidney disorders.
3. Collect both blood and urine specimens before the test and make sure that he or she has had a complete coagulation evaluation.

4. Obtain informed consent.
5. Ask the patient to void just before the test.
6. Following the procedure, check vital signs frequently as ordered, ensure that the hematocrit is determined frequently as ordered, examine all urine for blood (small amounts that may normally be present after the biopsy should disappear within 8 hours), encourage the patient to take fluids, and inform the patient of the need to rest in bed for 24 hours.

NURSING ALERT

Check the dressing frequently for signs of uncontrolled bleeding, and the urine for hematuria.

Monitor the patient's blood pressure.

Be alert to signs of infection.

8

Diagnostic tests for gastrointestinal disorders

ANATOMY AND PHYSIOLOGY

The gastrointestinal (GI) system (Fig. 8-1) extends from the mouth to the anus and allows the transportation, absorption, secretion, and excretion of various components. Sequentially, the gastrointestinal tract is made up of the pharynx, esophagus, stomach, small intestine, large intestine, and rectum. Organs such as the liver and pancreas manufacture and secrete components into the gastrointestinal tract that aid in digestion and absorption. Various diagnostic studies have been designed to evaluate the ability of the intestinal system to accomplish these four important functions. In addition, certain therapeutic modalities for possible treatment of pathologic conditions have also been developed. In this chapter we will discuss radiologic examinations, endoscopic procedures, including direct visualization and combined endoscopic and radiographic approaches, manometric and motility studies, and studies in reference to the secretive and absorptive functions of the gastrointestinal system.

OVERVIEW OF THE DIAGNOSTIC VALUE OF NEW AND OLD LABORATORY TESTS

Radiographic studies

Contrast studies can be performed by having the patient swallow barium or Gastrografin, which permits visualization of the upper gastrointestinal tract (esophagus, stomach, and small intestine). The

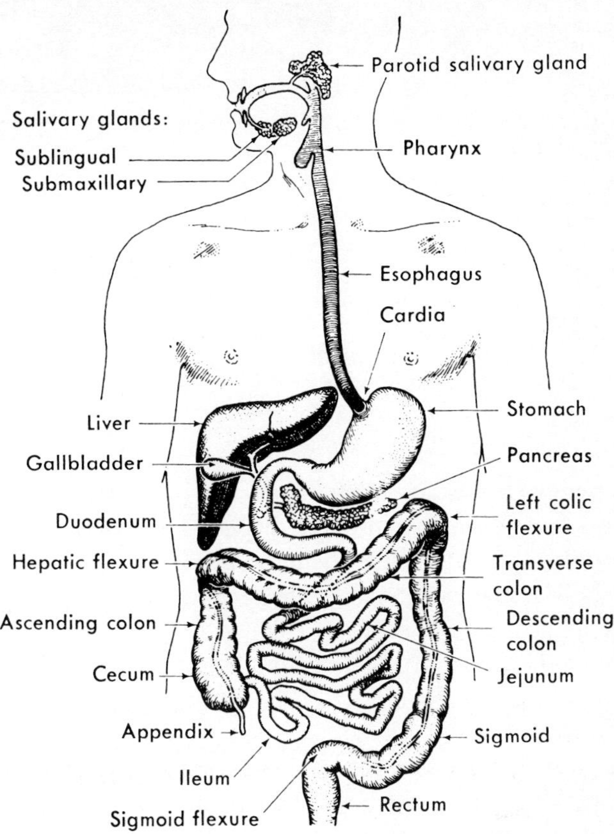

Fig. 8-1. *The gastrointestinal system and its accessory organs. (From Schottelius, B.A., and Schottelius, D.D.: Textbook of physiology, ed. 17, St. Louis, 1973, The C.V. Mosby Co.)*

large intestine can be evaluated by means of barium enema. *Ultrasound (sonography)* is available to evaluate the liver, biliary system (including the gallbladder), and pancreas. *CT scans* of the abdomen and pelvis can visualize the liver, biliary system, and, most importantly, the pancreas. Because of specialized studies such as *technetium-tagged red blood cell (RBC) studies* sites of bleeding can be visualized within the gastrointestinal system, and, in some very selective cases, *angiography* can be of value in visualizing sources of gastrointestinal bleeding or those rare cases of vascular anomalies.

Endoscopy

Endoscopic studies have revolutionized the field of gastroenterology. Endoscopy allows the direct visualization of the mucosa of various levels of the gastrointestinal tract including the esophagus, stomach, and duodenum, the ampulla of Vater, and the mucosa of the colon. In addition to direct visualization of the mucosa, it permits biopsies of visualized abnormalities, removal of polypoid lesions, injection of esophageal varices, sclerosing or cauterization of bleeding sites, and removal of foreign bodies. The ability to visualize the biliary and pancreatic system permits, in selected cases, treatment of diseases noted in these areas and the dilatation of various areas of narrowing or stricture.

Manometric and motility studies

Manometry is now available to evaluate progressive contractions of the esophagus, which allows the diagnosis of various diseases and therefore the ability to select the appropriate therapy for these diseases. Motility studies of the other levels of the gastrointestinal tract, such as the biliary system and the colon, have not been standardized for ready applicability at this time.

Secretory studies

Secretory studies, measurement of gastric acid levels both before and after stimulation, has allowed gastric analysis to be of value to suggest or document a diagnosis of Zollinger-Ellison syndrome. Collection and examination of duodenal drainage are of value in diagnosing such diseases as giardiasis and can suggest a possible diagnosis of biliary stones when cholesterol or calcium bilirubinate crystals are seen, and in selected cases it can be of value in diagnosing pancreatic cancer or insufficiency. Tests such as D-xylose absorption can be of value in diagnosing malabsorption; evaluation of the amount of fecal fat can aid in the diagnosis of pancreatic insufficiency.

THE ESOPHAGUS

ANATOMY AND PHYSIOLOGY

The esophagus is a muscular tube extending from the pharynx to the stomach and lying on the posterior wall of the thoracic cavity close to the midline. There are two esophageal sphincters, upper and lower. The esophagus serves no other function than the transmission of solids and liquids.

PATHOLOGY

Three symptoms can occur in relation to the esophagus: dysphagia (difficulty in swallowing), odynophagia (pain on swallowing), and bleeding. Dysphagia can occur because of direct esophageal obstruction from either an ingested foreign body, a malignancy, narrowing and stricture formation from reflux esophagus, anatomic abnormalities such as achalasia in which the lower esophageal sphincter is abnormal with a very high resting pressure, or esophageal dysmotility disorders. Painful swallowing can arise from ingested foreign bodies; ulcerations of the esophagus, either from reflux esophagitis or from ingested medications such as erythromycin; and motility disorders, such as diffuse esophageal spasm. Bleeding can occur from reflux esophagitis; malignancy; ulcerations; esophageal varices, seen in portal hypertension; and Mallory-Weiss tears, which occur at the lower esophageal sphincter area after forceful vomiting or coughing.

CLINICAL APPLICATION OF LABORATORY TESTS

The approach to the clinical evaluation of disorders of the esophagus are dependent on the exact symptoms, the clinical status of the patient, and the possible therapeutic approaches that are being considered. Radiologic studies, such as the *esophagram*, are of value for indirect visualization of the lumen and mucosa of the esophagus. *Endoscopy* is of value in that there is direct visualization of the esophageal mucosa. *Biopsy* can be obtained from mass lesions within the lumen, areas of friability (seen with esophagitis or early malignancy), areas of narrowing or strictures (seen either secondary to reflux esophagitis or from tumors), and direct dilatation of these areas of narrowing. Dilatation can be performed initially by using the endoscope itself or by passing instruments (through-the-scope [TTS] dilators). Selected bleeding esophageal varices can be sclerosed. *Esophageal manometry* is of value for dysphagia or odynophagia and chest pain from such motility disorders as diffuse esophageal spasm, achalasia, and esophageal dismotility. Acid perfusion tests, such as the *Bernstein test*, may be performed to see if there can be reproduction of the patient's symptomatology while a solution of hydrochloric acid is being administered.

Esophagitis

Esophagitis is irritation of the lining of the esophagus. When caused by reflux of gastric acid or bile into the esophagus, the patient suffers substernal burning sensation, usually when supine at night; a bitter, sour, or metallic taste in the mouth; and occasional episodes of vomiting, all of which are exacerbated after the ingestion of alcohol, salicylates, nicotine, or caffeine. Diagnosis is made by *barium swallow* or by *endoscopic visualization*, and confirmed by the *Bernstein test*.

Diffuse esophageal spasm (DES)

DES causes symptoms suggestive of coronary angina, both in terms of the symptoms presented and the fact that there is relief of the symptoms by ingestion of nitroglycerin. Before the diagnosis of DES is considered for evaluation, coronary artery disease *must* be excluded. The diagnosis of DES may be suggested by findings on *barium swallow* but can only be documented by esophageal *manometry*.

Achalasia

Achalasia is a motor disorder in which there is an increased resting pressure of the lower esophageal sphincter and abnormalities of motility of the body of the esophagus. Diagnosis is suggested by the findings of "bird beak" appearance on the *esophagram*. *Endoscopy* must then be performed to rule out the possibility of carcinoma at this level, which can also cause a similar type of appearance, and diagnosis can be confirmed by the application of esophageal *manometry*.

Barrett's esophagus

Barrett's esophagus is the condition in which there are areas in the esophagus consisting of mucosa that appears to be gastric in origin. This entity arises in those individuals who have persistent reflux into the esophagus and is of concern because it is considered precancerous in nature. Diagnosis is made both by *endoscopy* (gross appearance of the mucosa) and confirmed by biopsy material. Close follow-up and repeat biopsies of this condition are presently indicated.

Carcinoma of the esophagus

Cancer of the esophagus can be either squamous carcinoma arising from the esophageal mucosa itself or adenocarcinoma arising from the gastric mucosa. Diagnosis is made by *esophagogram* and confirmed by *endoscopic biopsy*. If surgical resection is not indicated, dilatation of the esophagus can be performed during endoscopy. New methods for dilatation are through-the-scope (TTS) lasers and heater probes.

LABORATORY TESTS FOR ESOPHAGEAL DISEASES

BERNSTEIN TEST

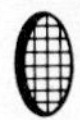

Normal results

Absence of pain or burning during perfusion of either saline or hydrochloric acid indicates a normal esophageal mucosa.

EXPLANATION OF THE TEST

The Bernstein test is an acid perfusion test in which alternating solutions of normal saline and hydrochloric acid are dripped into the esophagus to see if the patient's symptoms (chest pain) can be reproduced.

VALUE OF THE TEST

Distinguishes the chest pain of esophagitis from that of cardiac disease

NURSING ACTION

1. Instruct the patient not to take antacids for 24 hours before the test, as ordered, and to abstain from food for 12 hours and from fluids and smoking for 8 hours before the test.
2. Explain to the patient that the test will help to determine the cause of his or her chest pain.
3. Inform the patient that a narrow tube will be passed through the nose into the esophagus for the instillation of liquid and that he or she should report immediately any pain or burning during the instillation of the liquid.
4. After inserting a nasogastric tube, aspirate the stomach contents and withdraw the tube into the esophagus (to a 12-inch mark previously made on the tube).
5. Hang 0.9% normal saline and 0.1N hydrochloric acid solution on an intravenous pole situated behind the patient and connect the intravenous tubing to the nasogastric tube. Begin a drip of normal saline solution at 60 to 120 drops/minute for 5 to 10 minutes. Ask

the patient if he or she is experiencing any discomfort and record the answer. Without being observed by the patient switch solutions and permit the acidic solution to drip at the same rate for 30 minutes. Ask the patient if he or she is experiencing any discomfort and record the answer. If the patient complains of pain, close the line from the acidic solution and open the one from the saline solution, continuing to perfuse saline solution until the discomfort is gone.

6. Be sure to clamp the tube before removing it to prevent aspiration of the solution.

NURSING ALERT

Observe the patient for arrhythmias during intubation.

If, during intubation, the patient develops cyanosis or paroxysms of coughing, remove the tube because it may be in the trachea.

Note that cardiac disorders and esophageal varices are contraindications for the acid perfusion test.

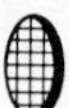

BARIUM SWALLOW, UPPER GI, AND SMALL BOWEL SERIES

NORMAL FINDINGS

The barium sulfate is propelled by peristaltic contraction through the esophagus in about 2 seconds. When the peristaltic wave reaches the base of the esophagus, the lower esophogeal sphincter opens and then closes after admitting the barium into the stomach. The pyloric sphincter relaxes and the barium empties into the duodenum, jejunum, and ileum. The mucosa of the pharynx and esophagus and the outline of the stomach are smooth and regular. The mucosa of the duodenal bulb is smooth giving way to circular folds in the duodenal loop, which deepen and increase in number in the jejunum and are less prominent in the ileum. A speckled pattern remains in the jejunum as the barium lodges in the deep folds.

EXPLANATION OF THE TEST

Barium sulfate or Gastrografin is swallowed by the patient so that the upper gastrointestinal tract and small bowel can be visualized under fluoroscopy.

VALUE AND LIMITATIONS OF THE TEST

Detects hiatal hernia, diverticula, varices, strictures, ulcers, tumors, polyps, and motility disorders

Definitive diagnosis may require endoscopic biopsy or manometric studies

NURSING ACTION

1. Instruct the patient to fast from midnight prior to the test.
2. Explain to the patient that the test evaluates the function of the upper gastrointestinal tract and that he or she will be asked to swallow a thick mixture followed by a thin one.
3. Explain that he or she will be secured to a tilting table and placed in different positions and that x-ray films will be taken.
4. Instruct the patient to remove all metal or radiopaque objects from the x-ray field.

NURSING ALERT

Inform the physician if the patient has not had a bowel movement for 2 or 3 days following the test. Barium retained in the intestine may harden and cause obstruction.

ESOPHAGOGASTRODUODENOSCOPY

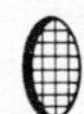

EXPLANATION OF THE TEST

Esophagogastroduodenoscopy is the insertion of a flexible fiber-optic endoscope through the mouth for the purpose of visualizing the lining of the esophagus, stomach, and upper duodenum. The procedure is indicated for patients with substernal or epigastric pain, melena, or hematemesis and for biopsy of gastric ulcers.

VALUE OF THE TEST

Provides direct visualization of the mucosa of the gastrointestinal tract from the esophagus to the duodenum

Detects small lesions not recorded by radiography

Permits biopsy or cytologic brushing of visualized abnormalities, removal of polypoid lesions, injection of esophageal varices, sclerosing of bleeding sites, removal of foreign bodies, dilatation of various areas of narrowing or stricture of the gastrointestinal tract, and, in selected cases, treatment of disease

Direct dilatation of areas of narrowing can be performed by using the endoscope itself or by passing a through-the-scope (TTS) dilator.

NURSING ACTION

1. Instruct the patient to fast for 6 to 12 hours before the test.
2. Inform the patient that this procedure permits visualization of the lining of the esophagus, stomach, and upper duodenum.
3. The patient should be instructed regarding every aspect of the procedure to alleviate fear or panic. Assure that he or she understands the following actions and reactions and that the endoscopic instrument will not interfere with breathing:
   a. A flexible tube will be inserted through the mouth, into the stomach, and beyond.
   b. A local anesthetic may be sprayed into the mouth to keep the patient from gagging. He or she will be asked to hold the breath while the spray is being used. This medication will take effect in about 10 minutes; it will be unpleasant to taste and will make the tongue and throat feel swollen so that is is difficult to swallow. The patient should let saliva drain from the side of the mouth or be suctioned away.
   c. A mouth guard will be used to protect the teeth and the endoscopic instrument. Dentures are removed.
   d. The patient will remain conscious but will be aided in relaxing by the administration of a sedative.
   e. He or she will experience fullness in the stomach when air is insufflated. This is necessary so that the stomach walls can be flattened for easier visualization.
4. Obtain a signed consent.

5. Instruct the patient to remove all metal or jewelry and to void before the procedure.
6. After spraying the throat, place the patient in left lateral position and provide an emesis basin and tissues. Insert the mouth guard.
7. During the procedure be alert for signs of respiratory depression, apnea, hypotension, diaphoresis, bradycardia, and laryngospasm.
8. Following the procedure
   a. Observe the patient for possible perforation.
   b. Withhold food and fluids until the gag reflex returns and then permit fluids and a light meal.
   c. Check vital signs every 15 minutes for 4 hours.

CLINICAL IMPLICATIONS

Note that documentation of gastric outlet obstruction can be made either by endoscopy or by the use of the *saline load test,* in which 700 ml of saline is infused into the stomach through a nasogastric tube; after 30 minutes has elapsed the remainder of the saline is removed from the stomach. If more than 400 ml of fluid is still present within the stomach, it is highly suggestive of gastric outlet obstruction.

ESOPHAGEAL MANOMETRY

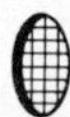

Normal baseline esophageal sphincter pressure

20 mm Hg

Relaxation pressure is at least 18 mm Hg.

Peristalsis is recorded as a series of peaks.

EXPLANATION OF THE TEST

Esophageal manometry is a diagnostic procedure that measures the pressure along the esophagus, determining esophageal sphincter pressure and recording the duration and sequence of peristaltic contractions.

VALUE OF THE TEST

Aids in the differential diagnosis of diffuse esophageal spasm, achalasia, and esophageal dysmotility

NURSING ACTION

1. Instruct the patient to fast for 4 hours before the test and to abstain from alcohol and smoking for 24 hours.
2. Inform the patient that this test evaluates the function of the esophagus and that he or she will be asked to swallow a catheter that has a small pressure transducer along its length.
3. Baseline measurements of pressures are recorded. Pressures in the lower esophageal sphincter are taken before and after swallowing and peristaltic contractions are recorded.

INTERFERING FACTORS

Failure to adhere to the dietary restrictions

CLINICAL IMPLICATIONS

Achalasia: Baseline sphincter pressure may reach 50 mm Hg; relaxation pressure is less than 25 mm Hg. Peristalsis is weak and nonpropulsive.

Diffuse esophageal spasm: Sphincter pressure is usually normal and peristalsis is disorganized (not sequential) and often occurs without the stimulus of swallowing.

Esophageal scleroderma: Baseline and relaxation pressures are depressed. Peristalsis is normal in the upper third but weak or absent in the lower two thirds of the esophagus.

THE STOMACH

PATHOLOGY

Digestion is initiated in the stomach, where food and liquid continue to be transported. Symptoms arising from abnormalities or disease within the stomach include abdominal pain, nausea, vomiting, and bleeding. However, disease can be completely asymptomatic. Abdominal pain can be caused by gastric ulcers, gastritis, which is inflammation of the lining of the gastric mucosa, and gastric carcinoma. Ulcers in the area of the pylorus or gastric malignancy can cause outlet obstruction, which obstructs the flow of food and liquid causing nausea and vomiting. Bleeding can occur in all three of the above entities.

CLINICAL APPLICATION OF LABORATORY TESTS

Evaluation of the stomach can be accomplished by radiologic studies such as *upper GI* or *endoscopic studies*. Endoscopy seems to be of greater applicability in that not only is there direct visualization of the gastric mucosa but biopsies can be obtained, bleeding can be stopped, and dilatation can be accomplished. *Gastric analysis* is of value to determine both basal and stimulated acid levels within the stomach, to document such entities as Zollinger-Ellison syndrome, or at the opposite extreme, achlorhydria as seen in pernicious anemia.

Gastritis

Irritation and inflammation of the lining of the stomach can occur after the ingestion of compounds such as salicylates or alcohol and in conjunction with diseases such as chronic renal failure or chronic obstructive pulmonary disease, or can be associated with stress or hyperacidity. Diagnosis is best made by *endoscopic evaluation*.

Gastric ulcer

Peptic ulcer disease includes both gastric and duodenal ulcers. A gastric ulcer is of great concern in that gastric carcinoma can initially present as a gastric ulcer. Thus, most gastric ulcers should be endoscopically evaluated and biopsied. Gastric ulcer in the face of achlorhydria, as seen in pernicious anemia, is highly suspicious for carcinoma.

Zollinger-Ellison (ZE) syndrome

Zollinger-Ellison sydrome is caused by hypersecretion of gastrin by adenomas found within the gastrointestinal tract, usually within the pancreas. These tumors produce gastrin independently of the normal feedback mechanism. Therefore, although there is high gastric acidity, which would normally suppress gastrin secretion, there is an extremely high serum gastrin level, which indicates an autonomous production of gastrin.

Diagnosis can be made on the findings of *gastric analysis*, in which both the basal and stimulated gastric acid levels are elevated, or by obtaining *serum gastrin* levels, which are markedly elevated.

Complications of peptic ulcer disease

There are four complications of peptic ulcer disease, which include persistent abdominal pain in spite of adequate therapy, bleeding, perforation, and gastric outlet obstruction.

1. Persistence of pain in spite of adequate therapy needs no further diagnostic studies performed and *surgical intervention* should be considered.
2. Perforation is diagnosed on *clinical evaluation* and by the observance of free air within the abdomen.
3. Bleeding can be evaluated both by *clinical presentation, CBC* (complete blood count), and *endoscopy*. Endoscopic intervention should be considered because of the treatment modalities now available (electrocautery, sclerotherapy, heater probes, and lasers).
4. Gastric outlet obstruction presents in those individuals with ulcer disease involving either the prepyloric area or pylorus of the stomach or the duodenal bulb. Documentation of outlet obstruction can be made either by *endoscopy* or by the use of the *saline load test*.

Bleeding in the alcoholic patient

A special concern is the presentation of upper gastrointestinal bleeding in the alcoholic patient. Diagnoses that should be considered include esophageal varices, bleeding esophagitis, Mallory-Weiss tears, gastritis, gastric ulcers, and duodenal ulcers. After stabilization of the patient, *endoscopy* should be performed to make the diagnosis and determine therapy.

LABORATORY TESTS FOR GASTRIC DISEASE

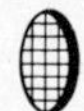

SERUM GASTRIN

Reference range

<300 pg/ml

EXPLANATION OF THE TEST

Gastrin is a polypeptide secreted by the gastric antrum. The secretion of gastrin in turn stimulates acid secretion by the parietal cells of the stomach. In the normal situation, gastric acid inhibits further secretion of gastrin by means of a feedback mechanism. Stimulation of gastrin production can be accomplished by means of intravenous infusions of calcium and secretin.

VALUE OF THE TEST

Confirms the diagnosis of Zollinger-Ellison syndrome
Aids in the differential diagnosis of gastric and duodenal ulcers and pernicious anemia

NURSING ACTION

1. Instruct the patient to abstain from alcohol for at least 24 hours and to fast for 12 hours before the test. The patient may drink water.
2. Withdraw venous blood in a 10 to 15 ml red-top tube. Handle the sample gently to prevent hemolysis.
3. Send the specimen to the laboratory immediately because proteolytic enzymes will destroy the gastrin. The serum should be separated and frozen immediately.

CLINICAL IMPLICATIONS

Zollinger-Ellison syndrome. There is a characteristically severe gastrinemia (>1000 pg/ml) in Zollinger-Ellison syndrome. The response to the infusion of calcium is a markedly elevated serum gastrin level.

Pernicious anemia. There is a marked elevation of serum gastrin level in pernicious anemia. This elevation reflects the characteristic failure of patients with this disorder to secrete gastric hydrochloric acid.

Increased gastrin levels may also occur in patients with duodenal ulceration (<1% increase), achlorhydria, or extensive stomach carcinoma.

GASTRIC ANALYSIS

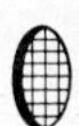

Gastric acid analysis is performed to determine:

1. Whether the patient is able to secrete acid. Such a determination

establishes the differential diagnosis of pernicious anemia and gastric ulcer, in which various amounts are secreted.

2. How much acid a patient secretes. A high basal secretion (10 mEq/hr or more) is suggestive of active peptic ulcer disease. Very high secretory rates of acid are seen in tumors that secrete gastrin (as in Zollinger-Ellison syndrome).
3. The type of surgery necessary. In hypersecretors, there is increased risk of stomach ulcer following ordinary gastric resection without vagotomy. If the patient is still having symptoms after a vagotomy for peptic ulcer, the completeness of the vagotomy should be ascertained by means of a Hollander test.

Gastric analysis includes determination of the basal secretion rate, the augmented gastric secretion test, the saline load test, the Hollander insulin test, and gastric acid stimulation with calcium and secretin.

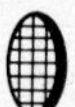

BASAL GASTRIC SECRETION RATE

Reference range

0-6 mEq/hr

EXPLANATION OF THE TEST

A nasogastric Levin tube is inserted into the stomach and the gastric residue aspirated continuously for 2 hours. The aspirate is titrated at half-hour intervals.

VALUE OF THE TEST

Ascertains how much acid a patient secretes without stimulation to do so

NURSING ACTION

1. Instruct the patient to restrict food for 12 hours and fluids and smoking for 8 hours before the test.
2. Describe the insertion of a nasogastric tube.
3. After inserting a nasogastric tube, aspirate the stomach contents with a 20-ml syringe, while the patient assumes different positions (supine, right and left lateral decubitus). Label the specimen "residual contents."

4. Connect the nasogastric tube to a continuous suction machine and aspirate with continuous low suction for 1½ hours.
5. Discard the first 30-minute specimen to eliminate the effects of stress and collect a specimen every 15 minutes after that.
6. Record the color, odor, and note the presence of food, mucus, bile, or blood in each specimen.

CLINICAL IMPLICATIONS

A secretion rate of more than 6 mEq/hr is indicative of hypersecretion. A secretion rate of 15 mEq/hr or more should lead one to suspect a hormonal abnormality affecting the parietal cells.

GASTRIC ACID STIMULATION TEST

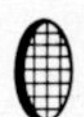

Reference range

Females: 11-21 mEq/hr
Males: 18-28 mEq/hr

EXPLANATION OF THE TEST

A gastric secretion stimulation test should immediately follow the basal secretion test since the capacity of the gastric cells to secrete on a particular occasion may not be significant in the basal state. In this test, gastric secretion is stimulated by means of an injection of histamine or Histalog (or Pentagastrin, which is safer than Histalog).

VALUE OF THE TEST

Useful to confirm the achlorhydria of pernicious anemia
Aids in the diagnosis of Zollinger-Ellison syndrome

NURSING ACTION

1. Instruct the patient to refrain from eating, drinking, and smoking from midnight prior to the test.
2. Describe the side effects (abdominal pain, flushing, dizziness, faintness, numbing of the extremities) and ask the patient to report these immediately.
3. The nasogastric tube will already be in place from the basal gastric secretion test. Pentagastrin is injected subcutaneously. After 15

minutes, collect a specimen and every 15 minutes for 1 hour collect specimens in separate containers.

4. Record the color, odor, and note the presence of food, mucus, bile, or blood in each specimen.
5. Label the specimens "stimulated contents" and number them in sequence.

CLINICAL IMPLICATIONS

A secretion rate of 50 mEq/hr or more indicates hypersecretion.

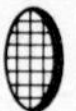

OTHER TESTS USED IN GASTRIC ANALYSIS

Diagnex Blue test. By means of a Diagnex Blue test, the presence or absence of acid can be determined without intubation. This test involves the ingestion of a tablet of caffeine followed by a dye (Diagnex Blue) and an exchange resin. If the gastric contents have a pH of 3 or less, dye is released from the resin and excreted in the urine. If the results of this test are negative or inconclusive, a gastric stimulation test is indicated.

Saline load test. This is a test to evaluate gastric outlet obstruction. A nasogastric Levin tube is inserted into the stomach. The gastric residue is aspirated and measured. Then 750 ml of 0.9% (normal) saline is instilled. After 30 minutes the gastric contents are again aspirated and measured. If more than 400 ml of fluid is still present in the stomach, gastric outlet obstruction should be suspected.

Hollander insulin test. This test is performed to determine whether a complete vagotomy has been performed or not. The test is based on the fact that insulin-induced hypoglycemia stimulates vagal centers because of their direct communication with the anterior hypothalamus. A 2-hour basal gastric analysis is performed, and a blood glucose analysis is done. The patient is then given an intravenous injection of insulin to produce hypoglycemia, and specimens of gastric juice are collected every 15 minutes for the next 2 hours. When symptoms of hypoglycemia appear, a second blood glucose analysis is done. The level should fall to 50% of the initial, fasting level. If any measurement of the gastric secretion in the first two postinsulin hours exceeds that of the higher of the 2 basal hours (preinsulin fasting stage, two determinations) the vagotomy is incomplete.

The safety of the Hollander test is in question; risk factors should be considered before patients are selected for this kind of stimulation.

Gastric analysis using calcium infusion. The differential diagnosis between hypersecretory states with and without inappropriate gastrin production can be made by performing the gastric analysis while the patient is receiving a calcium infusion. In this procedure serum gastrin levels are measured in the basal state and then again during calcium infusion. If the secretion of gastric acid approaches maximal levels and the serum gastrin levels rise appreciably with the calcium infusion, ectopic gastrin production, such as is seen in Zollinger-Ellison syndrome, should be suspected.

Gastric analysis using secretin. This is another test performed to differentiate Zollinger-Ellison syndrome from hypersecretory states that do not involve inappropriate secretion of gastrin. Secretin is given intravenously and should cause a decrease in acid secretion. However, in Zollinger-Ellison syndrome the acid secretion is increased and the serum gastrin level rises.

THE SMALL BOWEL

ANATOMY AND PHYSIOLOGY

The small intestine extends for approximately 23 feet from the stomach to the beginning of the large intestine at the ileocecal valve. This segment of the gastrointestinal tract facilitates transport through the gastrointestinal system and allows absorption of various nutrients across the intestinal mucosa. The total absorbing surface is markedly increased by fingerlike projections called villi and microvilli on the surface of the small intestine. Digestion, which was initiated in the stomach, continues in the small intestine with the addition of pancreatic enzymes and bile salts excreted from the liver. Secretion of bicarbonate from the pancreas produces a medium with a higher pH than that seen in the stomach. Abnormalities in the digestion and absorption of protein, fat, and carbohydrates can occur as a result of pathologic conditions arising from the small intestine, pancreas, or biliary system.

PATHOLOGY

Pathologic disorders can occur that interfere with the transportation aspect of the small intestine. Small bowel obstruction may be caused by adhesion, volvulus, intussusception, or mass lesions, such as lymphoma, strictures caused by regional enteritis, Crohn's disease, and rare malignancies. Bleeding may be the result of Crohn's disease, lymphomas, angiodysplasia, or the congenital finding of Meckel's diverticulum. Maldigestion within the small intestine is associated with pancreatic or biliary system abnormalities. Malabsorption results from diseases that interfere with the mucosal absorption of nutrients, such as celiac sprue (marked deformity in the configuration of the villi and microvilli), lymphoma, enzyme deficiencies, and change in the bacterial flora of the small intestine, which can occur with such diseases as bacterial overgrowth associated with diabetic enteropathy.

CLINICAL APPLICATION OF LABORATORY TESTS

The determination of the appropriate laboratory tests to evaluate the small bowel is dependent on the presenting signs and symptoms. In those patients who have an abnormality in transportation (i.e., an obstructive phenomena), initially *radiographic studies* such as a flat plate of the abdomen, or an abdominal series, which includes upright and decubitus films, should be performed. There are then *small bowel follow-throughs* with either barium or Gastrografin, if indicated. Bleeding disorders can be evaluated with *endoscopy* if the first and second portion of the duodenum is the area of concern, *technetium-tagged RBC scans* can be done to localize definitive bleeding sites, and *angiography* performed if bleeding is brisk enough (1 ml/min).

Malabsorption

The evaluation of malabsorption is instituted by obtaining some baseline blood studies. This can include a *CBC*, which can indicate whether anemia (iron deficiency or vitamin B_{12} and folic acid deficiency) is present, *serum albumin level*, and *prothrombin time*. An abnormal prothrombin time can be found in liver disease, inadequate intake of vitamin K, or mucosal abnormalities of the ileum interfering with absorption. If a patient's prothrombin time is abnormal, an injection of 10 mg of *aquamephyton* intramuscularly should be administered and a prothrombin time repeated 24 hours later. A prothrombin time that is still abnormal is consistent with liver disease; a prothrombin time that responds to a normal level is consistent with an inadequate amount of vitamin K intake or malabsorption of vitamin K in the ileum. Specialized blood tests such as *serum carotene* level can also be used to evaluate absorption in the ileum. *Stool evaluation* for ovum parasites can be of value to rule out causes of rare parasitic diseases, which can cause malabsorption. *Culture and sensitivity studies* sometimes are of value in determining the presence of bacterial overgrowth, and measurement of the *fecal fat content* over a 72-hour period can suggest whether malabsorption or maldigestion is present.

Assuming these baseline studies are performed and malabsorption is suspected, the next step would be to obtain a *small bowel follow-through study* to see if there are any classic findings such as flocculation of barium as seen in celiac disease, or mucosal abnormalities and strictures as seen in regional enteritis. *Biopsy* of the small intestine could then be performed.

Such diseases as giardiasis can be determined by *evaluation of the luminal contents* for presence of the parasite, or for detection of bacterial overgrowth from abnormal motility associated with diabetic enteropathy. Specialized tests can be performed such as the *D-xylose absorption test*. A *lactose tolerance test* can be performed when disaccharidase deficiency is suspected.

Inflammatory bowel disease (Crohn's disease)

Inflammatory bowel disease is a general term for a group of chronic inflammatory disorders of the gastrointestinal tract. The onset is insidious but ultimately the symptoms are chronic diarrhea, sometimes bloody in nature, abdominal pain, fever, and in some cases joint pains and skin lesions. On *physical examination*, apthous ulcers can be present in the mucous membranes of the mouth, and mass lesions may be found specifically in the right lower quadrant on abdominal examination. Occasionally, perirectal and perianal abscesses and fistulas may occur. Initially, *baseline blood studies* should be obtained, which may show anemia, either microcytic associated with iron deficiency, or macrocytic associated with *vitamin* B_{12} and *folic acid* deficiency, *leukocytosis* with a left shift, low levels of *albumin* and *calcium*, and an abnormal *prothrombin time* with correction after injection of aquamephyton. Radiologic studies such as flat plate study of the abdomen may be obtained if small bowel obstruction is suspected. Then either a *barium enema* in which there is reflux of barium into the terminal ileum may be used for diagnosis, or a *small bowel follow-through study* may be done.

For patients who are suspected of bacterial overgrowth syndrome in which there is persistent diarrhea and suspected malabsorption as documented by blood tests, one can attempt to make a specific diagnosis with the laboratory studies mentioned above followed by a therapeutic trial with an appropriate antibiotic such as tetracycline.

Celiac sprue or nontropical sprue

Celiac sprue or nontropical sprue is a disorder associated with malabsorption, abnormal small bowel structure, and intolerance to gluten, a protein found in wheat and wheat products. After obtaining a history and performing a physical examination, initial workup would include *blood studies;* depending on the findings of the *prothrombin time* test, and the response of the patient to an injection of aquamephyton, further evaluation would be made, using a *small bowel follow-through* study and perhaps a small bowel *biopsy*. The treatment of celiac disease is a gluten-free diet. In 2 to 3 months after the institution of the gluten-free diet repeat blood tests and small bowel follow-through studies are done. There should be normalization of the findings in the villi and microvilli of the small intestine on the repeat biopsy. The patient adheres to a lifelong gluten-free diet. Of concern in long-term follow-up of patients with celiac disease is the increased incidence of lymphoma. Therefore, recurrence or change of symptomatology, or change of findings on physical examination may require the repetition of the diagnostic workup.

LABORATORY TESTS FOR DISEASES OF THE SMALL BOWEL

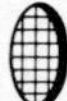

LACTOSE TOLERANCE TEST (ORAL)

Normal values

Within 15 to 60 minutes after ingestion of lactose, plasma glucose levels rise more than 20 mg/dl over fasting levels.

EXPLANATION OF THE TEST

This is a functional test that is performed when lactose intolerance resulting from lactase deficiency is suspected. Lactose is a disaccharide found in dairy products. The intestinal enzyme lactase breaks lactose down into glucose and galactose. If the lactase is absent, the lactose is not broken down and not absorbed by the small intestine, causing abdominal cramps and diarrhea.

VALUE OF THE TEST

Detection of lactose intolerance

NURSING ACTION

1. Instruct the patient to fast and to avoid strenuous activity for 8 hours before the test.
2. Explain to the patient that this test will help to determine or eliminate a cause of the symptoms.
3. Tell the patient that four blood samples will be taken over approximately 2 hours.
4. Withdraw venous blood into a 7-ml gray-top collection tube for a fasting blood sugar level.
5. Administer 100 g of lactose orally.
6. Withdraw venous blood into a 7-ml gray-top collection tube at 30, 60, and 120 minutes after the loading dose of lactose has been administered.

CLINICAL IMPLICATIONS

Over a 2-hour period the blood sugar level must increase at least 24 mg/L. Levels below this suggest intestinal lactose deficiency.

SMALL BOWEL BIOPSY

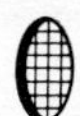

EXPLANATION OF THE TEST

Using a small bowel biopsy tube, which is passed and then followed fluoroscopically until its location within the jejunum is localized, both mucosal specimens and luminal contents can be obtained for evaluation. This can also be done with a long endoscope.

VALUE OF THE TEST

Aids in the diagnosis of diseases of the small intestine
Produces a larger specimen than does endoscopic biopsy
Allows removal of tissue from areas that cannot be reached by the endoscope

NURSING ACTION

1. Instruct the patient not to eat or drink for at least 8 hours before the test.
2. Explain to the patient that the test helps to evaluate disorders of the small bowel.
3. Obtain an informed consent.
4. Before the procedure check the tubing and mercury bag for leaks and assure that suction equipment is nearby. Lubricate the tube and capsule with a water-soluble lubricant.
5. Assist the physician in positioning and attending the patient during the procedure. You may spray the back of the patient's throat with a local anesthetic if ordered to reduce gag reflex.
6. When the specimen is seen in the capsule the mucosal side will be down. Use forceps to gently place it mucosal side up on a piece of mesh. Place it in a biopsy bottle with the recommended fixative and send it to the laboratory immediately.

CLINICAL IMPLICATIONS

Diseases that can be diagnosed by small bowel biopsy include celiac sprue (marked diminution of villi and flattening of the microvilli) or lymphoma, in which lymphatic infiltration can be evaluated.

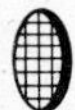

D-XYLOSE ABSORPTION TEST

Adult normal reference range

Blood levels of D-xylose peak 2 hours after ingestion (25 to 40 mg/dl); 80% to 95% is excreted in 5 hours (4 g in 5 hours).

Pediatric normal reference range

Blood levels of D-xylose peak 1 hour after ingestion (30 mg/dl); 16% to 33% is excreted in 5 hours.

EXPLANATION OF THE TEST

D-Xylose is administered orally and then its levels in the blood and urine are checked. D-Xylose is not metabolized and is excreted in the urine. Thus, its measurement in the urine and blood helps to evaluate the absorption qualities of the small intestine. The patient must have normal renal function and normal level of hydration for accurate results.

VALUE OF THE TEST

Aids in the differential diagnosis of malabsorption
Helps to determine the cause of malabsorption syndrome

NURSING ACTION

1. Instruct the patient to fast overnight before the test and during the test.
2. Explain to the patient that this test evaluates digestive function and that activity affects test results; thus he or she should remain in bed during the test.
3. Explain that several blood samples and a 24-hour urine specimen will be necessary.
4. Before the administration of D-xylose, withdraw venous blood in a 10-ml red-top tube and collect a first-voided morning urine specimen. Send both of these specimens to the laboratory immediately.
5. Give the patient 25 g D-xylose dissolved in 8 oz (240 ml) of water, followed by an additional 8 oz of water. For a child give 0.5 g D-xylose/lb body weight up to 25 g. Make a record of the time on ingestion.
6. Withdraw venous blood in a 10-ml red-top tube 2 hours after D-xylose ingestion (1 hour in a child).
7. Collect all urine following D-xylose intake for the time span ordered.

CLINICAL IMPLICATIONS

A decreased amount of D-xylose in the urine or in the blood implies malabsorption of D-xylose.

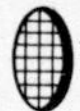

SERUM CAROTENE AND VITAMIN A

Reference ranges

Carotene: 70-300 μg/dl

Vitamin A: 9.15-9.60 μg/ml (SI units: 0.5-2.1 μmol/L)

EXPLANATION OF THE TEST

Carotene is a fat-soluble precursor of vitamin A and is supplied nutritionally through green and yellow vegetables. Absorption of these substances is compromised when fat is poorly absorbed.

VALUE OF THE TEST

Helps in the evaluation of absorption in the ileum

CLINICAL IMPLICATIONS

Decreased serum carotene and hypovitaminosis

Malabsorption syndrome
Febrile illness
Liver disease
Poor diet

Increased serum carotene levels

Myxedema
Diabetes mellitus
Hypothyroidism
Chronic nephritis
Hyperlipidemia
Excessive dietary intake (e.g., carrots)

THE COLON

ANATOMY AND PHYSIOLOGY

The colon or large intestine is approximately 5 feet long and extends from the ileocecal valve to the anus. It transports and eliminates the waste products of digestion and absorbs water and electrolytes.

PATHOLOGY

Symptoms of diseases of the colon are related to obstruction, pain, bleeding, or diarrhea. Patients who report a change in bowel habits (specifically constipation) must be evaluated for the possibility of malignancy, especially in the age group past 40. Gastrointestinal bleeding may be in the form of hematochezia (bright red blood per rectum), melena (black tarlike stool), or normal-appearing stool that tests positive for blood. Melena usually arises from an upper gastrointestinal source and can also be found in right-sided colonic bleeding sources. Diarrhea can be associated with inflammatory bowel disease such as ulcerative colitis or Crohn's colitis, with pseudomembranous colitis seen with antibiotic-associated colitis or bacterial infections such as *Salmonella, Shigella,* or *Campylobacter*. Other signs and symptoms that should direct suspicion toward the colon would be unusual weight loss seen with malignancy, lower abdominal pain in either the right or left lower quadrants, and anemia of unknown cause.

CLINICAL APPLICATION OF LABORATORY TESTS

Cancer of the colon

Patients with malignancy of the colon can present with changed bowel habits, evidence of rectal bleeding including stools positive for occult blood and unexplained weight loss or anemia, and should be evaluated by either *sigmoidoscopy* and *barium enema* or *colonoscopy*. Polypoid lesions of the colon, both benign and malignant, can be removed by colonoscopy in some instances. If the mass lesion cannot be safely removed by colonoscopy, surgical intervention is indicated.

Inflammatory bowel disease

Evaluation, as in any diarrheal disease, would include a *stool specimen* for ova, parasites, and culture and sensitivity studies. If negative, further evaluation by *sigmoidoscopy* and *barium enema* or *colonoscopy* would be indicated. Diagnosis can be made by direct observation of mucosal abnormalities. Biopsies of observed ulcerations can also be of value. The differentiation between ulcerative colitis and Crohn's disease includes distribution of the disease itself and involvement of the small bowel, the presence of fistulas, and the type of abnormalities seen on ulcer biopsy. Crohn's disease is characterized by "skip lesions" with rectal sparing of disease and the occurrence of fistula formation and the finding of noncaseating granulomas and lymphoid hyperplasia on biopsy.

Bacterial infections

Various bacterial infections can cause diarrhea. These include *Salmonella*, *Shigella*, and *Campylobacter*. Specific diagnosis is made after obtaining a *stool specimen* for culture and sensitivity.

LABORATORY TESTS FOR DISEASES OF THE COLON

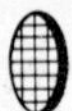

BARIUM ENEMA

Normal findings

In the single-contrast technique, the intestine uniformly fills with barium and colonic markings are clear. On the postevacuation film the mucosa has a regular, feathery appearance.

EXPLANATION OF THE TEST

Barium sulfate is given as an enema so that the lumen and mucosa of the colon can be studied through x-ray (single-contrast technique). It can be performed as a simple barium enema; the double-contrast technique, using barium and air, is more precise and diagnostic.

Of marked concern before performing the barium enema is a complete preparation of the colon, by the use of either cathartics or enemas. The presence of retained stool can interfere with the adequate performance of a barium enema.

VALUE OF THE TEST

Evaluation of the lumen and mucosa of the colon for malignancies, polyps, diverticulitis or bleeding from diverticulosis, and inflammatory bowel disease

NURSING ACTION

1. Explain to the patient that this test examines the large intestine and that x-ray films will be taken following a barium enema.
2. Impress upon the patient the importance of adhering to dietary restrictions. Ensure that he or she has written instructions in this regard. Usually there is a low-residue diet for 1 to 3 days before the test. Encourage the patient to take fluids (water or clear liquid) for 12 to 24 hours before the test. A cathartic is administered the

afternoon before the test and a cleansing enema both the evening before and the morning before the test. Repeat the enemas, but not more than 3 times, until the solution returns clear.

3. Explain to the patient the importance of keeping the anal sphincter tight around the rectal tube to prevent loss of barium.
4. Instruct the patient to breathe deeply through the mouth to ease the discomfort of cramping abdominal pain.
5. After completion of the barium enema, laxatives should be ordered or liquids encouraged to help evacuate the barium.

COLONOSCOPY

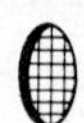

EXPLANATION OF THE TEST

Colonoscopy is the insertion of a flexible fiberoptic tube through the anus into the large bowel for a visual examination of the lining of the large intestine.

VALUE OF THE TEST

Evaluates the entire colon
An alternative to barium enema and sigmoidoscopy
Assess abnormalities seen on barium enema
Allows definitive evaluation of the mucosa of the colon
Allows biopsy of mucosa and mass lesions of the colon
Permits therapeutic intervention such as the removal of polypoid lesions and the sclerosing or electrocautery of bleeding lesions, such as angiodysplasia

NURSING ACTION

1. Instruct the patient to take only clear liquids for 48 hours before the test.
2. Explain to the patient that the test permits visualization of the lining of the large intestine.
3. Impress upon the patient the importance of thorough cleansing of the large intestine before the test. There are various purges available that allow complete cleansing of the colon before examination.

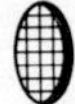

SIGMOIDOSCOPY

Normal

Green reaction (<2.5 ml of blood)

EXPLANATION OF THE TEST

For a complete examination of the gastrointestinal tract, barium enema is not totally adequate. If a barium enema is performed, the distal aspect of the colon and rectum should be examined with either a rigid sigmoidoscope, which can examine the area from the anus to 25 cm, or a flexible sigmoidoscope, which can examine the area from the anus to 60 cm.

VALUE OF THE TEST

Permits visualization of GI tract from the anus to up to 60 cm of the terminal colon

NURSING ACTION

1. Instruct the patient that he or she may have a light meal the evening before the test. An enema may be given the morning of the procedure.
2. Inform the patient that the examination will permit the physician to visualize the lower bowel.

OCCULT BLOOD TEST (FECES)

EXPLANATION OF THE TEST

No physical examination can be complete without obtaining a stool specimen, either at the completion of the rectal examination or as supplied by the patient, to evaluate for occult blood. If the findings are positive, further evaluation either by barium enema and sigmoidoscopy or by colonoscopy is indicated; if negative, further evaluation of the upper gastrointestinal tract should be completed.

VALUE OF THE TEST

Detects gastrointestinal bleeding
Aids in the early diagnosis of colorectal cancer

NURSING ACTION

1. Instruct the patient to eat a high-fiber diet and to avoid red meats, poultry, fish, turnips, and horseradish for 48 to 72 hours before the test and during the collection period.
2. Explain to the patient that the test helps to detect abnormal bleeding in the intestinal tract and that 3 stool specimens may be required.
3. Note on the laboratory slip if the patient has remained on medications before the test.
4. In order to test the stool specimen, place a small amount of stool from different areas of the stool on a piece of filter paper. Add 2 drops of tap water, glacial acetic acid, 1:60 solution of gum guaiac in 95% ethyl alcohol, and 3% hydrogen peroxide. Mix with a tongue blade and note the color immediately and in 5 minutes.

INTERFERING FACTORS

Ascorbic acid can produce normal results even though there is significant bleeding.

Ingestion of 1 to 5 ml of blood, such as with bleeding gums or following a dental procedure, can cause abnormal results.

Some drugs that may result in gastrointestinal bleeding are iron preparations, bromides, rauwolfia derivatives, indomethacin, colchicine, phenylbutazone, or steroids.

THE LIVER AND BILIARY SYSTEM

ANATOMY AND PHYSIOLOGY

The liver is the largest gland and the major metabolic factory in the human body. It lies immediately under the diaphragm, occupying most of the right upper quadrant. It is involved in metabolic functions, regulation of blood volume, immune mechanisms, formation and excretion of bile, and detoxification and excretion of toxic elements and is important in the synthesis, esterification, and excretion of cholesterol.

The biliary system includes the intrahepatic and extrahepatic biliary ducts, common bile duct, the gall bladder, and the cystic duct, which connects the common bile duct to the gallbladder (Fig. 8-2). Bile is produced by the liver, enters into the biliary system, and can

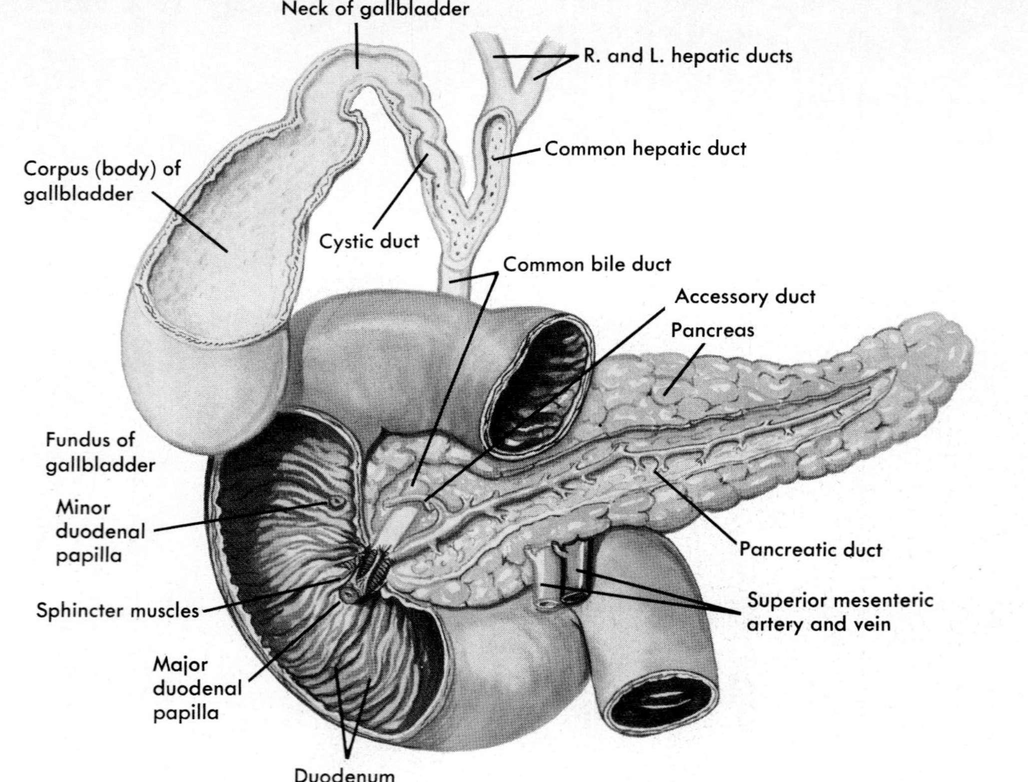

Fig. 8-2. *The gallbladder and its subdivisions: fundus, body, infundibulum, and neck. Obstruction of either the hepatic duct or the common bile duct by stone or spasm blocks the exit of bile from the liver, where it is formed, and prevents bile from being ejected into the duodenum. (From Thibodeau, G.A.: Textbook of anatomy and physiology, ed. 12, St. Louis, 1987, Times Mirror/Mosby College Publishing.)*

be stored in the gallbladder. Bile is transported through the common bile duct and enters the second portion of the duodenum by the ampulla of Vater.

CLINICAL APPLICATION OF LABORATORY TESTS

Hepatocellular carcinoma

Hepatocellular carcinoma is a primary tumor of the liver (as opposed to a metastatic tumor). It is frequently associated with an elevated *α-fetoprotein* level, occasionally with jaundice or an elevated *carcinoembryonic antigen (CEA)*. The tumor can be visualized by isotopic liver scanning, angiography, or computerized tomography. It is documented by liver biopsy.

Gallstones

For the patient with symptoms highly suggestive of gallstones such as right upper quadrant pain and nausea and vomiting, after initial history and physical examination are completed, laboratory studies would then be obtained, including a *CBC* to evaluate for leukocytosis and a *liver panel* to evaluate for abnormalities of *bilirubin level* and *transaminase levels*. *Ultrasound* would be the initial approach to rule out the presence of gallstones and/or obstruction of the biliary system. Further evaluation of the biliary system can then be accomplished using endoscopic retrograde choleangio-pancreatography (ERCP) or a *transhepatic cholangiogram* depending on the clinical situation.

Gallstones within the gallbladder are sometimes serendipitously diagnosed on *radiologic examination* of the abdomen (flat plate study of the abdomen), where the stones are seen as calcifications in the right upper quadrant. Suspicions concerning the presence of gallstones, however, are not completely alleviated by a flat plate study of the abdomen in that a large percentage of gallstones are not opaque and are not seen on such routine x-ray studies. Further evaluation in those individuals suspected of cholelithiasis requires the use of *ultrasound*. If the ultrasound findings are negative and there is a high suspicion of a possibility of disease of the gallbladder, *oral cholecystogram* may be of value. *Nuclear studies* have replaced intravenous cholangiograms and are used in those instances where obstructive lesions are of concern. *Percutaneous transhepatic cholan-*

giogram or ERCP is of value when direct visualization of the biliary tree is desired.

Obstructive jaundice

Obstruction of the biliary system, causing jaundice, would be approached in a similar manner to that of gallstones. One of the major causes of obstruction is gallstones. Other possible pathologic findings include carcinoma, either of the biliary system or of the ampulla of Vater.

Visualization of the biliary system after *ultrasound* would be accomplished by *endoscopic retrograde cholangiopancreatography (ERCP)* or *transhepatic cholangiogram*. The ampulla of Vater could be evaluated during the course of ERCP via the endoscope, and if indicated, biopsies could be obtained. Decompression of the biliary system may be treated with the application of biliary stents endoscopically. In addition, certain therapeutic modalities, such as sphincterotomy, in which the ampulla of Vater and sphincter of Oddi are cut, allowing spontaneous passage of gallstones retained within the common bile duct, or the endoscopic passage of balloon dilators to assist in the passage of gallstones can now be accomplished.

LABORATORY TESTS FOR THE LIVER AND BILIARY TRACT

The routine screening tests for liver and biliary tract disease have just been covered; they are listed here with their page number and the remainder are covered below. The immunoglobin and immunologic tests for viral hepatitis are on pp. 518-520. Liver function tests are selected in the light of the clinical setting and to assess different parameters of liver function, and they are used in the order that will permit the clinician to evaluate the course of the disease.

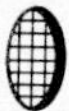

LIVER FUNCTION TESTS

- Serum bilirubin (page 14)
- Urine bilirubin (page 303)
- Serum enzyme assays
  - Alkaline phosphatase (page 10)
  - 5′-Nucleotidase (page 305)
  - Serum aspartate aminotransferase (AST, SGOT) (page 12)
  - Alanine aminotransferase (ALT, SGPT) (page 9)
- Albumin and globulins (page 43)
- Immunoglobulins and immunologic tests (pages 515-519, 526-528)

Clotting factors (page 418)
Plasma ammonia (page 304)
Blood lipids (page 135)
Urine urobilinogen (limited usefulness)
Bromsulphalein (BSP) excretion (rarely used)

URINE BILIRUBIN

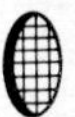

Normal

Bilirubin is not found in the urine in a routine screening test.

EXPLANATION OF THE TEST

Urine bilirubin causes the urine to become yellow, smoky, or tea-colored. The test detects high concentrations of conjugated bilirubin on the basis of (1) the color reaction with a dye-impregnated strip, (2) the foam test, (3) the Harrison spot test, or (4) the Ictotest tablet method. This differentiates the appearance of the urine from that caused by hemoglobin or myoglobin.

VALUE OF THE TEST

Establishes whether the cause of jaundice is due to conjugated or unconjugated bilirubin in the serum. When bilirubin is found in the urine it is of the conjugated type.

NURSING ACTION

1. Inform the patient that there are no dietary restrictions before this test.
2. Instruct the patient on the collection of a random urine specimen.
3. For bedside analysis for bilirubin (Dipstrip method or Ictotest tablet method), the urine should be tested while it is fresh since bilirubin disintegrates on exposure to light or room temperature after 30 minutes.

CLINICAL IMPLICATIONS

In the clinical setting of jaundice it is important to establish whether the jaundice is due to unconjugated or conjugated hyper-bilirubinemia. Since unconjugated bilirubin is tightly bound to albumin, it is not filtered by the renal glomeruli and not found in the urine. However, conjugated bilirubin, although not normally found in the urine with routine screening tests, is less tightly bound to albumin and approximately 5% remains unbound and more easily filtered by the glomeruli. In obstructive jaundice there is an elevated level of bile acids, which renders conjugated bilirubin more filterable.

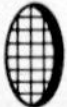

PLASMA AMMONIA

Reference ranges

12-55 μmol/L (SI units: 12-55 μmol/L)

EXPLANATION OF THE TEST

The normal liver synthesizes urea from ammonia, most of which comes from the gastrointestinal tract. This synthesis is critical to acid-base balance and normal brain function. The normal amount of ammonia found in the blood is in transit to the liver for synthesis. Elevations do not occur unless the liver is damaged or the blood flow to the liver is severely altered.

VALUE AND LIMITATIONS OF THE TEST

Aids in the diagnosis of hepatic encephalopathy or coma
No elevated levels until there is actual hepatic failure

NURSING ACTION

1. Inform the patient that he or she should fast overnight before the test.
2. Notify the laboratory so that preparations can be made before the blood sample is drawn.
3. Withdraw venous blood into a 10 ml green-top (heparinized) tube. Pack the specimen in ice and send it to the laboratory immediately. Handle gently to prevent hemolysis.

CLINICAL IMPLICATIONS

Elevated levels

Severe hepatic disease (cirrhosis and acute hepatic necrosis). In cirrhosis the extensive liver cell destruction and fibrosis distort the hepatic venous blood supply and cause an elevation of venous blood pressure, resulting in esophageal varices. Because the blood flow is altered, elevated blood ammonia levels appear with less severe decompensation than if the blood flow were normal.

Reye's syndrome
Severe congestive heart failure
Gastrointestinal hemorrhage
Erythroblastosis fetalis

5′-NUCLEOTIDASE

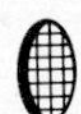

Reference range

1-11 U/L (SI units: 17-183 nmol/sec/L)

EXPLANATION OF THE TEST

This test measures serum levels of 5′-nucleotidase, an enzyme that originates mostly in the hepatobiliary tract.

VALUE AND LIMITATIONS OF THE TEST

Differentiates between hepatic disease and bone disease when alkaline phosphatase is elevated

When level is found to be elevated, other liver function tests are necessary to establish the presence of liver disease

NURSING ACTION

1. Inform the patient that there are no dietary restrictions before the test.
2. Withdraw venous blood into a 7-ml red-top tube. Handle the specimen gently to prevent hemolysis (this enzyme is in RBCs).

ULTRASONOGRAPHY (GALLBLADDER, BILIARY SYSTEM, LIVER, PANCREAS)

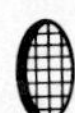

EXPLANATION OF THE TEST

Ultrasound is used to evaluate the liver, biliary system including the gallbladder, and pancreas. In this test high-frequency sound waves are directed into the area of the body to be examined. These sound waves produce echoes that are converted into electrical energy and appear on the oscilloscope as a pattern of spikes or dots. This pattern varies with tissue density and thus can depict organ size, shape, and position. Ultrasound has in most instances made oral cholecystogram and intravenous cholangiogram of little value.

VALUE AND LIMITATIONS OF THE TEST

Confirms the diagnosis of gallstones within the gallbladder or common bile duct, and distinguishes between obstructive and nonobstructive jaundice

Visualizes the pancreas in some instances and aids in evaluating the head of the pancreas for enlargement and the presence of pseudocysts

Screens for hepatocellular disease (metastases, hematoma, abscesses, or cysts)

NURSING ACTION

1. Instruct the patient regarding dietary restrictions:
   a. Fast for 8 to 12 hours before the procedure in order to reduce bowel gas, which can hinder the transmission of sound waves.
   b. If the gallbladder is to be evaluated, the evening meal before the test should be fat-free. Inform the patient that this promotes the accumulation of bile in the gallbladder and enhances ultrasonic visualization.
2. Assure the patient that this test is neither harmful nor painful and that he or she will simply feel the pressure of the transducer as it is pressed against the skin.
3. Instruct the patient to remain as motionless as possible during the procedure and that he or she will at times be asked to hold the breath.

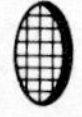

PERCUTANEOUS TRANSHEPATIC CHOLANGIOGRAM

Normal result

The biliary ducts fill with contrast media homogeneously and are seen as regular channels.

EXPLANATION OF THE TEST

Percutaneous transhepatic cholangiography is the injection of contrast media directly into a biliary radicle within the liver followed by fluoroscopic evaluation of the intrahepatic/extrahepatic common bile duct and cystic duct. This is accomplished by insertion of a Chiba skinny needle through the liver under fluoroscopic guidance. The contrast medium is injected as the needle is slowly withdrawn. When a biliary radicle has been entered the outline of the biliary tree is seen on fluoroscopy. A contraindication to performing this study is severe coagulopathy.

VALUE OF THE TEST

Permits direct visualization of the biliary tree

NURSING ACTION

1. Instruct the patient to fast for 8 hours before the test.
2. Explain to the patient that this test permits the physician to examine the biliary ducts through the use of a contrast media and x-ray viewing.
3. Inform the patient that he or she will be secured to a tilting table and be placed in vertical and horizontal positions during the procedure.
4. Obtain a signed consent.
5. Check the patient's laboratory tests for normal bleeding, clotting, and prothrombin times and a normal platelet count.

CLINICAL IMPLICATIONS

The ducts will be dilated in obstructive jaundice and normal in size in nonobstructive jaundice.

PERCUTANEOUS LIVER BIOPSY

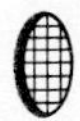

EXPLANATION OF THE TEST

Percutaneous biopsy is a method of establishing the pathologic and microscopic picture of the liver cells. Its major indications are:

1. Unexplained hepatomegaly and hepatosplenomegaly
2. Persistently abnormal results of liver function tests

3. Suspected systemic or infiltrative disease (e.g., sarcoidosis or miliary tuberculosis)
4. Suspected primary or metastatic liver malignancy

VALUE OF THE TEST

Useful in the diagnosis of diffuse parenchymal disorders of the liver
Helpful in differentiating disseminated granulomatous disease from tumors

NURSING ACTION

1. Inform the patient that he or she should take nothing by mouth for 4 to 8 hours before the test.
2. Explain the test to the patient and obtain a signed consent. Inform him or her that a local anesthetic will be administered.
3. Ask the patient to void just before the test.
4. Instruct the patient to lie on his right side for 2 to 4 hours following the biopsy. This is because hemorrhage, although uncommon, is the most serious complication of this procedure. Continue to check the patient's vital signs during this time.
5. Usually ambulation is not permitted for 24 hours.

NURSING ALERT

Check the prothrombin time and alert the physician if it is prolonged. Needle biopsy should not be performed if the prothrombin time is significantly prolonged.

Check the patient for ascites. This is a contraindication for the procedure.

Evaluate whether or not the patient can hold the breath or is uncooperative, both of which are contraindications to the procedure.

All of the above mentioned situations increase the risk of severe bleeding.

Needle biopsy is also contraindicated in obstructive jaundice, since bile leakage may ensue and cause peritonitis.

THE PANCREAS

ANATOMY AND PHYSIOLOGY

The pancreas is located posterior to the stomach. It is of importance in that it secretes both pancreatic enzymes and bicarbonate to facilitate digestion, it secretes insulin, and it is in a position where it can cause mechanical obstruction of the biliary system.

CLINICAL APPLICATION OF LABORATORY TESTS

Pancreatitis

Acute. The two most common causes of pancreatitis are alcoholism and gallstones. In individuals with acute pancreatitis evaluation would initially be performed by obtaining a *CBC* to evaluate for leukocytosis and *amylase and lipase* levels. In addition, *liver tests* should be performed. *Ultrasound* of the right upper quadrant should be performed to rule out the presence of gallstones. In those individuals without a history of alcoholism or the presence of stones and in which no other causation such as abdominal trauma or pancreatitis secondary to medications is evident, *endoscopic retrograde cholangiopancreatography (ERCP)* should be considered. However, as noted, one of the complications of ERCP itself is the occurrence or exacerbation of pancreatitis.

Chronic. Evaluation of recurrent episodes of pancreatitis can be made by the laboratory studies noted above. In addition, a *flat plate study of the abdomen* may show the presence of calcifications. *ERCP* is of value in that it demonstrates diagnostic changes including sacculations of the branches of the pancreatic duct or disruption of the pancreatic duct.

Pseudocysts of the pancreas

Pseudocysts of the pancreas occur when there is damage to the pancreatic duct itself, either in acute pancreatitis or in chronic pancreatitis.

Diagnosis can be made by *CT scan* of the abdomen, and in some instances by *ultrasound* study or by *ERCP*.

Pancreatic malignancy

Cancer of the pancreas is an insidious disease with vague initial symptoms. Usually by the time diagnosis is made, there is no therapy that can ensure complete cure. However, both *CT scan* of the abdomen and *ERCP* can be of value in making the diagnosis when indicated.

LABORATORY TESTS FOR PANCREATIC DISEASE

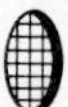

AMYLASE AND LIPASE (SERUM)

Normal

Amylase: 4-25 U/ml (SI units: 4-25 arb. unit)
Lipase: 2 U/ml or less (SI units: up to 2 arb. unit)

EXPLANATION OF THE TEST

Amylase is a digestive enzyme for carbohydrates. It is secreted by the pancreas, parotid glands, gynecologic system, and the bowel. Lipase is excreted specifically by the pancreas and parallels the elevation in amylase levels.

VALUE AND LIMITATIONS OF THE TEST

Diagnostic of acute pancreatitis
In chronic pancreatitis the serum amylase is not elevated.

NURSING ACTION

1. Inform the patient that it is not necessary to fast before the test.
2. Explain to the patient that this test assesses pancreatic function.
3. Note on the laboratory slip any drugs that the patient is taking.
4. Collect venous blood in a 7-ml red-top tube. Handle the specimen gently to avoid hemolysis.

INTERFERING FACTORS

Drugs that may cause false-positive results: aminosalicylic acid, asparaginase, azathioprine, corticosteroids, cyproheptadine, narcotic analgesics, oral contraceptives, rifampin, sulfasalazine, or thiazide and loop diuretics

CLINICAL IMPLICATIONS

Amylase can be elevated in mumps, acute pancreatitis, ischemic bowel disease, and pelvic inflammatory disease. In acute pancreatitis both amylase and lipase levels are elevated; in chronic pancreatitis these levels are not elevated. In the case of "burned-out" pancreas, the organ no longer has the ability to secrete amylase and lipase.

COMPUTED TOMOGRAPHY (CT) OF THE ABDOMEN

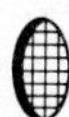

CT scans of the abdomen and pelvis visualize the liver, biliary system, and most importantly the pancreas. This is the only laboratory test available in which the complete pancreas can be evaluated, and it aids in the diagnosis of acute pancreatitis, pancreatic malignancy, and pseudocyst of the pancreas. This test is fully explained on p. 161.

ENDOSCOPIC RETROGRADE CHOLANGIOPANCREATOGRAPHY (ERCP)

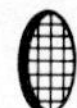

EXPLANATION OF THE TEST

ERCP is a procedure in which an endoscope is passed orally and ultimately localized within the second portion of the duodenum. The ampulla of Vater is then visualized and a catheter is inserted into the ampulla. Retrograde injection of contrast material into both the biliary system and pancreatic duct can then be accomplished. The choice of using ERCP versus percutaneous transhepatic cholangiogram depends on the patient's clinical presentation and the ability of the physician performing the test.

VALUE OF THE TEST

Enables evaluation of the biliary system and pancreatic duct
Evaluates for pancreatic malignancy and diagnoses pancreatic pseudocyst

NURSING ACTION

1. Instruct the patient to fast from midnight before the test.
2. Inform the patient that this procedure permits x-ray examination of the liver, gallbladder, and the pancreas following injection of a contrast medium.

3. The patient should be instructed regarding every aspect of the procedure to alleviate fear or panic. Assure that he or she understands the following actions and reactions and that the endoscopic instrument will not interfere with breathing:
   a. A long narrow tube will be inserted through the mouth, into the stomach and beyond.
   b. A local anesthetic may be sprayed into the mouth to keep the patient from gagging. The patient will be asked to hold the breath while the spray is being used. This medication will take effect in about 10 minutes; it will be unpleasant to taste and will make the tongue and throat feel swollen so that it is difficult to swallow. He or she should let saliva drain from the side of the mouth or be suctioned away.
   c. A mouth guard will be used to protect the teeth and the endoscopic instrument.
   d. The patient will remain conscious but will be aided in relaxing by the administration of a sedative intravenously.
   e. An anticholinergic or glucagon is also administered intravenously; each has possible side effects.
   f. The patient may experience transient flushing when the contrast medium is injected.
   g. At the completion of the procedure he or she is to remain prone until the films are reviewed.
4. Obtain a signed consent.
5. Obtain baseline vital signs.
6. Assure that emergency resuscitation equipment and a narcotic antagonist are at hand.
7. Instruct the patient to remove all metal or jewelry and to void before the procedure.
8. Establish an intravenous line with 150 ml of normal saline solution.
9. After spraying the throat, place the patient in left lateral posiion and provide an emesis basin and tissues. Insert the mouth guard.
10. Following the intravenous administration of 4 to 20 mg of diazepam midazolamHCL (versed), the physician commences the introduction of the endoscope.
11. During the procedure be alert for signs of respiratory depression, apnea, hypotension, diaphoresis, bradycardia, and laryngospasm.
12. Following the procedure

a. Be alert to the development of cholangitis (fever, chills, hyperbilirubinemia) and pancreatitis (pain in the upper left quadrant and transient hyperbilirubinemia), which is a complication following visualization of the pancreatic duct.
b. Withhold food and fluids until the gag reflex returns and then permit fluids and a light meal.
c. Check vital signs every 15 minutes for 4 hours.
d. Check for signs of urinary retention and notify the physician if it occurs.

QUANTITATIVE FECAL FAT

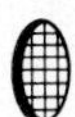

Normal

<7 g/24 hr

Fecal lipids normally constitute <20% of excreted solids.

EXPLANATION OF THE TEST

Normally, dietary lipids are emulsified by bile and almost completely absorbed in the small intestine. Fecal lipids are composed of unabsorbed dietary lipids, gastrointestinal secretions, intestinal bacterial cells, and epithelial cells. Excessive excretion of fecal lipids is called steatorrhea.

VALUE OF THE TEST

Aids in the diagnosis of malabsorption syndromes

NURSING ACTION

1. Instruct the patient regarding fat intake. At least 50 g of fat should be taken in each day for accurate test results. The patient should abstain from alcohol during the test.
2. Make sure that the patient understands that all stools must be collected for 3 full days and that the stool specimen should not contain urine or toilet tissue. Provide a nonwaxed collection container.
3. Refrigerate the collection container between collections and keep it tightly covered.

CLINICAL IMPLICATIONS

Steatorrhea and malabsorption in children are commonly the result of celiac disease and cystic fibrosis of the pancreas; in adults, the most common causes of steatorrhea and malabsorption are pancreatic insufficiency, tropical sprue, and nontropical sprue.

Ellen I. Tamagna, M.D.
Mary Conover, R.N.

9

Evaluation of endocrine disorders

The organs of the endocrine system produce small amounts of hormones, each manufactured by one particular organ and secreted into the circulation, exerting its influence on other organs or tissues ("target tissues"). The endocrine system is illustrated in Fig. 9-1; it is composed of the hypothalamus, anterior and posterior pituitary, thyroid, parathyroid, and adrenal glands, pancreatic islets of Langerhans, ovaries, testes, and placenta. Fig. 9-2 shows the interrelationships between the hypothalamus, endocrine glands, and target organs.

Since the endocrine system contains inherent checks and balances, endocrine function tests depend not only on overproduction or underproduction of a particular hormone but also on its reciprocal effects on other endocrine organs. For example, excess cortisone production by the adrenal glands suppresses adrenocorticotropic hormone (ACTH) production by the pituitary gland. Table 9-1 lists the hormones that are measured in certain endocrine disorders.

THE THYROID GLAND

ANATOMY AND PHYSIOLOGY

The thyroid gland is illustrated in Fig. 9-3. It consists of two lobes (one on each side of the trachea) and a connecting portion (isthmus), giving it an H-shaped appearance.

The principal thyroid hormones are thyroxine (T_4) and triiodothyronine (T_3). T_4 is produced only by the thyroid gland. T_3 is produced primarily (80%) by extrathyroidal deiodination of T_4; 20% of T_3 is secreted by the thyroid gland. T_4 is thought to be a prohormone, while T_3 exerts the major physiologic actions at the cellular level.

The first step in the synthesis of the thyroid hormones is absorption of dietary iodine from the small intestine into the circulation. The circulating iodine that is not taken up by the thyroid gland is cleared by the kidneys through glomerular filtration. After entering the thyroid, iodine is oxidized and combines with the amino acid tyrosine within a protein (thyroglobulin), where the thyroid hormones T_4 and T_3 are formed and stored.

The next step is the release primarily of T_4 from the thyroid gland. Under the influence of thyroid-stimulating hormone (TSH), which is secreted by the anterior pituitary gland, thyroglobulin is hydrolyzed and T_4 and T_3 are released into the circulation. Of the circulating thyroid hormones all but .05% are inactive because the hormones

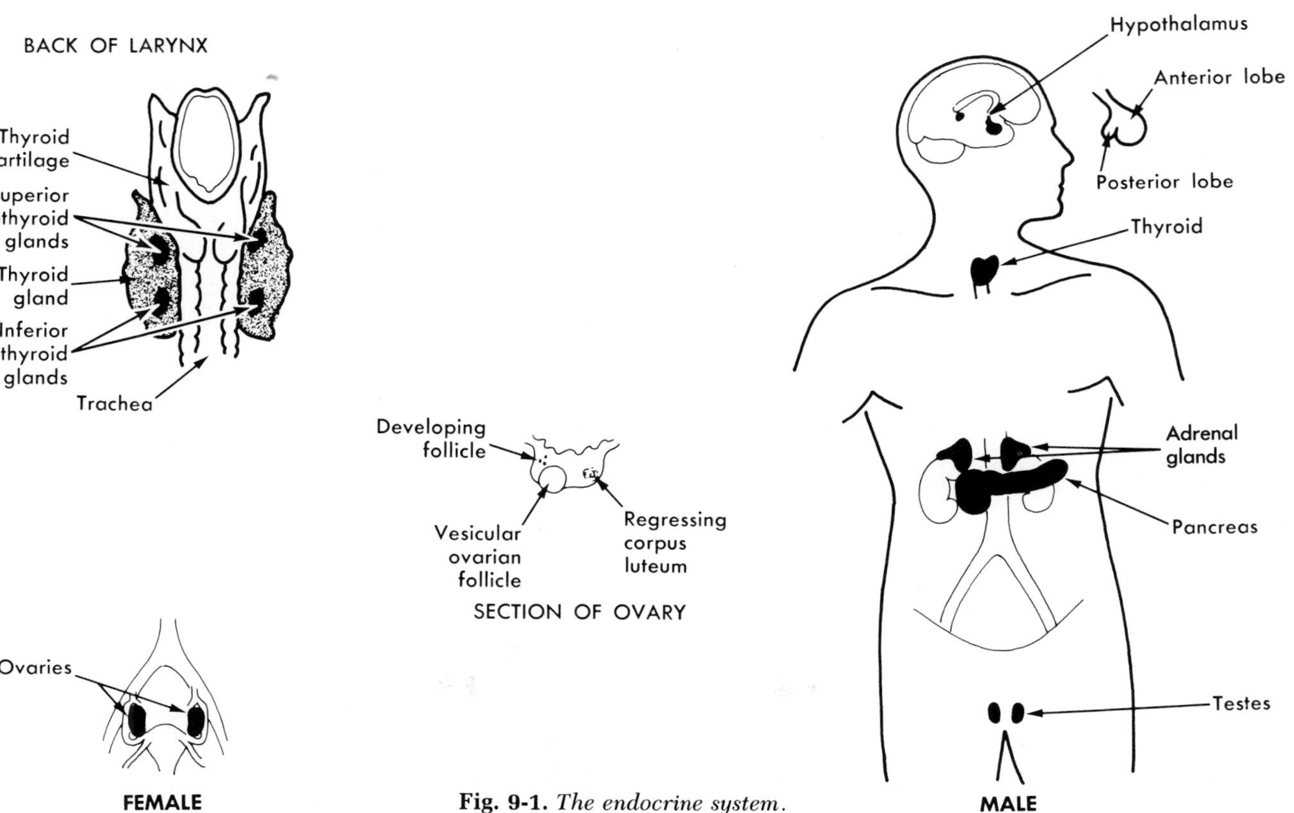

Fig. 9-1. *The endocrine system.*

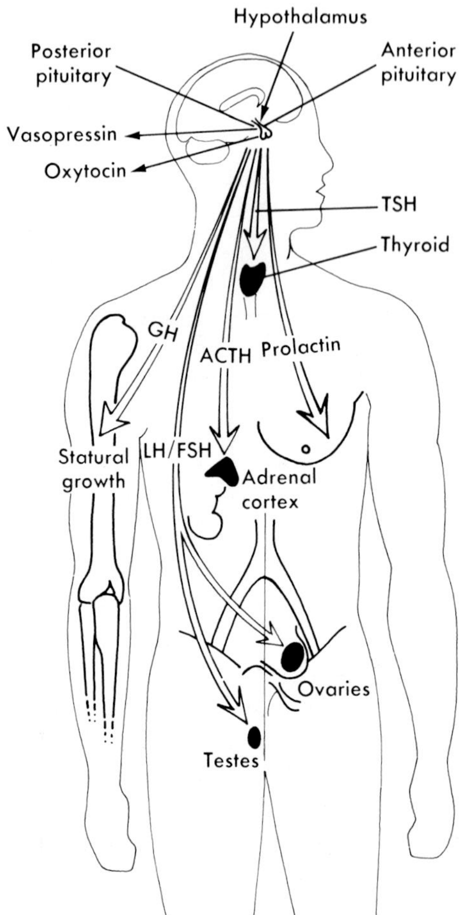

Fig. 9-2. *The interrelationships between the pituitary gland, the hypothalamus, and the target organs.*

are bound to serum proteins, particularly to thyroxine-binding globulin (TBG). Thus, only small amounts of unbound thyroid hormone circulate to provide biologic activity. The free T_4 is deiodinated in the liver and kidney to T_3. T_3 then exerts its action within the cell at the nuclear receptor level. It stimulates the oxidative reactions of the cells, helping to regulate lipid and carbohydrate metabolism, and is necessary for normal growth and development. Thyroid hormonal action is partially mediated through the sympathetic nervous system.

Table 9-1 Clinical indications for measuring serum hormones

Disease or disorder	Laboratory tests
Acromegaly or gigantism	GH, ACTH, FSH, LH, TSH, prolactin, T_4
Addison's disease	Cortisol, aldosterone, ACTH
Cushing's syndrome	ACTH, cortisol
Diabetes insipidus	ADH
Dwarfism	ACTH, GH, FSH, LH, TSH, T_4, prolactin
Hypogonadism	Estrogen, testosterone, FSH, LH, prolactin
Hyperthyroidism	T_4, free T_4 index, T_3, free T_3 index
Hypothyroidism	T_4, free T_4 index, TSH
Medullary thyroid carcinoma	Calcitonin
Pituitary tumor	Cortisol, ACTH, GH, prolactin, FSH, LH, estrogen or testosterone, TSH, T_4
Precocious puberty	FSH, LH, estrogen, androgens

Thus β-adrenergic blockers are effective modes of controlling the symptoms of hyperthyroidism.

The regulation of the thyroid gland occurs through a feedback system (Fig. 9-4) consisting of three main components: the thyroid gland (T_3 and T_4), the anterior pituitary gland (TSH), and the hypothalamus (thyrotropin-releasing hormone [TRH]). TRH stimulates the release of TSH and causes the synthesis of new TSH in the pituitary gland. Normal levels of unbound T_3 and T_4 are maintained by a negative feedback effect. Increased levels of free hormones cause decreased TSH secretion, and decreased levels of free hormones cause increased TSH secretion.

PATHOPHYSIOLOGY AND CLINICAL APPLICATION OF LABORATORY TESTS

Hyperthyroidism

Excess secretion of thyroid hormone (thyrotoxicosis) is most commonly caused by toxic goiter (Graves' disease). Other causes are subacute thyroiditis, hyperfunctioning thyroid nodule, toxic multinodular goiter, iodine-induced hyperthyroidism, factitious hyperthyroidism, or struma ovarii.

Thyroid function tests

Hyperthyroidism may be divided into three categories:

1. Standard T_4/T_3 toxicosis (T_4 and T_3 RIA elevated)

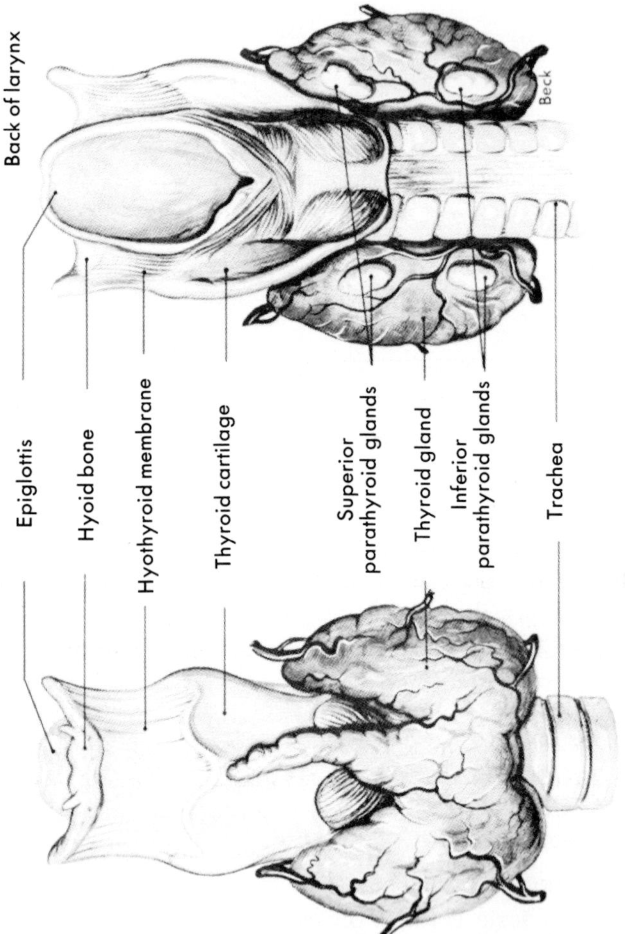

Fig. 9-3. *The thyroid and parathyroid glands.* (*From Thibodeau, G.A.: Anatomy and physiology, ed. 12, St. Louis, 1987, The C.V. Mosby Co.*)

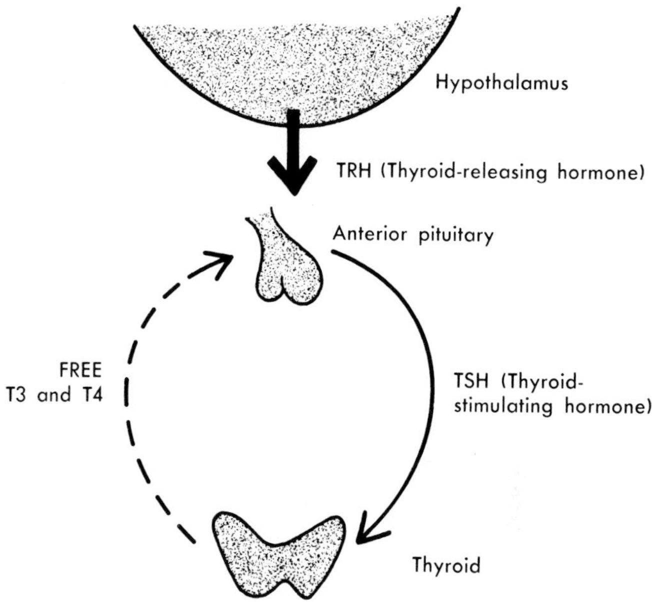

Fig. 9-4. *The regulation of the thyroid gland through a feedback system.*

2. T_3 toxicosis (only T_3 RIA elevated)
3. T_4 toxicosis (only T_4 elevated)

Other thyroid function tests useful in the diagnosis of hyperthyroidism are:

T_3 resin uptake, which corrects for most protein binding abnormalities

Free thyroxine index (FTI) and *free T_4 assay (FT_4)*, which negate the effects of thyroid-binding protein alterations on the T_4 assay

Radioactive iodine uptake (RAIU), used in conjunction with the *thyroid scan* to differentiate between diffuse hyperplasia (Graves' disease) and subacute thyroiditis, iodine-induced thyrotoxicosis, or factitious hyperthyroidism

Thyrotropin releasing hormone test, which is the most reliable test for confirmation or exclusion of the diagnosis of hyperthyroidism when the patient has normal thyroid hormone levels and symptoms suggestive of hyperthyroidism. It is also useful in evaluating hypothalamic or pituitary hypothyroidism.

Thyroid scan, which differentiates among toxic goiter (Graves' disease), hyperfunctioning nodule, or toxic multinodular goiter in patients with hyperthyroidism

Nonthyroid laboratory tests

Serum cholesterol and triglycerides (decreased)
Serum aminotransferases and alkaline phosphatase (increased)
Glucose/insulin relationship (altered)
Lymphocytes (increased)
Serum and urine calcium (increased)

Hypothyroidism

Hypothyroidism is divided into three types: (1) primary (95%) (failure of the thyroid to secrete hormone), (2) secondary (pituitary TSH secretion defect), and (3) tertiary (hypothalamic TRH secretion deficiency).

Thyroid laboratory tests

In primary hypothyroidism the *serum free* T_4 *index* is decreased and *TSH* is elevated, whereas in secondary and tertiary hypothyroidism the *free* T_4 *index* is decreased and the *TSH* is normal or decreased. T_3 *uptake* is not a screening test for hypothyroidism; however, it is useful in detecting thyroxine-binding globulin abnormalities.

Nonthyroid laboratory tests

Serum cholesterol and triglycerides (increased)
Serum carotene (increased)
CK (creatine kinase) and LD (lactic dehydrenase) (increased)
Serum prolactin (increased)
Hemoglobin (approximately 10 g/dl; normochromic anemia)
Capillary fragility (increased)

Neoplasms of the thyroid

Eighty to ninety percent of solitary thyroid nodules are benign adenomas. Malignant thyroid neoplasms are less frequent (generally 10% of all solitary cold thyroid nodules). Adenomas or carcinomas usually present as a solitary cold nodule in a euthyroid patient. If the adenoma is functioning autonomously it will accumulate radioactive iodine and the *thyroid scan* will show a hot nodule; these are rarely malignant. In carcinoma the thyroid scan generally demonstrates a cold (nonfunctioning) nodule.

There are no blood tests available to differentiate a benign adenoma from thyroid carcinoma except for medullary carcinoma of the thyroid. Elevation of the *serum calcitonin level* is the hallmark of the diagnosis of medullary thyroid carcinoma.

Ultrasound is helpful in differentiating cystic benign tumors from solid tumors, and *fine needle aspiration* is useful in the differential diagnosis of thyroid nodules.

Diffuse nontoxic goiter

A nontoxic goiter is associated with normal thyroid function tests. This is differentiated from Hashimoto's thyroiditis, which is an autoimmune, inflammatory process causing goiter and eventually hypothyroidism. The antithyroglobulin and/or antimicrosomal antibodies are elevated in Hashimoto's thyroiditis.

General nursing implications for elevated thyroid function tests

1. Assess for symptoms of hyperthyroidism and monitor for complications such as arrhythmias.
2. Assist with patient instruction and medical interventions.
3. Provide a cool, quiet environment and psychologic support for the patient.
4. Provide for daily weighing and an increase in calories.

General nursing implications for decreased thyroid function tests

1. Assess for symptoms of hypothyroidism. When checking temperature, shake the thermometer down well, since these patients may be hypothermic.
2. Assist with patient instruction and medical interventions.
3. Provide a warm, relaxed environment, psychologic support, and dietary counseling related to weight gain and constipation.

NURSING ALERT

Sedatives, tranquilizers, and narcotics are generally avoided in hypothyroid patients because of increased sensitivity to these medications and the possibility of precipitating myxedemic coma.

THYROID FUNCTION TESTS

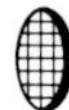

T_4, TOTAL SERUM

Adult reference range (radioimmunoassay [RIA])

4-12 μg/dl (SI units: 52-154 nmol/L)

Pediatric reference range

Newborn: 8-20 μg/dl
1-4 months: 7.5-16.5 μg/dl
4-12 months: 5.5-14.5 μg/dl
1-6 years: 5.5-13.5 μg/dl
6-10 years: 5-12.5 μg/dl

EXPLANATION OF THE TEST

T_4 (one of the thyroid hormones) is measured by radioimmunoassay and more recently by enzyme-linked assay. Since most of the T_4 is protein bound, the T_4 radioimmunoassay will be affected by alterations in T_4-binding proteins and the free T_4 assay may be done instead (see p. 329).

VALUE OF THE TEST

This is the basic screening test for thyroid disease.

NURSING ACTION

1. Note that thyroid hormone medication should be discontinued 4 to 6 weeks before the test to obtain a baseline sample. Otherwise, the blood can be measured for T_4 levels while the patient is taking thyroid medication to assess the dose.
2. Inform the patient that he or she may eat and drink before the test.
3. Collect 5 ml of venous blood in a red-top tube.

INTERFERING FACTORS

Severe illness decreases T_4 in 20% to 30% of cases.

Drugs causing increased levels of T_4: estrogens (pregnancy or oral contraceptives), amphetamine abuse, clofibrate, excess doses of thyroid hormones, methadone, iodine, and amiodarone

Drugs causing decreased levels of T_4: dopamine, iodine, lithium, methimazole (Tapazole), methylthiouracil, phenylbutazone, phenytoin, propylthiouracil, salicylates (high dose), steroids, sulfonamides, sulfonylureas, T_3 (Cytomel) therapy.

CLINICAL IMPLICATIONS

Elevated levels

Hyperthyroidism
Elevated thyroid-binding protein levels

Low levels

Hypothyroidism
Euthyroid sick state
Decreased thyroid-binding protein levels

> **NURSING ALERT**
>
> Decreased or mildly elevated T_4 levels are interpreted with caution when associated with severe nonthyroidal illness.

T_3 UPTAKE (T_3U)

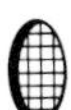

Adult reference range

25%-35% uptake (SI units: 0.25-0.35)

EXPLANATION OF THE TEST

The T_3U test indirectly estimates the amount of thyroid-binding globulin (TBG) in the patient's serum. This is an in vitro test; the patient does not receive radioactive material. In the test tube a hormone-binding resin and radioactive T_3 are added to the patient's serum. Radioactive T_3 will bind to sites on thyroid-binding proteins not already occupied by T_4 molecules; the remainder of the radioactive T_3 binds to the special hormone-binding resin. Thus, the amount of thyroid-binding protein can be estimated by the amount of radioactive T_3 taken up by the resin. With decreased TBG levels, increased amounts of radioactive T_3 will bind to the special resin, causing increased T_3RU levels. The reverse is true for increased TBG levels, resulting in decreased T_3U levels.

VALUE AND LIMITATIONS OF THE TEST

Confirms an elevated T_4
Used as an indicator of TBG-induced alterations in T_4
Must be interpreted in conjunction with T_4 value for clinical relevance

NURSING ACTION

1. Inform the patient that he or she may eat and drink before the test.
2. Collect 5 ml of venous blood in a red-top tube.

INTERFERING FACTORS

Any radioactive substances already taken could render the test invalid.
Drugs that cause increased levels: phenytoin, corticosteroid therapy, anabolic steroids
Drugs that cause decreased levels: oral contraceptives, estrogen replacement therapy, high-dose salicylates

CLINICAL IMPLICATIONS
Elevated level (>35%)

Hyperthyroidism
Protein malnutrition
Genetic TBG deficiency or absence
Chronic liver disease
Nephrotic syndrome
Uremia

Decreased level (<25%)

Hypothyroidism
Pregnancy
Genetic TBG excess
Acute hepatitis
Acute intermittent porphyria

FREE THYROXINE INDEX (FTI)

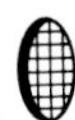

Reference range

1-4

EXPLANATION OF THE TEST

The free thyroxine index is derived from the serum T_4 multiplied by the T_3U ratio.

VALUE AND LIMITATIONS OF THE TEST

Negates the effects of thyroxine-binding protein alterations on the T_4 assay
Sensitivity in hyperthyroidism is approximately 95%.
Sensitivity in hypothyroidism is approximately 90% to 95%.
More reliable than a decreased T_4 in the diagnosis of hypothyroidism
May be decreased in severe nonthyroidal illness (10% to 15%)

FREE THYROXINE (FT_4) ASSAY

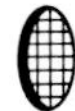

Reference range

0.9-2.3 ng/dl (SI units: 12-30 pmol/L)

EXPLANATION OF THE TEST

This test measures the metabolically active form of thyroid hormone, T_4. The test has recently become more available when several manufacturers introduced easy-to-use FT_4 kits, and it may be used instead of the total T_4. The FT_4 assay measures the small amount of T_4 present in the serum in the free state, about 5% of the total; the remainder of T_4 is bound to thyroxine-binding globulin (TBG) and other serum proteins. It is primarily the free T_3, and to some extent the free T_4, that affects cellular metabolism.

VALUE AND LIMITATIONS OF THE TEST

The measurement of FT_4 eliminates the inconsistencies in laboratory values associated with alterations in thyroxine-binding protein.
Has a sensitivity of about 95% in evaluating thyroid function

Used to aid in the diagnosis of hyperthyroidism and hypothyroidism and to monitor therapy

False test results may occur in seriously ill patients; however, the FT_4 is the most reliable assessment available in the evaluation of the euthyroid sick state (decreased T_4 in seriously ill patients).

NURSING ACTION

1. Inform the patient that he or she may eat and drink and be physically active before the test.
2. Collect 7 ml of venous blood in a red-top tube.

CLINICAL IMPLICATIONS

Normal levels

A normal FT_4 level does not guarantee normal thyroid function, since normal levels are associated with T_3 toxicosis. Further testing is indicated when the T_4 level is normal and there are clinical signs of hyperthyroidism (exophthalmos, lid lag, tachycardia, warm, moist skin, heat intolerance, hyperactivity, weight loss, tremor).

Elevated levels

Hyperthyroidism

Low levels

Hypothyroidism

Occasionally severe euthyroid sick state

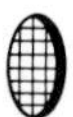

T_3, TOTAL SERUM (T_3 RIA)

Reference range

75-195 ng/dl (SI units: 1.16-3.00 nmol/L)

EXPLANATION OF THE TEST

This test measures both bound and free serum triiodothyronine (T_3). T_3 is the major physiologic thyroid hormone. Like T_4, it can be measured directly by radioimmunoassay. Since most of the T_3 is protein bound, this test will be affected by alterations in thyroid-binding proteins.

VALUE AND LIMITATIONS OF THE TEST

Evaluates hyperthyroidism
Detects T_3 toxicosis (T_3 is elevated but not T_4)
Not reliable in hypothyroidism because of the overlap with the low-normal levels

NURSING ACTION

1. Inform the patient that he or she may eat and drink before the test.
2. Collect 5 ml of venous blood in a red-top tube and send it to the laboratory.

INTERFERING FACTORS

Markedly increased or decreased TBG level
Drug effects: Drugs alter T_3 levels by affecting (1) thyroid-binding globulin levels, (2) T_4 production, or (3) peripheral T_4 deiodination and conversion to T_3. Levels are increased by estrogen and Cytomel and decreased by dopamine, methimazole (Tapazole), methylthiouracil, phenylbutazone, phenytoin, propranolol, propylthiouracil, salicylates (high dose), steroids, certain iodinated radiographic agents (Oragrafin, Telepaque), and amiodarone.

CLINICAL IMPLICATIONS

Elevated levels

Thyrotoxicosis

Normal or reduced levels

Interpreted with caution when associated with severe nonthyroidal illness or when the patient is over 60 years of age

THYROID-STIMULATING HORMONE (TSH) 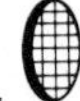

ASSAY, SERUM

Reference range

0.5-5.0 μU/ml (SI units: 0.5-5.0 arb. unit)

EXPLANATION OF THE TEST

The TSH assay is performed by radioimmunoassay.

VALUE AND LIMITATIONS OF THE TEST

It is the most useful single test to confirm primary hypothyroidism.

It helps to differentiate primary from secondary or tertiary hypothyroidism (pituitary or hypothalamic dysfunction).

It helps to monitor drug therapy in patients with primary hypothyroidism or in patients undergoing thyroid suppression therapy for a thyroid nodule or thyroid cancer.

Most patients with secondary or tertiary hypothyroidism have normal TSH values.

Some of the TSH kits do not differentiate low (suppressed) from low-normal values.

TSH values may be inappropriately elevated in the presence of elevated free-T_4 levels caused by a TSH-producing pituitary tumor or in pituitary or peripheral tissue resistance to thyroid hormone. However, these conditions are quite rare.

NURSING ACTION

1. Inform the patient that there are no dietary restrictions before the test.
2. Collect 5 ml of venous blood in a red-top tube.

CLINICAL IMPLICATIONS

Elevated levels

Primary hypothyroidism
Thyroiditis—subacute hypothyroid phase or Hashimoto's thyroiditis
After thyroidectomy
After ^{131}I therapy
Iodine deficiency goiter
Euthyroid goiter with enzyme defect

Low or low-normal levels

Secondary (pituitary or hypothalamic) hypothyroidism
Thyroid hormone therapy
Corticosteroid therapy
Dopamine infusion
Hyperthyroidism
Euthyroid sick state
Primary hypothyroidism generally ruled out by a normal value

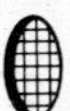

THYROTROPIN RELEASING HORMONE (TRH) TEST

Reference (negative)

Twenty to thirty minutes after administration of TRH intravenously there is a significant rise in serum TSH levels (see Fig. 9-5); serum prolactin also increases.

EXPLANATION OF THE TEST

TRH is a tripeptide hormone from the hypothalamus that regulates TSH secretion from the pituitary. This test evaluates the ability of injected synthetic TRH (Thypinone) to directly stimulate the pituitary to release TSH and prolactin.

VALUE AND LIMITATIONS OF THE TEST

This is the most reliable test for confirmation or exclusion of the diagnosis of hyperthyroidism when the patient has normal or bor-

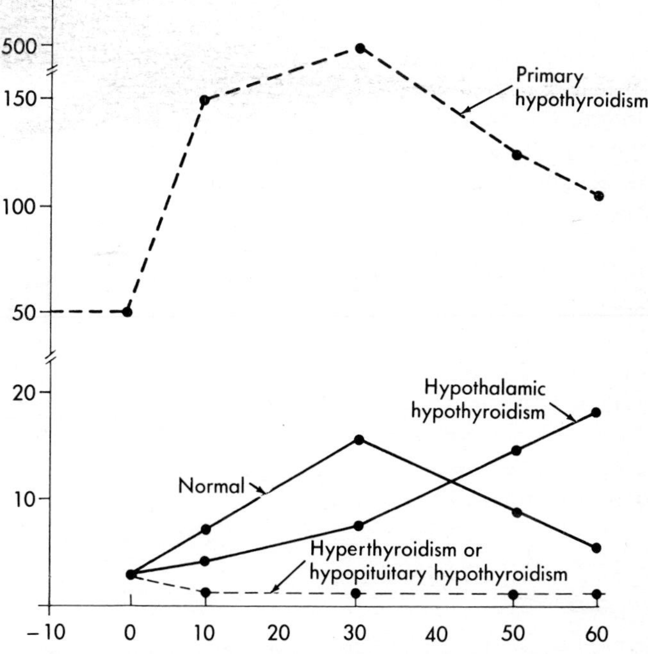

Fig. 9-5. *TSH response to administration of TRH.*

derline serum FT_1I and T_3 levels and clinical evidence of hyperthyroidism.

The test may be helpful in differentiating pituitary or hypothalamic hypothyroidism from euthyroid sick state (with low FT_4I and low TSH levels).

It is useful in assessing thyroid suppressive treatment in patients with a history of thyroid cancer.

The test is reported to be useful in differentiating primary depression (TSH response is blunted) from manic-depressive psychiatric illness (TSH response is normal) and from secondary types of depression.

The TSH response to TRH may be blunted with aging, acute illness, and corticosteroid or dopamine therapy.

NURSING ACTION

1. Inform the patient that there are no dietary restrictions before this test.
2. Note that thyroid hormone therapy should be discontinued 4 to 6 weeks before the TRH test for baseline evaluation. However, to enable the physician to assess the adequacy of thyroid hormone treatment, the test is performed while the patient is on a given dose of T_4.
3. Inform the patient that 2 blood samples will be required and that the physician will administer a hormone to aid in evaluating thyroid function. Warn the patient that he or she may experience transient flushing, nausea, and urinary urgency, and assure the patient that these side effects are self-limited and that they will resolve several minutes after the intravenous injection.
4. Note that the blood pressure may rise temporarily following the injection of TRH.
5. Withdraw venous blood for baseline TSH and prolactin levels. TRH 500 μg is then administered intravenously. Twenty to thirty minutes later another blood sample is collected for serum TSH and prolactin levels.

CLINICAL IMPLICATIONS

Negative test

Normal degree of TSH elevation after injection of TRH; excludes thyrotoxicosis

Positive test

Abnormally low TSH response

1. Suggestive but not conclusive of hyperthyroidism
2. Suggestive of pituitary hypothyroidism
3. Confirms adequate TSH suppression by dose of T_4 in the treatment of thyroid cancers

Exaggerated TSH response

Primary hypothyroidism

RADIOACTIVE IODINE UPTAKE (RAIU)

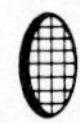

Reference range

12%-20% absorbed by the thyroid gland after 6 hr
15%-35% absorbed by the thyroid gland after 24 hr

EXPLANATION OF THE TEST

The RAIU test is based on the thyroid gland's uptake of iodine to produce thyroid hormone. When a small dose of radioactive iodine is ingested the ability of the thyroid gland to concentrate iodine can be measured, providing an indirect evaluation of thyroid activity. The test measures the amount of radioactive iodine accumulated in the thyroid gland after 6 and 24 hours. Although it is not used as a screening test, in conjunction with the thyroid scan it is helpful in the evaluation of patients with laboratory evidence of hyperthyroidism.

VALUE AND LIMITATIONS OF THE TEST

Used in conjunction with the thyroid scan to differentiate between Graves' disease, subacute thyroiditis, hyperfunctioning nodule, or factitious hyperthyroidism

Diagnoses causes of hyperthyroidism (approximately 90% accuracy) but is not as useful in the diagnosis or evaluation of hypothyroidism

NURSING ACTION

1. Instruct the patient to abstain from food and drink from 8 hours before the test until 1 hour after ingestion of the radioiodide capsule or liquid.

2. The patient will return to the nuclear medicine laboratory after 6 and 24 hours.
3. Note that this test should precede tests using contrast media.
4. This test is contraindicated during pregnancy because radioactive iodine may affect the fetus.

INTERFERING FACTORS

Drugs causing decreased uptake: thyroid hormones or their antagonists (thioureas), iodine ingestion, iodinated contrast studies, and amiodarone

CLINICAL IMPLICATIONS
Elevated levels

Usually indicates Graves' disease

Low levels

Occurs with elevated T_3, T_4, and free thyroxine levels
Hyperthyroidism induced by excessive amounts of dietary iodine
Factitious hyperthyroidism
Subacute thyroiditis
Certain forms of chronic thyroiditis

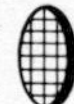

THYROID SCAN

Normal scan

The thyroid gland is seen as butterfly-shaped and approximately 5 cm long and 3 cm wide. The uptake of the radioisotope is uniform and no tumors are visualized.

EXPLANATION OF THE TEST

The thyroid scan evaluates the thyroid's uptake of radioactive isotopes of iodine or technetium, enabling visualization of localized hyperactive or hypoactive areas. The thyroid is visualized by a scintiscanner.

VALUE AND LIMITATIONS OF THE TEST

Differentiates between diffuse hyperplasia (Graves' disease), hyperfunctioning nodule, or toxic multinodular goiter in patients with hyperthyroidism

NURSING ACTION

1. Seven to fourteen days before the test the patient should discontinue medications containing iodine, which may interfere with the accuracy of the test. If the patient is taking thyroid medications, these should be discontinued 4 to 6 weeks before the scan. The patient should not have received radiographic contrast agents for 3 months before the scan.
2. Instruct the patient to fast from midnight before the test.
3. The radioisotope (usually Iodine 123) is taken orally and fasting continued for another 45 minutes.
4. In 24 hours the scan is performed. When technetium is used, Tc-99m-pertechnetate is given 30 minutes before the scan.

INTERFERING FACTORS

Increased uptake

Renal disease, iodine-deficient diet, phenothiazines

Decreased uptake

Thyroid hormones or their antagonists, multivitamins, cough syrup containing iodides (SSKI), iodine preparations, radiographic contrast agents

CLINICAL IMPLICATIONS

A characteristic nonuniform appearance may suggest the diagnosis of chronic lymphocytic thyroiditis (Hashimoto's thyroiditis) or multinodular goiter.

Hyperactive areas. Fig. 9-6, *B*, is a thyroid scan of a hyperfunctioning nodule (hot nodule) in the left lower lobe, which suppresses the remainder of the thyroid gland. This permits a differentiation between diffuse hyperplasia and toxic nodule as a cause of thyrotoxicosis. Hot nodules are generally benign.

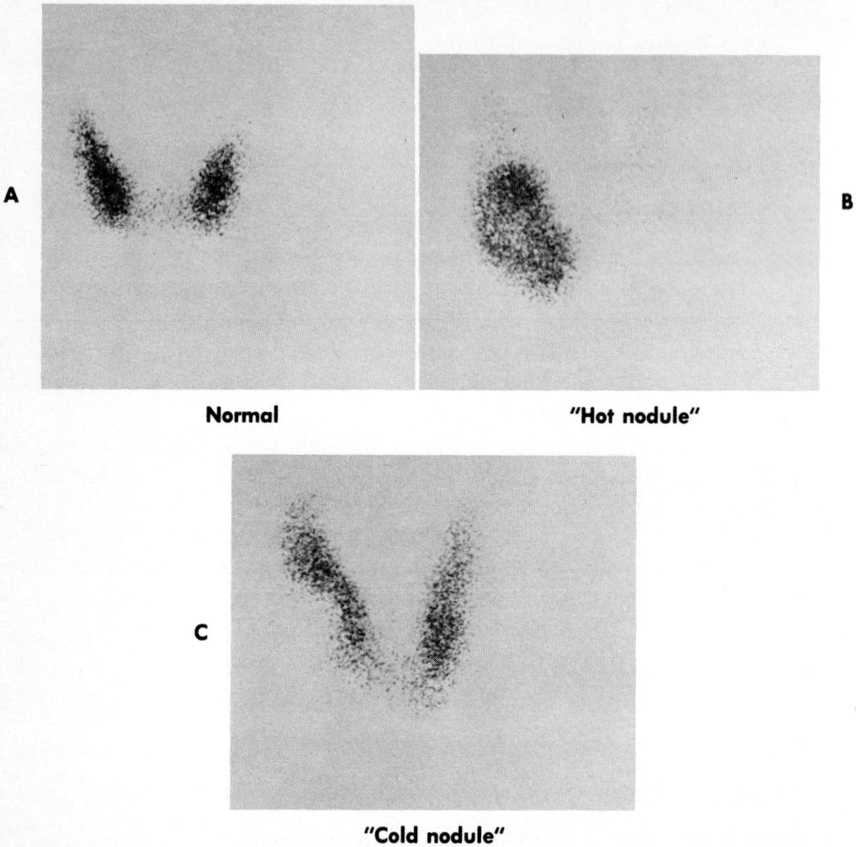

A

B

Normal

"Hot nodule"

C

"Cold nodule"

Fig. 9-6. *Normal and abnormal thyroid scans.* ***B,*** *Hot nodule, right lobe, with suppression of remainder of thyroid.* **C,** *Solitary cold nodule, right lower lobe.*

Hypoactive areas. The lack of radioactivity in Fig. 9-6, *C* (compare with the normal in *A*) indicates a hypofunctioning nodule (cold nodule), increasing the suspicion of carcinoma.

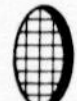

THYROID ULTRASONOGRAPHY

Normal findings

The normal thyroid is reflected by a uniform echo pattern throughout the thyroid gland.

EXPLANATION OF THE TEST

Ultrasonic pulses are directed at the thyroid gland and echoes from the interfaces of the gland are reflected back and displayed on an oscilloscope.

VALUE OF THE TEST

Permits noninvasive evaluation of the thyroid gland
Differentiates between a cyst and a solid tumor

NURSING ACTION

1. Inform the patient that there are no dietary restrictions before this test.
2. Tell the patient that the test uses harmless sound waves to evaluate the size and shape of the thyroid gland.

CLINICAL IMPLICATIONS

Cysts have a smooth border and are echo-free areas with enhanced sound transmission.

Adenomas and carcinomas are solid or well-demarcated areas. If a tumor is suspected, the definitive diagnosis is made with fine needle aspiration or a biopsy.

FINE NEEDLE ASPIRATION

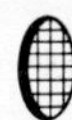

EXPLANATION OF THE TEST

A 21-gauge needle is used to obtain a small amount of thyroid tissue. After insertion of the needle into the thyroid nodule, negative pressure is exerted to draw material into the needle core. While negative pressure is maintained, various areas of the nodule are sampled. The vacuum is released and the needle withdrawn. The syringe is removed from the needle, filled with air, and reattached to force the cells onto a slide.

VALUE AND LIMITATIONS OF THE TEST

Allows cytologic evaluation of thyroid nodules
Allows cytologic diagnosis of benign lesions such as colloid goiter,

Hashimoto's or subacute thyroiditis, or cysts
Allows diagnosis of malignant lesions such as papillary, follicular, anaplastic, or medullary carcinomas
Few complications are noted with the procedure (rarely there may be local bleeding).
Unfortunately, benign follicular adenomas often are difficult to distinguish from well-differentiated follicular carcinomas by needle aspiration.
Cytologic interpretation of thyroid aspirate requires special training and experience.
Well-differentiated follicular carcinoma is difficult to diagnose on aspirate as well as needle biopsy.

NURSING ACTION

1. Inform the patient that there are no dietary restrictions before this test.
2. Explain the procedure to the patient.
3. The nurse generally assists the physician during the procedure by placing light pressure on the aspiration site to prevent local bleeding after the needle is removed from the nodule.

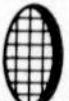

THYROGLOBULIN LEVEL

Reference range

<2-30 ng/ml (increases following TSH stimulation)

EXPLANATION OF THE TEST

Thyroglobulin is a glycoprotein produced by the follicular cells. T_4 and T_3 are formed within the thyroglobulin molecule, which serves as storage or prohormone. Thyroglobulin is released into the bloodstream in cases of carcinoma and several other thyroid disorders. It is measured in the serum by radioimmunoassay.

VALUE AND LIMITATIONS OF THE TEST

Assesses the adequacy of therapy for thyroid carcinoma
Monitors for recurrence or dissemination of thyroid carcinoma
Is too nonspecific to be diagnostic of thyroid carcinoma

NURSING ACTION

1. Inform the patient that there are no dietary restrictions before the test.
2. Withdraw venous blood in a 7-ml red-top tube.

CLINICAL IMPLICATIONS
Elevated levels

Active thyrotoxicosis (diffuse or nodular)
Thyroiditis
Benign thyroid adenomas
Differentiated thyroid carcinomas (usually elevated in papillary, follicular, and mixed papillary-follicular neoplasms)

THE PARATHYROID GLANDS
ANATOMY AND PHYSIOLOGY

The four, small parathyroid glands (Fig. 9-3) are so closely associated with the thyroid that in the past they were often removed during thyroidectomy. Parathyroid hormone is essential for life; it is responsible for the maintenance of ionized calcium in the blood, the renal reabsorption of calcium and excretion of phosphate, and the control of bone mineralization.

The serum calcium level is controlled in part by the parathyroid hormone through a feedback mechanism. When serum calcium levels fall there is an increased secretion of *parathyroid hormone (PTH)*, which causes calcium levels to rise by several different mechanisms.

PTH causes serum calcium levels to rise by its direct action on bone and through the enzyme *cyclic adenosine monophosphate (cAMP)*. Bone resorption and release of bone calcium and phosphorus are increased. PTH stimulates cAMP production in the renal tubules, controlling renal excretion of phosphorus. PTH also mediates the conversion of 25-hydroxycholecalciferol (25-OHD_3) to 1,25-dihydroxycholecalciferol (25-OHD_3), the active vitamin D compound that controls gastrointestinal absorption of calcium.

Calcitonin, which is produced by the C cells of the thyroid, is a hypocalcemic hormone. When serum calcium levels are acutely elevated there is an increased secretion of calcitonin, which inhibits bone resorption of calcium. However, the physiologic role of calcitonin in mineral homeostasis remains unclear.

PATHOPHYSIOLOGY AND CLINICAL APPLICATION OF LABORATORY TESTS

Primary hyperparathyroidism

Primary hyperparathyroidism is characterized by excessive secretion of parathyroid hormone, usually caused by parathyroid adenomas, and less commonly by parathyroid hyperplasia. This results in disorders of calcium, phosphate, bone metabolism, and excess renal calcium excretion. The most common laboratory manifestation of hyperparathyroidism is *hypercalcemia;* the serum *phosphorus* is usually low but may be normal, and *hypercalciuria* is common.

Secondary hyperparathyroidism

Secondary hyperparathyroidism results from chronic hypocalcemia, usually secondary to vitamin D deficiency or renal disease. Vitamin D deficiency results in decreased intestinal absorption of *calcium* and *phosphate* with associated hypocalcemia and hypophosphatemia. Hypocalcemia stimulates PTH secretion, which in turn increases the calcium level toward normal while it decreases the phosphorous level more.

Hypoparathyroidism

Hypoparathyroidism is usually the inadvertent result of thyroidectomy, but rarely it may be due to autoimmune disease or may be idiopathic. *PTH* and *calcium* levels decrease while *phosphorous* levels increase.

Pseudohypoparathyroidism

Pseudohypoparathyroidism is a rare genetic disorder with end-organ (kidney and bone) resistance to the action of PTH. As with hypoparathyroidism, *calcium* levels decrease and *phosphorous* levels increase. However, unlike hypoparathyroidism, the *PTH* level is elevated.

PARATHYROID FUNCTION TESTS

Parathyroid function is evaluated first of all with the measurement of serum calcium and serum phosphorus (pp 17 and 37), and PTH. Other tests include acid-base balance and renal and gastrointestinal function.

PARATHYROID HORMONE (PTH) ASSAY

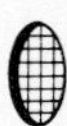

Reference range

<25 pg/ml (SI units:<2.94 pmol/L)

EXPLANATION OF THE TEST

PTH is measured by radioimmunoassay. Once secreted by the parathyroid gland, PTH is metabolized into several fragments, among which are N-terminal, C-terminal, and midregion groups; the radioimmunoassay antisera (anti-N, anti-C, and anti-M) react with these groups, allowing them to be measured directly. Serum calcium is usually done concurrently with the PTH.

VALUE AND LIMITATIONS OF THE TEST

When compared to serum calcium levels, PTH levels differentiate between the hypercalcemia caused by neoplasm or other causes and that caused by primary hyperparathyroidism.

N-terminal antisera measures the fragments with a short half-life and thus evaluates acute changes in PTH secretion. It is more useful than C-terminal assay in measuring PTH from the neck vein. It is also more reliable in assessing PTH secretion in patients with renal insufficiency.

C-terminal antisera measures the chronic changes in PTH secretion.

Anti-M sera is similar in its results to C-terminal antisera, although each detects different molecular fragments.

NURSING ACTION

1. Inform the patient that there are no dietary restrictions before the test.
2. Withdraw 7 ml of venous blood into a red-top tube.

CLINICAL IMPLICATIONS

Clinical implications will not be divided into anti-N, anti-C, and anti-M antisera since the clinical results differ among laboratories.

Normal to high levels

X-linked familial hypophosphatemic rickets (defect in renal phosphate reabsorption and intestinal phosphate absorption; may also occur with magnesium deficiency)

Increased levels

Primary hyperparathyroidism. There is substantial overlap in the PTH values of patients with primary hyperparathyroidism in which theoretically serum PTH should be increased, and those with hypercalcemia of other causes, in which PTH should be decreased. This limitation can be overcome if individual laboratories construct a nomogram for each PTH antiserum, correlating serum PTH and calcium values with the calcium values from patients with surgically proven primary hyperparathyroidism.

Pseudohypoparathyroidism (nonresponse of kidney and bone to PTH). Calcium is low, phosphorus high.

Secondary hyperparathyroidism (severe renal disease and failure of 1, 25-dihydroxycholecalciferol [25-OHD_3] formation). Calcium low, phosphorus high, and 25-OHD_3 low.

Vitamin D deficiency (dietary malabsorption). Both calcium and phosphorus low.

Severe liver disease causing decreased 25-hydroxycholecalciferol formation. Calcium, phosphorus, and 25-OHD_3 low.

Type I vitamin D–dependent rickets (pseudo–vitamin D deficiency; caused by decreased renal α_1-hydroxylase enzyme)

Type II vitamin D–dependent rickets with alopecia (bone nonresponsive to calcitriol)

Decreased levels

Ectopic PTH secretion by tumors (lung, renal cell, pancreas)

Primary hypoparathyroidism. The diagnosis of hypoparathyroidism is usually made when a patient presents with neuromuscular symptoms of hypocalcemia and is then found to be hypocalcemic and hyperphosphatemic with normal renal function. If, in spite of the stimulus of the hypocalcemia, no PTH is found by radioimmunoassay, hypoparathyroidism is the most likely diagnosis. If, however, high concentrations of PTH are detected by radioimmunoassay, a diagnosis of pseudohypoparathyroidism is strongly suggested.

Nonparathyroid hypercalcemia (sarcoidosis, hypervitaminosis A or D, acute alkali syndrome)

CHLORIDE-PHOSPHATE RATIO (C/P)

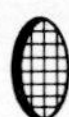

Reference range

30:1

EXPLANATION OF THE TEST

The serum chloride value (mEq/L) is divided by serum phosphorous value (mg/dl).

VALUE AND LIMITATIONS OF THE TEST

Helps to differentiate primary hyperparathyroidism from hypercalcemia resulting from other causes
Not useful when serum calcium is normal
Not useful in significant renal failure
Produces false results in ectopic PTH syndrome
Some reports of overlap between the hypercalcemia of primary hyperparathyroidism and that from other causes.

CLINICAL IMPLICATIONS

In primary hyperparathyroidism the C/P ratio is less than 33.

URINE ADENOSINE 3′,5′-MONOPHOSPHATE ASSAY (CYCLIC AMP OR cAMP)

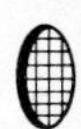

EXPLANATION OF THE TEST

PTH causes cyclic adenosine monophosphate (cAMP) to be produced in the renal tubules. cAMP mediates the conversion of 25-*hydroxycholecalciferol to 125-dihidroxycholecalciferol,* which causes increased renal reabsorption and gastrointestinal tract absorption of calcium, as well as enhancing release of calcium from bone, increasing serum calcium levels. Serum calcium and creatinine values are determined at the end of the collection period. The results are expressed as a function of glomerular filtration (GF) rate (nanomoles/dl GF), using the urine cAMP, urine creatinine, and serum creatinine to calculate the results.

VALUE AND LIMITATIONS OF THE TEST

Used to differentiate primary hyperparathyroidism from pseudohypoparathyroidism
Not useful to detect renal failure
Little data on cAMP levels in metastatic tumor to bone

NURSING ACTION

1. Inform the patient that there are no dietary restrictions before this test.
2. The urine must be collected in acid solution. Make certain that the appropriate preservative is in the collection bottle.

CLINICAL IMPLICATIONS

Increased levels

Primary hyperparathyroidism (in approximately 70% of patients); hypercalcemia and hypercalciuria complete the clinical picture.

Decreased or normal levels

Hypercalcemia from other causes.

Normal levels following injection of PTH

Pseudohypoparathyroidism

Increased levels following injection of PTH

Normal, idiopathic, or postsurgical hypoparathyroidism

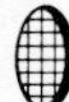

GLUCOCORTICOID SUPPRESSION

EXPLANATION OF THE TEST

A large dose of corticosteroids (100 to 200 mg hydrocortisone daily) is administered for 7 to 10 days and its effect on the serum calcium level is evaluated.

VALUE OF THE TEST

Generally replaced by the PTH assay, but sometimes useful in evaluation of sarcoidosis or vitamin A or D intoxication

Helps differentiate primary hyperparathyroidism from other causes of hypercalcemia (sarcoidosis, hypervitaminosis A or D, multiple myeloma)

CLINICAL IMPLICATIONS

Patients with primary hyperparathyroidism rarely suppress serum calcium with steroid administration, whereas patients with sarcoidosis, hypervitaminosis A and D, or hematologic malignancies generally show a reduction to normal serum calcium.

THE ADRENAL GLANDS

ANATOMY AND PHYSIOLOGY

The adrenal glands are located on the upper poles of the kidneys. Each gland is composed of two distinct parts, the medullary or inner portion and the cortical or outer portion (Fig. 9-7). The adrenal medulla secretes catecholamines (epinephrine and norepinephrine) and is a part of the sympathetic nervous system. It differs from other ganglia of the sympathetic nervous system because it secretes more epinephrine (adrenaline) than norepinephrine, and it secretes its hormones directly into the bloodstream, classifying it as an endocrine organ. The adrenal cortex secretes the steroid hormones.

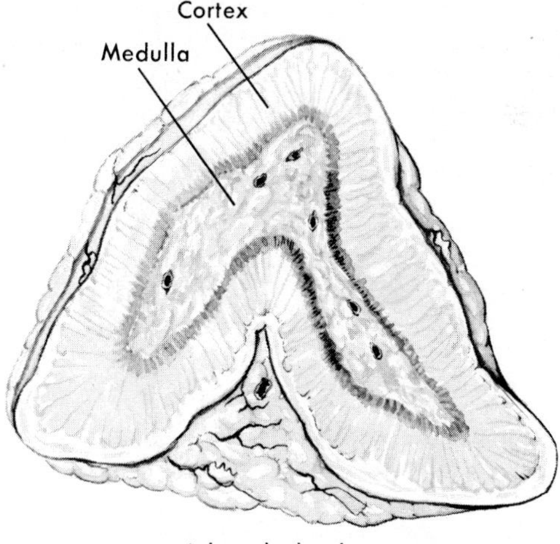

Fig. 9-7. *The adrenal gland. (From Schottelius, B.A., and Schottelius, D.D.: Textbook of physiology, ed. 18, St. Louis, 1978, The C.V. Mosby Co.)*

The adrenocortical hormones

The steroid hormones of the adrenal cortex and their physiologic effects (Fig. 9-8) are as follows:

1. The glucocorticoids *cortisol* and *corticosterone*, which affect metabolism of proteins, carbohydrates, and lipids
2. The mineralocorticoid *aldosterone*, which predominantly affects sodium and potassium excretion
3. The sex steroids, *androgens* and *estrogens*, which primarily affect secondary sex characteristics

Cortisol, most of which is bound to globulin and albumin, represents 75% to 90% of the plasma corticoids, and its plasma level usually parallels the total corticoid level. Less than 5% of circulating cortisol is free and physiologically active. The free cortisol is filterable by the renal glomerulus, and its level in the plasma regulates ad-

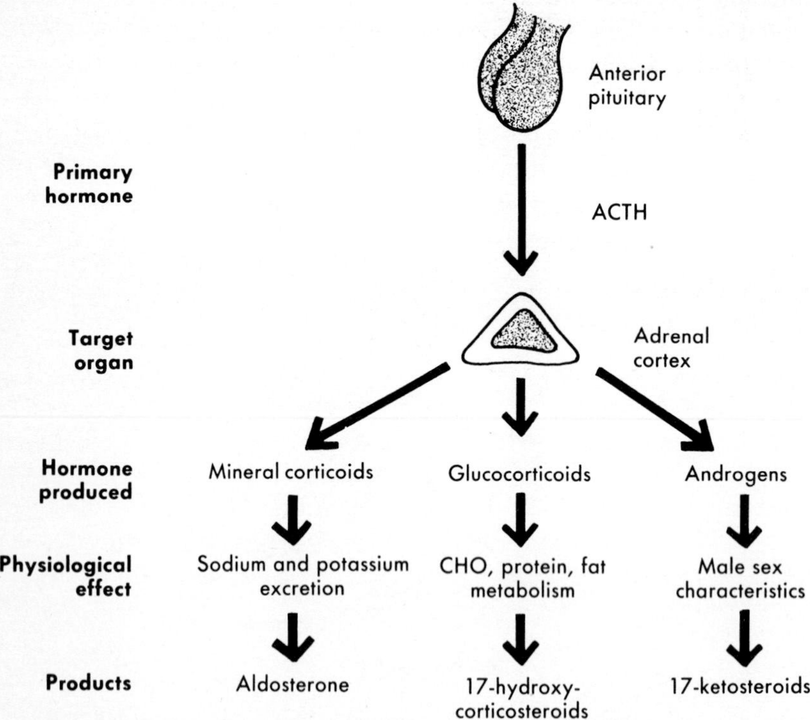

Fig. 9-8. *The steroid hormones of the adrenal cortex, their physiologic effects and products.*

renocorticotropic hormone (ACTH) release. If cortisol levels are reduced, such as in the adrenogenital syndromes, the secretion of ACTH is increased and the levels of total corticoids and deoxycorticoids increase.

Aldosterone (see also Chapter 7) is the chief electrolyte-regulating hormone of the adrenal gland and the most potent of the mineralocorticoids. The kidneys require aldosterone for the normal reabsorption of sodium and chloride, which leads to a loss of potassium and hydrogen. Normally, an increase in total body sodium triggers a decrease in the rate of aldosterone secretion, causing the kidneys to lose large quantities of sodium until the total body sodium level returns to normal. If the total body sodium level falls below normal or if serum potassium levels rise, the rate of aldosterone secretion increases so that sodium is retained and potassium lost.

Aldosterone is also important in the maintenance of blood pressure and blood volume. Aldosterone secretion is believed to be regulated primarily by the hormone renin, which is secreted by the kidney cells in hypovolemic or hyponatremic states, and by stimulation of sympathetic outflow to the kidney.

The carbon atoms on the basic steroid nucleus are numbered in sequence from 1 to 17. The steroids derived from this basic nucleus are of two structural types, the C-19 steroids and the C-21 steroids.

The C-19 steroids have predominantly androgenic activity and carry methyl groups at positions C-18 and C-10. If there is also a ketone group at the C-17 position, they are called *17-ketosteroids (17-KS)*.

The C-21 steroids have predominantly glucocorticoid or mineralocorticoid properties. These steroids have two carbon side chains (C-20 and C-21) attached at position 17 of the molecule. There are also methyl groups at C-18 and C-19. The C-21 steroids that also possess a hydroxyl group at position 17 of the steroid nucleus are called *17-hydroxycorticosteroids (17-OHCS)* or *17-hydroxycorticoids*.

Adrenocorticotropic hormone (ACTH)

The role of the anterior pituitary gland in adrenocortical secretion is shown in Fig. 9-9. Adrenocorticotropic hormone is stored in and

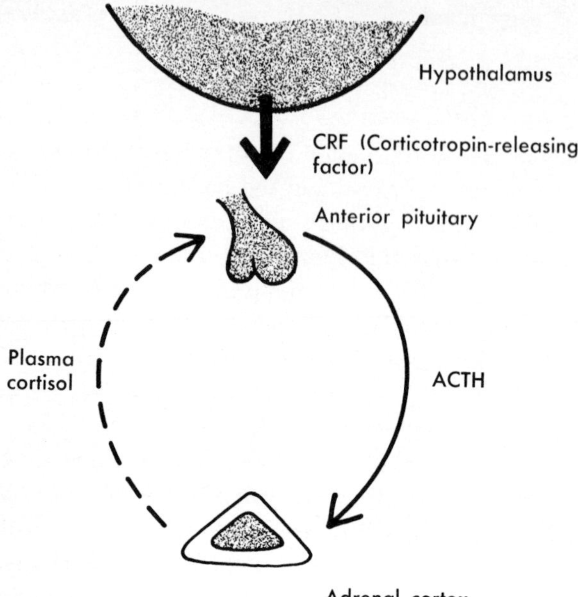

Fig. 9-9. *The roles of the hypothalamus and the anterior pituitary gland in adrenocortical secretion.*

released from the anterior pituitary gland. The release of stored ACTH is governed by a corticotropin releasing factor (CRF) in the hypothalamus, which in turn is governed by plasma cortisol levels, stress, and the sleep-wake cycle. The plasma ACTH level roughly follows a diurnal pattern, being highest just before waking and lowest just before retiring. In certain types of stress (emotional trauma, surgery, pyrogens) the ACTH levels rise. However, the circulating cortisol is the principal regulator of ACTH and CRF release. This is a negative feedback mechanism (Fig. 9-7): a low plasma cortisol level causes an increase in the rate of release of CRF; a high plasma cortisol level causes a decrease in the rate of release of CRF. A low plasma cortisol level increases the responsiveness of the anterior pituitary adrenocorticotropic cells to CRF. Thus a smaller amount of CRF, in the absence of cortisol, will cause an inappropriate increase in the secretion of ACTH.

PATHOPHYSIOLOGY AND CLINICAL APPLICATION OF LABORATORY TESTS

Cushing's syndrome

Cushing's syndrome is caused by increased production of cortisol by the adrenal gland, owing to bilateral adrenal hyperplasia (Cushing's disease) secondary to hypersecretion of pituitary ACTH (80%), an adrenal adenoma or carcinoma (15%), or ectopic ACTH production (5%). Pituitary ACTH overproduction may in turn be secondary to either pituitary-hypothalamic dysfunction or pituitary microadenomas or macroadenomas that produce ACTH. Ectopic ACTH-producing tumors may be oat cell bronchogenic carcinoma, thymoma, pancreatic islet tumors, bronchial adenoma, carcinoid, or medullary thyroid carcinoma.

The most frequently used tests to screen for Cushing's syndrome are the *overnight dexamethasone suppression test* or the 24-hour *urine free cortisol test*. Tests useful to differentiate the various causes of primary hyperadrenalism are the *standard dexamethasone suppression test*, serum *ACTH assay*, and *computerized tomography* of the adrenals.

Laboratory findings are increased plasma *cortisol*, urinary *17-OHCS*, and *free cortisol*. There may also be hyperglycemia, hypokalemia, hypochloremia, metabolic alkalosis, leukocytosis and, on x-ray examination, osteoporosis.

Primary aldosteronism

Primary aldosteronism (Conn's syndrome) results from the overproduction of aldosterone, caused by an aldosterone-secreting adenoma, adrenal hyperplasia (including bilateral nodular hyperplasia and glucocorticoid-suppressible aldosteronism), or rarely adrenal carcinoma.

The diagnosis is suspected because of diastolic hypertension, hypokalemia, absence of edema, and low *plasma renin activity*, which does not increase during volume depletion (upright posture, sodium depletion). Elevated 24-hour *urinary aldosterone* excretion that does not decrease during volume expansion (salt loading) confirms the diagnosis in this clinical setting. Once the diagnosis of primary aldosteronism is established by these tests, the adenoma is located by *CT scan* or by bilateral adrenal vein catheterization, to measure *plasma aldosterone* concentrations, and to perform *adrenal venography*.

Adrenocortical insufficiency

Adrenocortical insufficiency may be primary or secondary. Primary insufficiency (Addison's disease) results from progressive bilateral adrenocortical destruction; secondary insufficiency is the result of pituitary ACTH deficiency.

Clinical signs of Addison's disease may not appear until more than 90% of the adrenal cortex is destroyed bilaterally. The definitive diagnosis is made by evaluating adrenal reserve capacity for steroid production (*ACTH stimulation test, metyrapone stimulation test*, or *insulin-induced hypoglycemia test*). If the adrenal insufficiency is severe, 24-hour *urine cortisol, 17-OHCS*, and *17-KS* are low or absent.

Pheochromocytoma

Pheochromocytoma is a catecholamine-producing tumor most commonly located in the adrenal medulla. It releases abnormally large amounts of catecholamines into the circulation, causing hypertension and marked vasomotor changes. A small percentage of the excess catecholamines is excreted unchanged in the urine. Some of the adrenal medullary hormones appear in the urine as metanephrine or vanillylmandelic acid (VMA), metabolic by-products of catecholamine degradation.

A complete workup for a patient with a possible pheochromocytoma includes a *24-hour urine collection* with determinations of levels of VMA, catecholamines, and metanephrine, any one of which might be elevated in a given case of pheochromocytoma. *Computerized tomography* generally localizes the tumor; however, occasionally venography or arteriography is necessary for localization.

ADRENAL FUNCTION TESTS

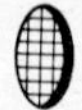

PLASMA CORTISOL

Adult reference range

8 AM: 8-19 μg/dl (SI units: 0.22-0.52 μmol/L)

4 PM: 4-11 μg/dl (SI units: 0.11-0.30 μmol/L)

Pediatric reference range

8 AM: 3-21 μg/dl (SI units: 0.08-0.69 μmol/L)
4 PM: 5-10 μg/dl (SI units: 0.14-0.28 μmol/L)

EXPLANATION OF THE TEST

Plasma cortisol levels are evaluated by radioimmunoassay. The test is ordered for patients with suspected adrenal dysfunction; however, the definitive diagnosis is made with stimulation and suppression tests.

Cortisol is released from the adrenal cortex in response to ACTH stimulation. This potent glucocorticoid affects the metabolism of carbohydrates, protein, and lipids; is an antiinflammatory agent; maintains blood pressure; inhibits the action of insulin; and stimulates gluconeogenesis in the liver. Normally, plasma cortisol levels are higher in the morning and lower in the evening, with the lowest values about 11 PM. Normally the evening value is less than 50% of the morning value. Single determinations are not reliable for screening for Cushing's syndrome.

Total cortisol is measured by three basic assay techniques: competitive protein-binding assay, radioimmunoassay, and fluorimetric assay. For correct interpretation of results in some clinical situations (such as the metyrapone test and congenital adrenal hyperplasia), it is important to know which method is being used to measure cortisol levels.

The competitive protein-binding assay measures cortisol, cortisone, compound S, progesterone, and 17-hydroxyprogesterone. The fluorescent procedure measures cortisone and compound S. Radioimmunoassay is almost completely specific for cortisol.

VALUE AND LIMITATIONS OF THE TEST

The clinical value of this test is limited because of the manner in which the hormone is secreted—episodically.

The fluorescent procedure is faster and requires less blood than the competitive protein-binding assay.

Various medications may interfere with the fluorescence assay.

Radioimmunoassay requires small volumes of blood and is not interfered with by other medications.

All techniques used measure total blood cortisol; bound and free plasma cortisol levels are thus falsely increased if the patient is pregnant or taking estrogens for birth control. In such cases, a urine free cortisol assay will reflect the blood levels of unbound cortisol.

NURSING ACTION

1. Inform the patient that there are no dietary restrictions before the test.
2. The patient should be relaxed and recumbent for 30 minutes before the test.
3. It is important to note the time of sample drawing, since cortisol has a diurnal rhythm.

INTERFERING FACTORS

Ketosis
Various drugs (estrogens, steroid therapy)
Marked decrease in serum albumin level and cortisol-binding globulin
Stress
Severe depression or psychiatric disease
Obesity
Severe hepatic or renal disease
Increased androgens
Pregnancy
Various medications (spironolactone, niacin, quinidine, and heparin) may interfere with the fluorescence assay.

CLINICAL IMPLICATIONS

Because so many factors alter the diurnal pattern of cortisol secretion, a normal circadian rhythm is probably more significant than is an abnormal one. In Cushing's syndrome diurnal variation is absent in approximately 90% of patients. Although a single determination may be misleading, a definite reversal in the diurnal variation may help in the diagnosis of an adrenal disorder.

Increased levels

Adrenocortical hyperfunction (Cushing's syndrome)
Carcinoma of the adrenal gland
Benign adenomas of the adrenal cortex

Stress
Pregnancy
Obesity
Acute myocardial infarction or other major illness
Acute alcoholic intoxication
Diabetic acidosis
Hyperthyroidism
Severe depression or psychiatric disease

Decreased levels

Anterior pituitary hypofunction (ACTH deficiency)
Adrenal cortical hypofunction (Addison's disease)
Hypothyroidism

URINE FREE CORTISOL

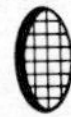

Adult reference range

24-108 μg/24 hr

EXPLANATION OF THE TEST

This test measures the level of active urinary free cortisol by radioimmunoassay. Its level in the urine correlates well with the level of circulating free cortisol.

VALUE OF THE TEST

A sensitive test for the diagnosis of adrenocortical hyperfunction
Especially useful in evaluating obese individuals (the serum cortisol may be lower as a result of decreased cortisol-binding globulins and the urinary 17-hydroxycorticosteroids may be elevated)
The determination of urinary free cortisol is more useful in the diagnosis of adrenal hyperfunction than are random plasma cortisol determinations.

NURSING ACTION

1. Inform the patient that there are no dietary restrictions before and during the collection of the specimen.
2. Collect an accurate 24-hour urine specimen.

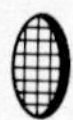

URINARY ASSAY OF 17-HYDROXYCORTICOSTEROIDS (17-OHCS) AND 17-KETOSTEROIDS (17-KS)

Reference range 17-KS/24 hr urine

Adult male: 10-25 mg (SI units: 6-14 mg)
Adult female: 35-88 μmol/day (SI units: 23-49 μmol/24 hr)

Reference range 17-OHCS/24 hr urine

Adult male: 3-6 mg/24 hr (SI units: 2-6 mg/24 hr)
Adult female: 10-35 μmol/day (SI units: 7-21 μmol/day)
(as tetrahydrocortisol)

Normal response to IM injection of 25 USP units ACTH

17-OHCS and 17-KS increase 200% to 400% the day of injection and return to normal in the next 24 hours.

EXPLANATION OF THE TEST

These tests measure urine levels of 17-OHCS and 17-KS. The urinary concentration of 17-OHCS is an indirect indicator of the secretory rate of cortisol. 17-KS measures primarily androgen by-products secreted by the adrenal glands and the testes and aids in the diagnosis of adrenal and gonadal dysfunction.

VALUE AND LIMITATIONS OF THE TEST

Urine assays of 17-OHCS and 17-KS assay are not considered reliable enough to screen for Cushing's syndrome because of many false positives, false negatives, and interfering factors. However, if a patient is hospitalized for a definitive dexamethasone suppression test, prolonged ACTH infusion, or metyrapone stimulation, the 24-hour urinary excretion of 17-OHCS and 17-KS is determined in response to suppression or stimulation.

NURSING ACTION

1. Inform the patient that there are no dietary restrictions, except for coffee, during and before the collection of the specimen.
2. Collect urine in a 24-hour specimen bottle that is kept refrigerated or on ice during collection. In lieu of refrigeration or icing the

bottle, a preservative may be added to the bottle before collection of the specimen.

3. Three days before the test withhold drugs that may interfere with results (meprobamate, chlorpromazine and related drugs). If drugs are not withheld, inform the laboratory.

CLINICAL IMPLICATIONS

Elevated levels

Cushing's syndrome
Extreme stress
Adrenal cancer
Eclampsia
Hyperpituitarism
Hyperthyroidism
Obesity

Decreased levels

Addison's disease
Androgenital syndrome
Hypopituitarism
Myxedema

SERUM ACTH

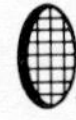

Reference range

15-70 pg/ml (SI units: 3.3-15.4 pmol/L)

EXPLANATION OF THE TEST

Plasma adrenocorticotropic hormone (ACTH) level is determined by radioimmunoassay in reference laboratories. ACTH is produced and secreted by the anterior pituitary gland, being regulated by the blood levels of cortisol. When plasma cortisol levels are too high, pituitary production of ACTH is inhibited. When plasma cortisol levels are low, pituitary production of ACTH is increased. There is a diurnal variation in serum ACTH level parallel to cortisol secretion. Highest levels are between 8 and 10 AM, lowest near midnight.

VALUE AND LIMITATIONS OF THE TEST

Useful in differentiating primary from secondary adrenal insufficiency

Useful in differentiating Cushing's syndrome secondary to a pituitary adenoma from adrenal adenoma or carcinoma and ectopic ACTH syndrome

The assay technique for measuring serum ACTH is difficult and is performed only in reference laboratories.

NURSING ACTION

Note that ACTH is inactivated at room temperature and adheres to glass; thus, careful collection is essential. The specimen is collected in a plastic, heparinized test tube on ice and immediately spun in a refrigerated centrifuge and frozen until the assay is run.

INTERFERING FACTORS

Stress and other factors affecting cortisol secretion may eliminate diurnal variation of ACTH.

CLINICAL IMPLICATIONS

Primary versus secondary adrenal insufficiency. Both are characterized by low cortisol concentrations. However, the serum ACTH level is high in primary adrenal insufficiency (Addison's disease) and low or normal in secondary adrenal insufficiency.

Cushing's syndrome. In Cushing's syndrome secondary to a pituitary adenoma, serum ACTH is normal to slightly elevated. In adrenal adenoma or carcinoma, ACTH levels are suppressed and in ectopic ACTH syndrome, they are markedly elevated. In Cushing's syndrome caused by adrenal tumor, the cortisol produced by the tumor suppresses the pituitary production of ACTH; diurnal variation is absent.

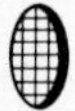

SINGLE-DOSE DEXAMETHASONE SUPPRESSION TEST (ACTH SUPPRESSION TEST)

Adult reference range

Following an 11 PM oral dose of 1 mg dexamethasone (Decadron), cortisol production is suppressed and the normal 8 AM peak of plasma cortisol does not occur (serum cortisol <5 μg/dl (SI units: 138 nmol/L).

EXPLANATION OF THE TEST

This test documents cortisol hypersecretion. In normal individuals dexamethasone, a cortisone analog that is about 30 times more potent than cortisone, suppresses pituitary ACTH release, which in turn suppresses the release of the adrenocortical hormone cortisol. Dexamethasone is used because it does not interfere in the measurement of serum cortisol or its urinary metabolites. There is failure to suppress cortisol secretion in more than 95% of Cushing's syndrome patients.

VALUE AND LIMITATIONS OF THE TEST

This is an accurate and simple screening test for Cushing's syndrome. It may produce false-positive results in obese persons (about 13%), in the chronically ill (25%), and in severely depressed patients.

NURSING ACTION

1. Inform the patient that there are no dietary restrictions before this test and that he or she should have a good night's sleep after taking the dexamethasone.
2. At 11 PM the patient takes 1 mg of dexamethasone.
3. At 8 AM collect 5 to 10 ml of venous blood in a heparinized tube for cortisol.

INTERFERING FACTORS

Hyperthyroidism
Acromegaly
Estrogens
Phenytoin, phenobarbital
Certain psychiatric medications
Obesity
Chronic illness
Stress
Psychiatric depression
Acute and substantial alcohol intake
Malnutrition

CLINICAL IMPLICATIONS

A negative response (serum cortisol less than 5 μg/dl) rules out Cushing's syndrome in most cases.

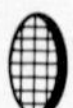

STANDARD DEXAMETHASONE SUPPRESSION TEST (LOW-DOSE AND HIGH-DOSE TESTS)

Low-dose test reference range

Urinary 17-OHCS is suppressed to <4 mg/24 hr (SI units: 8.3 μmoles/dl).
Urinary free cortisol is suppressed to <20 μg (SI units: 552 nmol/24 hr).

High-dose test reference range

Following larger doses (8 mg/day) of dexamethasone, urine 17-OHCS is significantly depressed (usually 50% or less of basal value).

EXPLANATION OF THE TEST

The serum level of glucocorticoids (primarily cortisol) determines the amount of ACTH released from the anterior pituitary, which in turn determines the amount of steroid produced by the adrenal gland. Therefore dexamethasone, a potent glucocorticoid analog of cortisol, is given to test this feedback mechanism.

VALUE AND LIMITATIONS OF THE TEST

Confirms the diagnosis of Cushing's syndrome
Differentiates between adrenocortical hyperplasia (Cushing's disease) and other types of hypercortisolism

NURSING ACTION

1. Explain the test to the patient and inform him or her that there are no dietary restrictions for the test.
2. Before the test collect a 24-hour urine specimen for 17-OHCS and free cortisol to determine a baseline value.
3. Dexamethasone is administered as follows:
   a. For the low-dose test, dexamethasone 0.5 mg is given orally every 6 hours for 2 days and the response of urinary 17-OHCS and free cortisol and serum cortisol are measured (in Cushing's disease there is no decrease).
   b. For the high-dose test, dexamethasone 2 mg is given orally every 6 hours for 2 days, and the urine 17-OHCS and free cortisol and serum cortisol values measured. In patients with bilateral hyperplasia (Cushing's disease), this value falls to 50% or less of the baseline measurement. In patients with ade-

nomas, carcinomas, or ectopic ACTH production there is no change.

4. Discontinue all medications for 24 to 48 hours before the test.
5. Collect a 24-hour urine specimen during the 2 days of the test. This is tested for 17-OHCS and free cortisol levels. Each 24-hour urine sample should be collected in separate containers and the times and dates of each sample carefully recorded on the bottle.

CLINICAL IMPLICATIONS (LOW-DOSE TEST)

In Cushing's disease and Cushing's syndrome, the urinary 17-OHCS and free cortisol do not suppress appropriately following administration of dexamethasone 0.5 mg orally every 6 hours for 2 days.

CLINICAL IMPLICATIONS (HIGH-DOSE TEST)

There is no suppression with adrenal adenoma or carcinoma, or ectopic ACTH-producing tumor. However, patients with Cushing's disease (bilateral adrenal hyperplasia secondary to hypersecretion of pituitary ACTH) suppress adequately with the higher dose of dexamethasone. Thus, this phase of the test helps differentiate Cushing's disease from the other causes of hypercortisolism.

ACTH STIMULATION TEST

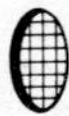

Reference range

Rapid Screening Test: Serum cortisol level is stimulated to double the baseline level or peak cortisol level is >20 μg/dl.

24-Hour Test: An increase in plasma cortisol of >40 μg/dl; urine 17-OHCS increases by at least 25 mg/24 hr.

EXPLANATION OF THE TEST

When ACTH is injected, the adrenal cortex is stimulated. In the normal person there are increased plasma cortisol and urine 17-OHCS levels the day of the injection, returning to normal within the next 24 hours.

VALUE AND LIMITATIONS OF THE TEST

The 8-hour infusion test enables differentiation between primary and secondary adrenal insufficiency.

Provides an index of the functional reserve of the adrenal gland to produce cortisol, especially in cases in which cortisol production has been suppressed because of exogenous corticoid administration
Assists in diagnosis of Addison's disease

NURSING ACTION

Rapid screening test

1. Collect venous blood in a green-top tube and send it to the laboratory for measurement of plasma cortisol level.
2. A synthetic ACTH analog (cosyntropin [Cortrosyn]) 0.25 mg is then injected intramuscularly or intravenously.
3. At 30 and 60 minutes after the injection of cosyntropin collect another blood specimen for cortisol measurement.
4. If plasma cortisol levels have not increased, a 24-hour test should be performed (see below).

8-Hour infusion test

1. Collect a 24-hour urine specimen the day before the test.
2. Check the physician's orders. Bovine ACTH may cause severe allergic reactions and is no longer used. Instead the synthetic ACTH analog is used.
3. Administer 25 units of ACTH intravenously in 500 ml of normal saline during 8 hours.
4. During the infusion and over a span of 24 hours, collect another urine specimen (to be evaluated for cortisol or 17-OHCS).

CLINICAL IMPLICATIONS

Normally, the cortisol or 17-OHCS levels are stimulated to twice baseline levels during the 8-hour infusion test. In Addison's disease there is no response. Patients with secondary adrenal insufficiency (hypothalamic or pituitary insufficiency) have an intermediate response of cortisol or 17-OHCS levels.

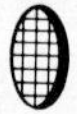

METYRAPONE TEST

Reference range (24-hour metyrapone test)

The urinary excretion of 17-hydroxycorticosteroids is stimulated to at least twice basal level (or a rise of 8 to 10 mg/24 hr).

Reference range (overnight test)

Cortisol levels <10 μg/dl and compound S levels >7 μg/dl.

EXPLANATION OF THE TEST

The metyrapone test measures the ability of the pituitary gland to correct a decrease in circulating cortisol. Metyrapone (metapyrone) blocks the conversion of compound S (11-deoxycortisol) to cortisol. With metyrapone administration, the result is a decline in cortisol level, stimulating the pituitary to secrete more ACTH in an attempt to increase the cortisol production. Since cortisol production is blocked, the precursor compound S (11-deoxycortisol) increases with ACTH stimulation. Thus, in normal persons (or those with adrenal cortex hyperplasia) urinary 17-OHCS levels sharply increase as a result of the increase in compound S. If serum cortisol and compound S are measured separately (RIA method), the ability to evaluate the status of the pituitary reserve capacity is improved. The metyrapone overnight test is a simpler outpatient procedure for assessing adrenal pituitary reserve.

VALUE OF THE TEST

Assesses pituitary adrenal reserve

NURSING ACTION (24-HOUR METYRAPONE TEST)

1. Before the test collect a 24-hour urine specimen to establish a baseline 24-hour excretion of 17-OHCS.
2. Continue collecting urine for two more 24-hour periods (during and 1 day following ingestion of metyrapone).
3. Metyrapone 500 mg is taken orally every 4 hours for 24 hours.

NURSING ACTION (OVERNIGHT TEST)

1. Metyrapone 2 to 3 g (depending on the patient's weight) is given at midnight with a snack to minimize nausea.
2. The following morning at 8 AM, blood is drawn for compound S and cortisol levels.

INTERFERING FACTORS

Chlorpromazine
Phenobarbital
Estrogens
Phenytoin (Dilantin) (overnight test)

CLINICAL IMPLICATIONS

A poor response indicates primary or secondary adrenal insufficiency.

> **NURSING ALERT**
>
> The metyrapone suppression test may occasionally induce an adrenal crisis in patients with insufficient adrenal or pituitary reserve. Patients with a high suspicion of pituitary or adrenal insufficiency should be hospitalized for the 24-hour test and observed closely for signs of postural hypotension, nausea, vomiting, tachycardia, or diaphoresis.

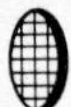

ALDOSTERONE ASSAY (PLASMA AND URINE)

Reference ranges

Urine
Excretion: 5-19 μg/24 hr (SI units, 14-53 nmol/24 hr)
Plasma (AM samples on ad lib. sodium intake)
Supine: 3-16 ng/dl (SI units, 133 ± 80 pmol/L)
Upright: (2 hr) 7-30 ng/dl (SI units 180 ± 64 pmol/L)

EXPLANATION OF THE TEST

Aldosterone is the major electrolyte-regulating steroid of the adrenal cortex. It is instrumental in sodium and potassium homeostasis and in maintenance of blood pressure. Although the production of aldosterone is stimulated by ACTH, it is not dependent on this since the renin-angiotensin system is the primary regulator of aldosterone production and secretion. Aldosterone levels are also influenced by sodium, potassium, and magnesium. Aldosterone production is decreased by high-sodium intake, hypokalemia, and licorice ingestion;

it is increased by low-sodium intake, hypomagnesemia, and hyperkalemia. Aldosterone promotes tubular reabsorption of sodium and chloride in exchange for potassium and hydrogen ions, thus maintaining blood pressure and blood volume and regulating fluid and electrolyte balance.

VALUE OF THE TEST

Aids in the diagnosis of aldosteronism

Along with plasma renin levels, distinguishes between primary and secondary aldosteronism

Aids in the diagnosis of adrenal adenoma and adrenal hyperplasia

NURSING ACTION

Serum

1. Before the patient arises in the morning (the patient must be supine for several hours before the test), withdraw venous blood in a 7-ml red-top collection tube. Draw another sample 4 hours later after the patient has been up and around and while the patient is standing.
2. If aldosterone levels are increased, monitor electrolytes and blood pressure. If low, monitor electrolytes.

Urine

1. Collect 24-hour urine specimen, refrigerating during collection.
2. If the patient has been on sodium restriction or diuretics, the physician will probably order sodium supplements (3 to 9 g/day for 4 days) to be given before beginning the collection of the 24-hour urine specimen. The sodium and creatinine content of the 24-hour urine specimen or a random specimen may be measured as a further check.

INTERFERING FACTORS

Hydralazine (Apresoline), diazoxide (Hyperstat), nitroprusside, and diuretics (furosemide) increase aldosterone secretion.

Glucose ingestion decreases aldosterone secretion.

CLINICAL IMPLICATIONS

Elevated levels of aldosterone occur in primary aldosteronism (adenoma or bilateral hyperplasia). Aldosterone levels are also secondarily increased in congestive heart failure, cirrhosis with ascites, nephrotic syndrome, or hypovolemia (sodium excretion is decreased with resultant sodium and fluid retention). This may or may not be associated with hypertension and/or hypokalemia. However, in primary or secondary aldosteronism associated with hypertension, after a steady state the urine sodium is usually high and there is urinary loss of potassium, causing hypokalemia. The reverse can occur in conditions of low aldosterone secretion. Table 9-2 lists typical renin-aldosterone patterns in various clinical conditions.

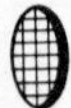

PLASMA RENIN ACTIVITY (PRA)

Reference range

Normal diet
Supine: 1.1 ± 0.8 ng/ml/hr (SI units: 0.9 ± 0.6 nmol/L/hr)
Upright: 1.9 ± 1.7 ng/ml/hr (SI units: 1.5 ± 1.3 nmol/L/hr)

Low-sodium diet
Supine: 2.7 ± 1.8 ng/ml/hr (SI units: 2.1 ± 1.4 nmol/L/hr)
Upright: 6.6 ± 2.5 ng/ml/hr (SI units: 5.1 ± 1.9 nmol/L/hr)

Table 9-2 Typical renin-aldosterone patterns

Clinical conditions	Plasma renin	Aldosterone
Primary aldosteronism	Low	High
Low-renin essential hypertension	Low	Normal
Cushing's syndrome	Low	Normal/elevated
Licorice ingestion syndrome	Low	Low
High-salt diet	Low	Low
Oral contraceptives	High	Normal
Cirrhosis	High	High
Malignant hypertension	High	High
Unilateral renal disease	High	High
High-renin essential hypertension	High	High
Pregnancy	High	High
Diuretic overuse	High	High
Juxtaglomerular tumor	High	High
Low-salt diet	High	High
Addison's disease	High	Low
Hypokalemia	High	Low

Adapted from Ravel, R.: Clinical laboratory medicine, Chicago, 1984, Year Book Medical Publishers.

Note: When renal function is normal, urinary sodium levels are related to the fluid volume and inversely related to the plasma concentration of renin.

EXPLANATION OF THE TEST

Renin is an enzyme secreted by the kidney in response to a fall in glomerular flow, a reduction in the level of sodium at the distal tubule, or sympathetic stimulation. Renin converts angiotensinogen to angiotensin I, which is in turn converted to angiotensin II, a potent vasopressor that also stimulates the adrenal cortex to release aldosterone.

VALUE AND LIMITATIONS OF THE TEST

Screens for renal origin of hypertension

Aids in the identification of primary aldosteronism

Aids in the identification of hypertension linked to unilateral renovascular disease by renal vein catheterization

Confirms the diagnosis of primary aldosteronism (sodium-depleted plasma renin test)

Renin release is influenced by many variables (posture, diuretics, sodium in diet).

Procedural differences exist among laboratories, making comparison of results impossible.

Commercially available kits vary in their results on the same plasma sample.

NURSING ACTION (SUGGESTED PROTOCOL)

High-sodium diet—recumbent position

1. A high-sodium diet is ordered for 4 days and medications are withheld.
2. The morning of the fourth day blood is drawn for plasma renin activity and aldosterone and a 24-hour urine specimen is collected for aldosterone and sodium assays.
3. The patient should remain recumbent before and during the withdrawal of blood; plasma renin activity is increased by upright posture among other things.
4. Remove the tourniquet before drawing the blood sample, since stasis may lower renin level.
5. Collect 5 to 7 ml of venous blood in a cold tube without heparin

The six known hormones secreted by the anterior lobe of the pituitary gland are:

1. Growth hormone (GH), which has a general effect on growth
2. Prolactin, which controls the secretion of milk by the mammary glands
3. Thyroid-stimulating hormone (TSH), which stimulates the formation and release of thyroid hormones
4. Adrenocorticotropic hormone (ACTH), which controls the secretion of the adrenal cortex
5. Luteinizing hormone (LH), which initiates ovulation and luteinization in the ovary and testosterone production and secretion in the testes
6. Follicle-stimulating hormone (FSH), which stimulates estrogen secretion and the growth of the graafian follicle in women and spermatogenesis in men

The releasing factors secreted by the hypothalamus are as follows: corticotropin releasing factor (CRF), gonadotropin releasing factor (GRF), thyrotropin releasing hormone (TRH), and growth hormone releasing factor (GHRF). In addition, three known inhibiting factors are secreted by the hypothalamus: prolactin inhibiting factor, melanocyte inhibiting factor, and growth hormone inhibiting factor (somatostatin).

The releasing factors stimulate the synthesis and release of the specific pituitary hormones. These factors reach the pituitary gland by way of the hypothalamic-pituitary venous plexus. The pituitary hormones ACTH, FSH, LH, and TSH are also controlled by a negative feedback loop, in which the concentration of the circulating hormone secreted from the target gland suppresses the elaboration of the corresponding pituitary hormone.

The posterior pituitary hormones are vasopressin (antidiuretic hormone, ADH) and oxytocin; both are manufactured in the hypothalamus and stored in and released from the posterior pituitary gland.

Vasopressin and oxytocin are synthesized in the hypothalamus and reach the posterior pituitary for storage by traveling along the supraopticohypophyseal tract (Fig. 9-10). Vasopressin is stored bound to a protein (neurophysine); both are released into the circulation mainly in response to serum osmolality. Some of the stimulators of ADH release are dehydration, saline infusion, isomolar injection of carbohydrate solutions, decrease in plasma volume or blood pressure, pain, stress, sleep, exercise, and certain drugs (nicotine, morphine,

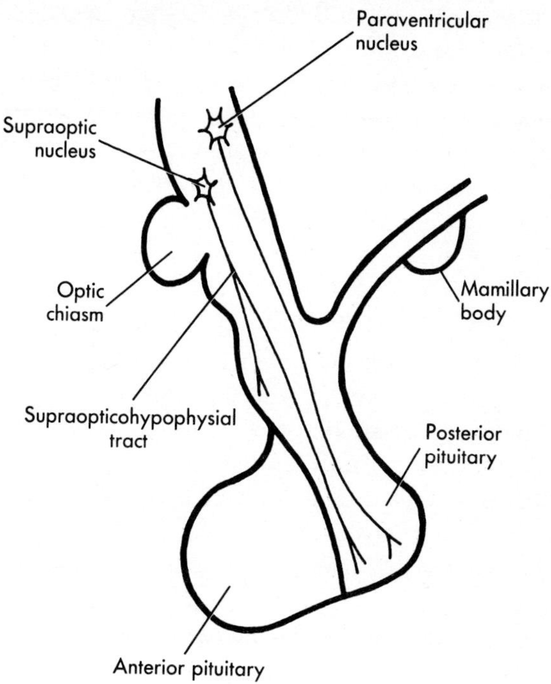

Fig. 9-10. *Posterior pituitary gland and the supraopticohypophyseal tract. Vasopressin and oxytocin, synthesized in the hypothalamus, travel along the supraopticohypophyseal tract to be stored in the posterior pituitary.*

and barbiturates). The following are some of the inhibitors of ADH release: increase in plasma volume, hypoosmolality, exposure to cold, alcohol, and some drugs (phenytoin and glucocorticoids).

ADH stimulates water reabsorption by the distal tubules and collecting ducts. This major physiologic effect determines the final concentration of urine. In the presence of ADH more water is reabsorbed, resulting in concentrated urine; in the absence of ADH less water is reabsorbed, resulting in dilute urine.

PATHOPHYSIOLOGY AND CLINICAL APPLICATION OF LABORATORY TESTS

Pituitary insufficiency

Deficiencies of anterior pituitary hormones may result from pituitary tumors, hypothalamic disorders, and idiopathic or congenital deficiencies of a single or many hormones, vascular problems such as occlusion, aneurysm, vasculitis, or postpartum necrosis (Sheehan's syndrome), infections, surgery, trauma, and autoimmune or idiopathic disorders. Diagnostic laboratory tests will differentiate between problems with the hypothalamic-pituitary system and end organs. Evaluation consists in various suppression and stimulation tests such as the *metyrapone test* and *thyrotropin releasing hormone test* (pp. 362 and 333), and tests evaluating pituitary gonadotropins and hypothalamic function.

Growth hormone (GH) deficiency

Growth hormone (GH) deficiency is suspected when a child fails to grow appropriately. Not only is the growth hormone from the anterior pituitary necessary for normal growth, but also insulin, thyroxine, testosterone, estrogens, somatomedins, and good nutrition are essential for adequate growth. GH is stimulated by sleep, exercise, stress, and hypoglycemia. Provocative tests are generally necessary to evaluate GH deficiency and to assess growth hormone reserve.

Many provocative tests have been developed to test GH release. The simplest one is to have the fasting patient *exercise* before drawing a blood sample. A GH level of greater than 6 ng/ml is normal. Other stimulation tests are *insulin-induced hypoglycemia, arginine infusion,* and ingestion of *levodopa* (L-*dopa*), *or propranolol*. Other recommended tests for suspected growth disorders are *hand-wrist x-ray study,* and *somatomedin-C assay*.

Hyperprolactinemia

Prolactin normally stimulates lactation in females. Prolactin levels are elevated in patients with prolactin-secreting microadenomas or macroadenomas (prolactinomas), in 20% of patients with postpubertal amenorrhea, and occasionally in cases of male infertility. Various medications can also increase prolactin levels (phenothiazianes, cimetidine, haloperidol, estrogens, morphine). The laboratory diagnosis of prolactinomas is made with evaluation of *basal prolactin levels* and pituitary *CT scanning*.

Growth hormone excess

An excess of GH is usually due to a pituitary eosinophilic adenoma. If this occurs before the epiphyses have sealed it results in gigantism; after epiphyseal fusion it results in acromegaly.

The laboratory diagnosis of acromegaly is made by the finding of *elevated GH levels,* sometimes measured after a suppression test such as the *glucose tolerance test* and/or after administration of *TRH*. An elevated *plasma somatomedin-C* level (RIA) may confirm the diagnosis.

Diabetes insipidus

Diabetes insipidus is characterized by the production of large quantities of urine caused by (1) deficient vasopressin (ADH) release (central type) in response to normal physiologic stimuli, (2) the abnormal response of the renal tubules to the action of vasopressin (nephrogenic type), or (3) reaction to a drug or drugs.

Vasopressin is responsible for the reabsorption of water from the distal tubules. When it is absent or when the renal tubules do not respond to its presence, there is a massive polyuria, with urine production sometimes approaching 15 to 20 L per day. After several hours of water deprivation, the patient with diabetes insipidus is unable to concentrate urine. In central diabetes insipidus (deficient ADH), the renal response to ADH is normal. Thus the individual will respond to an injection of ADH with a decrease in urine output.

PITUITARY FUNCTION TESTS

The tests for thyroid stimulating hormone (TSH), adrenocorticotropic hormone (ACTH), the metyrapone test, and thyrotropin releasing hormone (TRH) test have already been discussed.

GROWTH HORMONE (GH) (SERUM)

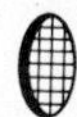

Adult reference range

<0.7-5 ng/ml (SI units: <233 pmol/L)

Note: GH is low to nondetectable in unstressed individuals; increases occur during sleep (especially during the first 2 hours) and exercise, postprandially, and during major surgery or stress.

EXPLANATION OF THE TEST

Serum growth hormone (somatotropin) is measured by radioimmunoassay. In patients with low or normal GH values a GH stimulation test should be performed to rule out deficiency.

VALUE AND LIMITATIONS OF THE TEST

Aids in the differential diagnosis of dwarfism or delayed growth
Confirms the diagnosis of acromegaly and gigantism
Aids in the diagnosis of pituitary or hypothalamic disease
Low values may be seen in normal persons or in patients with GH deficiency.

NURSING ACTION

1. Explain to the patient that this test helps to evaluate growth patterns.
2. Instruct the patient to fast overnight and to limit physical activity for 10 to 12 hours before the test.
3. Inform the patient that a fasting blood specimen is collected before he or she arises.
4. Screening tests include:
   a. Withdrawing the blood sample (7 ml of venous blood into a red-top tube) 60 to 90 minutes after the onset of deep sleep; this is when the highest levels of GH are secreted.
   b. Withdrawing the blood sample 20 to 30 minutes after the end of a vigorous 20 to 30 minutes of exercise.

CLINICAL IMPLICATIONS

Increased levels

Gigantism and acromegaly (increased levels cause gigantism in children and acromegaly in adults and adolescents and may indicate a pituitary or hypothalamic tumor, usually an adenoma)
Diabetes mellitus (patient may have increased GH levels without acromegaly; suppression testing determines the cause of the increased GH)
Anorexia nervosa (may have elevated levels)

Decreased levels

Pituitary insufficiency
Pituitary tumors (other than GH-secreting tumors)
Dwarfism (may be caused by low GH levels; a definitive diagnosis is made with stimulation testing with arginine or insulin)

INSULIN TOLERANCE TEST

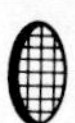

Reference range

A 50% reduction from the basal glucose level should be enough to cause a 10 to 20 ng/ml increase of GH and an increase of 10 μg/dl (a value equal to or more than 20 μg/dl) of cortisol, with peak levels at 60 to 90 minutes after the administration of insulin.

EXPLANATION OF THE TEST

Just as growth hormone secretion is suppressed by glucose administration, it is stimulated by insulin-induced hypoglycemia. Insulin-induced hypoglycemia and arginine infusion are the major procedures used to stimulate GH secretion. The insulin-induced hypoglycemic test is used to assess ACTH reserve in evaluating pituitary disease. However, 20% of normal individuals will not respond to either of these tests alone. Some investigators have been more successful with the arginine test when estrogen is administered.

Note: The use of levodopa as a GH stimulation test is thought to be as accurate and safer than either insulin or arginine. If propranolol is given with the levodopa, stimulation of GH secretion is enhanced. False low results with levodopa alone are 25% to 30%; with propranolol and levodopa they are only 10%.

NURSING ACTION

1. Instruct the patient to fast and to restrict physical activity for 10 to 12 hours before the test.
2. Explain that this test helps to evaluate hormonal secretion. Tell the patient that an indwelling venous catheter will be in place to avoid repeated venipunctures.
3. Before the patient rises in the morning collect 3 specimens of venous blood for basal levels: the specimens should be 5 ml each, one in a gray-top tube (for blood glucose), two in green-top tubes (for GH and cortisol).
4. Administer regular insulin as ordered intravenously over 1 to 2 minutes (0.05 to 0.15 units/kg) (see nursing alert).
5. Withdraw venous blood as described in step no. 3 at 15, 30, 45, 60, 90, and 120 minutes after administration of insulin.

6. At the end of the test a meal or intravenous feeding with dextrose in water should be given immediately.
7. If levodopa is used as a stimulation test, it is given orally 60 to 90 minutes before the blood sample is drawn; if arginine is used, an intravenous infusion is begun following secural of basal blood sample and continued for 30 minutes.
8. When the arginine infusion is completed three 6-ml blood samples are collected at 30-minute intervals in red-top tubes.

INTERFERING FACTORS

An adequate response may not be obtained if the glucose is not reduced sufficiently.

Impaired GH responses are seen in obesity, depression, hypothyroidism or hyperthyroidism, steroid therapy, and chronic renal failure.

CLINICAL IMPLICATIONS

Failure of stimulation or a blunted response

Suggests dysfunction of the hypothalamic-pituitary-adrenal axis

Increase in GH of <10 ng/dl

Suggests GH deficiency; an arginine test should be done to confirm the diagnosis

Increase in cortisol of <10 μg/dl

Suggests adrenal or pituitary insufficiency; an ACTH stimulation test will determine if the cause is primary or secondary adrenal insufficiency. Serum ACTH levels will also make the differential diagnosis between primary and secondary adrenal insufficiency.

NURSING ALERT

Use lower doses of insulin when hypopituitarism is strongly suspected, since these patients are very sensitive to the effects of insulin. Higher doses are used in patients with diabetes mellitus, obesity, and Cushing's disease, since these patients are relatively resistant to the effects of insulin.

During the insulin tolerance test the patient should be closely monitored by both physician and nurse, because the patient may have profound hypoglycemia during the test. Concentrated glucose solution should be available in case of a severe hypoglycemic reaction.

GH SUPPRESSION TEST

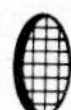

Reference range

Growth hormone level following a glucose load for male and female: <2 ng/ml (SI units: <93 pmol/L)

EXPLANATION OF THE TEST

The baseline serum GH levels are compared with those obtained following a loading dose of glucose, which suppresses GH secretion, unless the basal level is excessive.

VALUE OF THE TEST

Evaluates acromegaly or gigantism

NURSING ACTION

1. Instruct the patient to fast and limit physical activity for 10 to 12 hours before the test. Explain that several blood samples will be drawn.
2. Explain to the patient that this test helps to evaluate growth patterns.
3. Withdraw venous blood into a 10-ml red-top tube.
4. Administer 75 g of glucose solution orally; venous blood (6 ml in the red-top tube) is drawn every 30 minutes for 2 hours for growth hormone assay.

INTERFERING FACTORS

Failure to adhere to dietary restrictions and physical activity

GH levels may be decreased by corticosteroids and phenothiazines (chlorpromazine) and increased by arginine, levodopa, amphetamines, glucagon, niacin, or estrogens.

CLINICAL IMPLICATIONS

GH is generally suppressed 1 hour after glucose loading. In active acromegaly basal levels are above 5 ng/ml and are not suppressed after glucose loading to less than 5 ng/ml. In acromegaly or gigantism the GH levels may remain unchanged or rise following glucose loading.

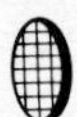

HAND-WRIST X-RAY

EXPLANATION OF THE TEST

When there is a suspected growth disorder a hand-wrist x-ray study allows evaluation of bone age and comparison of chronologic age with linear growth.

CLINICAL IMPLICATIONS

Retarded bone age

Hypopituitarism with GH deficiency
Cushing's syndrome or steroid therapy
Severe chronic disease
Hypothyroidism
Gonadal dysgenesis (Turner's syndrome)
Constitutional growth delay
Type I diabetes mellitus that is poorly controlled and severe

Accelerated bone age

Excess androgens
Excess estrogens
Albright's syndrome (polyostotic fibrous dysplasia)
Hyperthyroidism

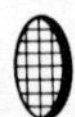

SOMATOMEDIN-C ASSAY

Reference ranges

Prepubertal: 0.08-2.8 U/ml (SI units: 0.08-2.8 arb. unit)
During puberty: 0.9-5.9 U/ml (SI units: 0.9-5.9 arb. unit)
Adult males: 0.34-1.9 U/ml (SI units: 0.34-1.9 arb. unit)
Adult females: 0.45-2.2 U/ml (SI units: 0.45-2.2 arb. unit)

EXPLANATION OF THE TEST

Somatomedins are a group of peptides produced in the liver with insulin-like activity, controlled by the secretion of GH, and carried in the plasma bound to proteins. They induce increased protein production and increased sulfation of cartilage constituents. Somatomedin-C is measured by radioreceptor and immunoassay in only a few laboratories.

VALUE AND LIMITATIONS OF THE TEST

This is a screening test for GH deficiency, pituitary insufficiency, and acromegaly, but does not replace GH testing.

Somatomedin serum levels are not influenced by diurnal variations and food intake.

Depressed serum levels may also be found in nonpituitary conditions such as decreased caloric intake, malabsorption, severe chronic illness, liver disease, hypothyroidism, and Laron dwarfism.

CLINICAL IMPLICATIONS

Increased concentrations

Acromegaly

Decreased concentrations

Deficient growth hormone with hypopituitarism
Hypothyroidism
Chronic illness
Nutritional deficiency

SERUM PROLACTIN

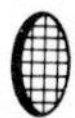

Reference range

2-15 ng/ml (SI units: 0.08-6.0 nmol/L)

EXPLANATION OF THE TEST

Prolactin stimulates lactation in postpartum females. Prolactin release is stimulated by thyrotropin releasing hormone (TRH) or chlorpromazine and suppressed by levodopa. Serum prolactin is measured by radioimmunoassay.

VALUE AND LIMITATIONS OF THE TEST

Used to screen for pituitary adenomas, especially in patients with postpubertal amenorrhea

Aids in the diagnosis of hypothalamic dysfunction

TRH or chlorpromazine stimulation tests or levodopa suppression tests have conflicting results in the evaluation of pituitary and hypothalamic disease; therefore, the stimulation and suppression tests are rarely performed in the evaluation of hyperprolactinemias.

NURSING ACTION

1. Inform the patient that there are no dietary restrictions before this test.
2. Tell the patient that the test helps the physician to evaluate hormonal secretion.
3. If possible, withhold drugs that may influence the test.
4. Collect 5 ml of venous blood in a red-top tube. Handle the specimen gently.

INTERFERING FACTORS

Breast stimulation may increase prolactin levels.

Drugs that decrease secretion of prolactin: dopaminergic antagonists (i.e., chlorpromazine, reserpine), cimetidine, haloperidol, morphine, estrogens

Drugs that decrease secretion of prolactin: dopaminergic agonists (L-dopa, bromocriptine)

CLINICAL IMPLICATIONS

Elevated levels

Pituitary microadenomas and adenomas (often acidophil cell adenoma, but also chromophobe adenomas). Very high prolactin levels are due to this more than to any other cause. The majority of patients (45% to 81%) with pituitary adenomas have prolactin levels greater than 100 ng/ml. However, not all patients with pituitary adenomas have serum prolactin elevation above 100 ng/ml (25% to 57%).

Postpubertal amenorrhea (20% to 30%), in which the incidence of pituitary tumors is 35% to 45%

Prolactin is also elevated in major stress, during pregnancy and nursing, breast stimulation, and by certain medications (see interfering factors). Other causes of elevation are hypothalamic space-occupying lesions such as granulomatous diseases or destructive diseases, hypothyroidism, chronic renal failure, cirrhosis, chest wall trauma and thoracic operations (related to effect on nerves from the areolar area), hypoglycemia, and polycystic ovarian disease.

TESTOSTERONE (SERUM)

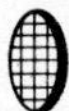

Reference ranges

Adult male: 300-1100 ng/dl (SI units: 10.4-38.1 nmol/L)
Adult female: 25-90 ng/dl (SI units: 0.87-3.12 nmol/L)

EXPLANATION OF THE TEST

Testosterone is the main androgen secreted by the testes; in the male it induces puberty and maintains secondary sex characteristics. Its production is under the control of luteinizing hormone from the anterior pituitary. In males most of the circulating testosterone is from the testes and a small amount from the adrenals, whereas in females it is secreted by the ovaries and adrenals.

VALUES OF THE TEST

Evaluates testicular function

NURSING ACTION

1. Inform the patient that there are no dietary restrictions before this test.
2. Withdraw an AM sample of venous blood in a 7-ml red-top tube. On the laboratory slip record the patient's age, sex, and hormonal therapy.

CLINICAL IMPLICATIONS

Increased levels (in males)

Testicular tumors

Increased levels (in females)

Stein-Leventhal syndrome (polycystic ovarian disease)
Ovarian tumors
Adrenal tumors
Adrenal hyperplasia

Decreased levels

Secondary hypogonadism in males (secondary to hypopituitarism, prolactinomas, or hypothalamic disease)
Primary hypogonadism in males (testicular failure, orchidectomy, Klinefelter's syndrome)
Estrogen therapy
Steroid therapy
Alcoholism

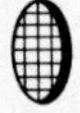

ESTRADIOL (SERUM)

Reference ranges

Male: <50 pg/ml (SI units: <184 pmol/L)
Adult female: 23-361 pg/ml (SI units: 84-1325 pmol/L)
Postmenopausal: <30 pg/ml (SI units: <110 pmol/L)
Prepubertal female: <20 pg/ml (SI units: <73 pmol/L)

EXPLANATION OF THE TEST

Estradiol is the most potent and the major estrogen secreted during the nonpregnant state (there is more estriol secreted during pregnancy). In the nonpregnant state, estrogens are secreted primarily by the ovarian follicles during the first half of the menstrual cycle and by the corpus luteum during the luteal phase of the menstrual cycle and during pregnancy. The level of estradiol varies depending on the time during the menstrual cycle.

VALUE OF THE TEST

Determines sexual maturation
Aids in the diagnosis of gonadal dysfunction
Aids in the diagnosis of ovarian and testicular tumors

NURSING ACTION

1. Inform the patient that there are no dietary restrictions before this test.
2. Withdraw venous blood into a 10-ml red-top tube. Indicate the phase of the patient's menstrual cycle on the laboratory slip.

CLINICAL IMPLICATIONS

Increased levels

Certain types of ovarian, testicular, or adrenal tumors
Polycystic ovarian disease

Decreased levels

Primary ovarian malfunction
Dysfunction of the pituitary or hypothalamus
Postmenopausal states

PROGESTERONE (PLASMA)

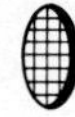

Reference ranges

Male: <1.0 ng/ml (SI units: <3.2 nmol/L)

Female

Follicular phase: 0.2-0.6 ng/ml (SI units: 0.6-1.9 nmol/L)
Midcycle peak: 0.3-3.5 ng/ml (SI units: 0.95-11 nmol/L)
Postovulatory: 6.5-32.2 ng/ml (SI units: 21-102 nmol/L)

EXPLANATION OF THE TEST

Progesterone is a major female steroid hormone involved in preparation of the uterus for and maintenance during pregnancy and in the preparation of the breasts during lactation. In the nonpregnant state it is synthesized by the corpus luteum, in the pregnant state by the placenta. In males it is produced in small amounts by the testes and the adrenals as a precursor for androgens and corticosteroids.

VALUE OF THE TEST

Aids in the detection of luteal insufficiency, defective ovulation, or malfunctioning placenta

NURSING ACTION

1. Inform the patient that there are no dietary restrictions before this test.
2. Withdraw venous blood in a 7-ml green-top tube.
3. For nonpregnant patients, indicate the date of the patient's last menstrual period and the phase of her cycle on the laboratory slip. For pregnant patients, indicate the week of gestation.

CLINICAL IMPLICATIONS
Elevated levels

Ovulation (during and after)
Luteinizing tumors
Adrenocortical hyperplasia

Decreased levels

Amenorrhea (nonovulatory)
Toxemia of pregnancy
Threatened abortion
Fetal death

GONADOTROPIN HORMONES (FSH AND LH)

Reference ranges for follicle-stimulating hormone (FSH)

Adult males: 4-25 mIU/ml

Adult females
Follicular phase: 5-30 mIU/ml
Midcycle peak: 15-90 mIU/ml
Luteal phase: 5-18 mIU/ml
Menopausal phase: 50-250 mIU/ml

Reference ranges for luteinizing hormone (LH)

10-14 years of age: 4-20 mIU/L
Adult males: 6-23 mIU/L

Adult females
Follicular phase: 5-30 mIU/L
Midcycle peak: 75-150 mIU/L
Luteal phase: 5-40 mIU/L
Menopausal phase: 30-200 mIU/L

EXPLANATION OF THE TEST

The two gonadotropins secreted by the anterior pituitary are luteinizing hormone (LH) and follicle-stimulating hormone (FSH). Gonadotropin releasing hormone, secreted by the hypothalamus, stimulates secretion of LH and, to a lesser degree, FSH. LH induces ovulation and maintains the corpus luteum in women and stimulates testosterone secretion in men. FSH stimulates the growth of ovarian follicles in women and spermatogenesis in men. After stimulation by FSH, the ovarian follicles secrete estrogen, which in turn suppresses the secretion of FSH. LH secretion is suppressed by testosterone and to a lesser degree by estrogen.

VALUE OF THE TEST

FSH and LH levels aid in the diagnosis of infertility, amenorrhea, precocious puberty, and the differential diagnosis of hypogonadism.

NURSING ACTION

1. Inform the patient that there are no dietary restrictions before the test.
2. Withdraw venous blood into a 7-ml red-top collection tube.

CLINICAL IMPLICATIONS

Increased levels of FSH

Primary gonadal failure
Ovarian or testicular agenesis
Klinefelter's syndrome
FSH-secreting tumors
Menopausal state

Decreased levels of FSH

Panhypopituitarism
Pituitary tumors
Prolactinomas
Hypogonadotropic hypogonadism or other hypothalamic diseases
Anorexia nervosa
Prepuberty
Estrogen administration

Increased levels of LH (females)

Primary ovarian failure
Ovariectomy
Menopausal state
Polycystic ovarian disease

Decreased levels of LH (females)

Secondary ovarian failure (pituitary or hypothalamic insufficiency)
Pituitary or hypothalamic tumors or disease
Hypophysectomy
Following administrations of oral contraceptives or estrogen

Increased levels of LH (males)

Primary testicular failure
Seminiferous tubule dysgenesis (Klinefelter's syndrome)
Anorchia
Testicular feminizing syndrome

Decreased levels of LH (males)

Secondary testicular failure (pituitary or hypothalamic failure)
Testosterone administration
Hypophysectomy
Pituitary tumors
Prolactinomas

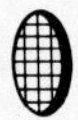

WATER DEPRIVATION AND VASOPRESSIN INJECTION TEST

EXPLANATION OF THE TEST

After several hours of controlled water deprivation, the urine of a patient with diabetes insipidus will not be concentrated and the serum osmolality will be high since the renal tubules are unable to reabsorb water. The presence of diabetes insipidus may be further documented by an injection of antidiuretic hormone (ADH). Because of ADH (vasopressin) deficiency, patients with central diabetes insipidus produce excessive urine. However, an injection of vasopressin will correct the massive polyuria and document the deficiency as well as the normal responsiveness of the renal tubules to the hormone.

VALUE OF THE TEST

Diagnostic of diabetes insipidus

NURSING ACTION

1. Explain to the patient that it will be necessary to abstain from fluids for several hours. Depending on the severity of diabetes insipidus, the patient may be kept NPO for 4 to 20 hours until a plateau of urine osmolality is reached. At the end of that time a urine specimen will be collected for osmolality and a blood sample drawn for osmolality, sodium, and ADH level.
2. Vasopressin is then injected subcutaneously. One hour after the injection, urine and plasma are collected for sodium and osmolality.

NURSING ALERT

If the patient has severe central diabetes insipidus, he or she may become quite dehydrated with water deprivation. Patients should be hospitalized and observed closely during this test. Monitor vital signs (pulse and blood pressure), urine output, and urine osmolality hourly. Weigh the patient every 3 hours to observe for excess volume loss. Report a change in vital signs (tachycardia, hypotension) or excess weight loss (greater than or equal to 3% loss of total body weight) to the physician.

HYPOGLYCEMIA

Plasma glucose concentration below 60 mg/dl after an overnight fast or below 55 mg/dl in males and below 45 mg/dl in premenopausal women after a *72-hour fast* is suggestive of significant hypoglycemia. The blood glucose concentration is dependent on the interaction between glucose production (dietary intake and liver glycogenolysis and gluconeogenesis) and glucose utilization (liver and peripheral tissues).

Hypoglycemia may be either reactive or organic. The reactive type develops in response to a high-carbohydrate meal, is transient, and involves inappropriate insulin response. The organic type occurs spontaneously in the fasting state and suggests a significant disease process. Causes of fasting hypoglycemia include insulin-producing islet cell tumors, nonpancreatic tumors, growth hormone or cortisol deficiency, severe hepatic or renal disease, severe malnutrition, or drugs (alcohol, insulin, oral hypoglycemic agents, high-dose aspirin).

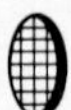

SERUM INSULIN

Reference range

Fasting: <2-20 μU/ml (SI units: 14-144 pmol/L)

EXPLANATION OF THE TEST

Glucose elevations stimulate insulin secretion and cause a rise in serum insulin levels. When plasma glucose concentrations fall, insulin release is inhibited and serum insulin levels fall. Thus the two levels are measured together, and the insulin level is evaluated in the light of the glucose value.

VALUE AND LIMITATIONS OF THE TEST

Aids in the differential diagnosis of hypoglycemia resulting from nonpancreatic tumors, islet cell hyperplasia or tumors, glucocorticoid deficiency, severe hepatic disease, or other causes

NURSING ACTION

1. Instruct the patient to fast for 10 to 12 hours before the test.
2. Withhold ACTH, steroids, oral contraceptives, thyroid supplements, and epinephrine.
3. Collect venous blood in a 7-ml red-top tube and in a fluoride tube (for glucose).
4. If the results after an overnight fast are inconclusive, fasting can be prolonged to 72 hours and the insulin/glucose ratio determined again.

CLINICAL IMPLICATIONS

Insulin levels tend to be suppressed in normal individuals after a fast and are normal or elevated in patients with insulinomas.

C-PEPTIDE

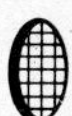

Reference range

1-2 ng/ml (fasting)
Levels rise 5- to 6-fold following glucose load.

EXPLANATION OF THE TEST

C-peptide is a 31-amino acid residue that is biologically inactive. It is formed in the pancreatic beta-cells where proinsulin is enzymatically degraded to C-peptide and insulin. Although secreted into the circulation in equal amounts, the ratio of C-peptide to insulin in the serum is about 5 to 15:1. This is due to the rapid removal of insulin and negligible extraction of C-peptide in their initial passage through the liver. In spite of the different catabolism, C-peptide levels correlate well with insulin values in that if one decreases, so does the other. C-peptide is measured by radioimmunoassay.

VALUE OF THE TEST

Measured with serum insulin and glucose in the evaluation of hypoglycemia
Permits assessment of pancreatic beta-cell secretory function, especially in cases in which insulin antibodies that are present interfere with insulin determinations
Useful in the diagnosis of self-injection of insulin, which results in "factitious" hypoglycemia
Detection of insulinoma in diabetic patients requiring insulin therapy
May demonstrate remission phase of diabetes

NURSING ACTION

1. Explain the purpose of the test to the patient.
2. Instruct the patient to fast from food from 8 to 12 hours before the test.
3. A fasting venous blood sample is obtained.

CLINICAL IMPLICATIONS
Increased levels

Endogenous hyperinsulinism

Decreased levels

Surreptitious injection of insulin with hypoglycemia and high insulin levels

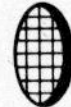

PROLONGED (72-HOUR) FAST

Normal findings

In normal individuals, plasma insulin levels fall steadily as the glucose levels fall during a prolonged fast.

EXPLANATION OF THE TEST

When fasting hypoglycemia is suspected but cannot be definitely diagnosed by overnight fasting, glucose, insulin, and C-peptide levels, a prolonged fast (72 hours for adults, 24 to 36 hours for children depending on age) is performed.

The patient must be hospitalized during the fast to observe for complications and to assure adequate blood drawing. Blood for plasma glucose, serum insulin, and C-peptide levels is drawn every 6 hours and also when the patient has hypoglycemic symptoms.

VALUE OF THE TEST

Establishes whether the patient has hypoglycemia in the fasting state
Determines whether or not the hypoglycemia is due to excessive insulin secretion
Aids in the diagnosis of hypoglycemia when other tests are equivocal

NURSING ACTION

1. Instruct the patient that he or she will be fasting for 3 days and will be permitted to take only water.
2. During the fast observe the patient closely for symptoms of hypoglycemia.
3. Withdraw venous blood for glucose, insulin, and C-peptide levels every 6 hours and if the patient has symptoms during the fast.

CLINICAL IMPLICATIONS

Blood glucose levels below 55 mg/dl in men and below 45 mg/dl in women are significant but must be correlated with the serum insulin level. In normal individuals, serum insulin levels fall to suppressed levels as the glucose levels fall during the fast. However, in patients with insulinomas or factitious insulin administration, the serum insulin level does not fall, and remains in the normal or elevated range in the presence of hypoglycemia. A normal insulin/glucose ratio is equal to or less than 0.3. Patients with insulinomas or factitious insulin administration have insulin/glucose ratios greater than 0.3. C-peptide levels measured with the insulin and glucose levels during the test can differentiate patients with insulinomas from those injecting insulin surreptitiously.

DIABETES MELLITUS

Diabetes mellitus is a disease associated with fasting hyperglycemia and/or postprandial hyperglycemia. It is characterized by metabolic abnormalities and long-term complications involving the eyes, kidneys, nerves, and blood vessels. The endocrine function of the pancreatic islets of Langerhans is to secrete glucagon and insulin directly into the bloodstream. The primary abnormalities causing diabetes mellitus are (1) failure of the beta cells to produce insulin or (2) subnormal insulin production with abnormal insulin release and a peripheral resistance to the action of insulin. A *fasting blood glucose level* of 140 mg/dl or above found on 2 determinations is diagnostic, and no further testing is necessary. However, if the fasting blood glucose level is equivocal (110 to 130 mg/dl), an oral *glucose tolerance test* is ordered. A normal result is strong evidence against diabetes. However, a positive test is not necessarily diagnostic of diabetes, since other conditions such as stress, illness, inadequate diet, and various medications may produce an abnormal response.

FASTING BLOOD GLUCOSE

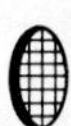

Adult reference range

Serum and plasma: 70-110 mg/dl (SI units: 3.85-6.05 mmol/L)
Whole blood: 60-100 mg/dl (SI units: 3.30-5.50 mmol/L)

EXPLANATION OF THE TEST

Dietary carbohydrates in the diet are digested and transported by the portal vein to the liver, where they are converted to glucose.

The utilization of glucose by the body cells is intimately related to (1) the circulating level of insulin secreted from the islets of Langerhans in the pancreas and (2) the effectiveness of insulin's actions on the cell to metabolize glucose.

VALUE OF THE TEST

Helps to detect diabetes mellitus, but a normal level does not rule out diabetes mellitus

Helps to evaluate the clinical status of those patients with diabetes mellitus

NURSING ACTION

1. Instruct the patient not to eat or drink for 12 hours before collection of the specimen.
2. Explain to the patient that this test measures the blood sugar levels.
3. Collect 5 to 10 ml of venous blood in a gray-top tube (contains fluoride to diminish glycolysis) or red-top tube (for serum measurement). Insulin may be given as ordered after the blood sample is taken.

INTERFERING FACTORS

Drugs that may cause increased levels: ACTH, cortisone medications, thiazide and loop diuretics, anesthesic drugs, oral contraceptives, diazoxide

Insulin excess, excessive doses of oral hypoglycemic agents (decreased glucose levels)

Trauma or other major illness (elevated blood sugar)

CLINICAL IMPLICATIONS OF HYPERGLYCEMIA

Diabetes
Cushing's disease
Pheochromocytoma
Hyperthyroidism
Pancreatic carcinoma (non–islet cell tumors)
Acute or chronic pancreatic insufficiency
Pancreatitis

ORAL GLUCOSE TOLERANCE TEST

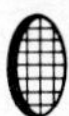

Reference range

Following ingestion of 75 g of glucose, fasting venous plasma glucose concentration is less than 115 mg/dl.
At 30, 60, and 90 minutes it is less than 200 mg/dl.
At 120 minutes it is less than 140 mg/dl.

EXPLANATION OF THE TEST

This test challenges the ability of the pancreas to secrete insulin in response to hyperglycemia and the body's response to insulin action. These are reflected by the rise and fall of blood glucose following ingestion of glucose.

VALUE AND LIMITATIONS OF THE TEST

Aids in the assessment of patients with signs, symptoms, or complications suggestive of diabetes but with normal fasting and random blood glucose

Useful in the diagnosis of gestational diabetes (diabetes with onset during pregnancy)

Limited in its clinical usefulness because (1) the results are often not reproducible on repeat tests in the same individuals and (2) borderline results (impaired glucose tolerance) do not necessarily predict the development of overt diabetes

NURSING ACTION

1. Instruct the patient to maintain a normal diet with approximately 300 g of carbohydrate per day for 3 days before the test.
2. Instruct the patient to fast for 10 to 16 hours before the test. A fasting blood specimen is taken. Withdraw venous blood into a 7-ml gray-top tube and collect a urine specimen at the same time. Send specimens to the laboratory immediately or refrigerate them. Record all pertinent information on the laboratory slip such as when the patient had the last meal, any medications, and the time of specimen collection.
3. Instruct the patient to take the 75 g dose of glucose (100 g for pregnant women) within 5 minutes. The glucose can be mixed in up to 300 ml of water and flavored with lemon juice. Timing begins when the patient starts to drink.

4. Instruct the patient to remain seated during the test period and to refrain from smoking; he or she may lie down if feeling faint.
5. Draw venous blood samples at ½, 1, 1½, and 2 hours after the patient ingests the glucose. Use 7-ml gray-top tubes.
6. If ordered in the clinical setting of suspected gestational diabetes, 100 g of glucose is given and blood is drawn immediately and at 1, 2, and 3 hours for glucose.

INTERFERING FACTORS

False-positive responses may occur because of low carbohydrate and caloric intake for as few as 3 days before the test, inactivity, obesity, illness, fever, or stress, or alcohol ingestion.

Medication that could affect the test results are oral contraceptives, steroids, diuretics, anticonvulsants, and diazoxide.

CLINICAL IMPLICATIONS

Low or flat responses

Hypothyroidism
Hypopituitarism
Panhypopituitarism
Insulinoma
Malabsorption
Addison's disease

Elevated responses

Diabetes mellitus
Cushing's disease
Hemochromatosis
Pheochromocytoma
Acromegaly

Impaired glucose tolerance

For a diagnosis of impaired glucose tolerance, three criteria must be met (see Table 9-3):

1. Fasting glucose less than 140 mg/dl
2. Two-hour glucose between 140 and 200 mg/dl
3. At least one value between 30 to 90 minutes equal to or greater than 200 mg/dl

Table 9-3 Diagnostic criteria of diabetes mellitus and glucose intolerance by oral glucose tolerance test (venous plasma levels) (National Diabetes Data Group) (mg/dl)

	Normal	Impaired glucose tolerance	Diabetes mellitus
Fasting	<115	<140	<140*
½, 1, 1½ hr	<200	>200	>200
2 hr	<140	140-200	>200

*If the fasting glucose is >140 mg/dl on 2 occasions, the diagnosis of diabetes mellitus can be made without the oral glucose tolerance test.

The long-term significance of this diagnosis is still to be determined, since these patients may or may not develop overt diabetes mellitus.

Diabetes mellitus

If the fasting blood glucose is equal to or greater than 140 mg/dl on at least 2 occasions, the diagnosis of diabetes mellitus can be made without an oral glucose tolerance test.

If the fasting glucose is less than 140 mg/dl, a glucose tolerance test can be done. Both the 2-hour and at least 1 other sample (at 30, 60, and 90 minutes) equal to or greater than 200 mg/dl is diagnostic of diabetes mellitus (see Table 9-3).

10

Diagnostic tests for hematologic disorders

LEUKEMIA

Leukemia is a progressive, malignant disease characterized by abnormal proliferation of the precursors of lymphocytes, granulocytes, or monocytes. It is classified as acute or chronic, according to cell type and the duration of the disease. The diagnosis is based on clinical signs, examination of the *peripheral blood smear, bone marrow aspirate,* and *bone marrow biopsy* (when aspirates are not attainable). Further characterization may necessitate additional cytochemical and histochemical studies. In 1976 hematologists from France, America, and Britain classified acute leukemia based on morphologic and cytochemical criteria (Table 10-1).

ANEMIAS

Anemia is a symptom of a disease process and is usually first recognized because of a low *hemoglobin* level or low *hematocrit* count. If a repeat hemoglobin and hematocrit are still abnormal, and if the patient is not receiving intravenous fluids (hemodilution), these tests are usually ordered: *white blood cell count (WBC), WBC differential, platelet count, red blood cell (RBC) indices* (including red cell distribution width [RDW], *reticulocyte count,* and a *peripheral*

Table 10-1 French-American-British (FAB) classification of acute leukemia

Designation/Description	Appearance
M1: Acute myelocytic without differentiation	Predominantly myeloblasts; other immature granulocytes absent
M2: Acute myelocytic with differentiation	Myeloblasts with other immature granulocytes
M3: Acute promyelocytic	Predominantly promyelocytes with heavy granulation
M4: Acute myelomonocytic	Predominantly blastic cells with both myelocytic and monocytic differentiation
M5A: Acute monocytic without differentiation	Predominantly monoblasts
M5B: Acute monocytic with differentiation	Predominantly blasts with monocytic characteristics ("pure monocytic")
M6: Erythroleukemia	Megaloblastoid pronormoblasts and myeloblasts
L1: Homogeneous small blast type	Predominantly small blasts, fairly uniform appearance
L2: Heterogeneous blast type	Mixed blast size and appearance; typically with nuclear clefting or irregularity
L3: Homogeneous large blast type ("Burkitt cell")	Uniformly large blasts with intensely basophilic cytoplasm that usually contains vacuoles

M, myeloid; L, lymphoid.

smear (for morphologic evaluation of the RBCs and platelets). A combination of tests that is particularly helpful in the differential diagnosis of anemic disorders is based on the *mean cell volume (MCV), RDW,* and the *reticulocyte count*.

Anemias may be classified according to pathogenesis (factor deficiency, production defect, depletion) or according to RBC morphology (microcytic, normocytic, or macrocytic). Factor deficiency anemia is usually the result of a deficiency either of iron or vitamin B_{12} or folic acid. Production defect anemia may be due to replacement of bone marrow by fibrosis or neoplasm, hypoplasia of the bone marrow (usually caused by chemicals), or toxic suppression of marrow production or delivery without hypoplasia. Depletion anemia is usually due to hemorrhage, hemolytic anemia, or hypersplenism.

Iron store depletion

Early on, iron store depletion may be asymptomatic. However, even at early stages the patient may have symptoms of fatigue, weakness, and dyspnea associated with the anemia. There may also be koilonychia, tongue soreness, angular stomatitis, and dysphagia.

When the iron deficiency is in its early stage, the *MCV* tends to be on the low side of normal and the *reticulocyte count* is not abnormal as it would be in the hemolytic anemias and anemias resulting from acute blood loss. However, the *RDW* is high, and this finding leads the clinician to order determinations of *transferrin saturation* and *plasma ferritin* levels. In some cases it is only the plasma ferritin level that is decreased, but the diagnosis of early iron deficiency is made from the findings of normal MCV, high RDW, and low ferritin values. This laboratory picture indicates depleted body stores of iron. If there is also hypersegmentation of neutrophils, the *serum vitamin* B_{12} and *serum folic acid* levels should also be measured.

Megaloblastic anemia

Megaloblastic anemia is an anemia that is characterized by macrocytes in the circulation and megaloblasts in the bone marrow. Megaloblasts are early precursors of erythrocytes that have characteristic immature nuclei. Their typical appearance on stained smears of bone marrow is diagnostic.

The megaloblastic anemias are usually caused by deficiencies of vitamin B_{12} or folate, or they are secondary to other defects of nucleoprotein metabolism, such as chemotherapy or inherent metabolic defects of the erythroid cells.

Laboratory tests for megaloblastic anemia

The routine blood smear

Macrocytosis (which may be masked by associated iron deficiency or thalassemia minor)

Deformed red cells

Multilobed neutrophils, with increased cell volume noted in their precursors (especially bands and metamyelocytes)

Severe neutropenia and infection

Thrombocytopenia, which may be severe enough to cause life-threatening hemorrhage

Bone marrow examination

Nuclei on stained smears with fine chromatin separated by abundant parachromatin are diagnostic of megaloblastic anemia

Giant band neutrophils and late metamyelocytes, which have cell diameters twice that of other cells at the same period and maturation

Serum vitamin B_{12}: deficient (and there may be neurologic manifestations of this)

Serum folate: low

Erythrocyte folate: low

Platelets: may be fewer in number owing to abnormal or fewer than normal megakaryocytes

Special studies for megaloblastic anemia

Schilling's test is the most important special study performed for megaloblastic anemia (it also tests absorption).

In covert folate or vitamin B_{12} deficiency the diagnosis is sometimes uncovered using the *deoxyuridine (dU) suppression test* on bone marrow and on peripheral blood lymphocytes.

Measurement of antibody to intrinsic factor in serum (seen in 55% to 60% of pernicious anemia cases; very uncommon in others)

Vitamin B_{12} binding protein may be useful in assessing megaloblastic states.

Normochromic-normocytic anemias

Normochromic-normocytic anemia may be due to acute blood loss or hemolytic anemia, in which bone marrow production of erythrocytes may be multiplied 6 to 8 times normal. In some forms of normochromic-normocytic anemia, the bone marrow does not deliver enough erythrocytes to the peripheral blood to sustain an adequate hemoglobin level and hematocrit. However, the actual hemoglobin content of the red cells is normal ("normochromic") and the size of the red blood cells is not abnormal.

These anemias of insufficient erythropoiesis are diverse in etiology and pathology and include anemia of chronic diseases, aplastic anemia, and pure red cell aplasia. Their shared laboratory findings are a normal MCV (usually), RDW, and mean corpuscular hemoglobin concentration (MCHC), low reticulocyte count, and hypocellular or normocellular bone marrow.

LABORATORY TESTS FOR LEUKEMIAS AND ANEMIAS

Many diagnostic tests for leukemia and anemia have already been covered in Chapter 2, such as hemoglobin, hematocrit, WBC, differential, RBC indices (including RDW), reticulocyte count, and a *peripheral smear* (for morphologic evaluation of the RBCs).

BONE MARROW ASPIRATION

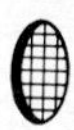

Reference ranges for bone marrow differential cell count (%)

Hemocytoblasts	0.1-1.0
Myeloblasts	0.1-5.0
Promyelocytes	0.5-8.0
Myelocytes	
Neutrophilic	4.2-8.9
Eosinophilic	0.1-3.0
Basophilic	Up to 0.5
Metamyelocytes	
Neutrophilic	10.0-32.0
Eosinophilic	0.3-3.7
Basophilic	Up to 0.3
Band cells	
Neutrophilic	10.0-35.0
Eosinophilic	0.2-2.0
Basophilic	Up to 0.3
Segmented cells	
Neutrophilic	7.0-30
Eosinophilic	0.2-4.0
Basophilic	Up to 0.7
Lymphocytes (all stages)	12.7-24
Monocytes (all stages)	Up to 2.7
Plasmacytes	0.1-1.5

Megakaryocytes	0.1-0.5
Pronormoblasts	0.2-4.0
Basophilic normoblasts	1.5-5.8
Polychromatophilic normoblasts	5.0-26.4
Orthochromic normoblasts	1.6-21
Reticulum cells	0.1-2.0
Myeloid (WBC)/erythroid (RBC) ratio or M:E ratio	
Adult	3:1 (range 4:1 to 2:1)

EXPLANATION OF THE TEST

At birth, the bone marrow is the only site of active hematopoiesis. During development, active hematopoietic sites are the liver, the spleen, and the marrow cavities of nearly all bones. In healthy adults this function takes place in only a few places: the sternum, ribs, vertebral bodies, pelvic bones, and the proximal portions of the humerus and femur. However, under conditions of hematopoietic stress, the liver and spleen may resume blood cell production.

The bone marrow may be removed by aspiration or needle biopsy under local anesthetic. The aspiration site is chosen and the overlying area and periosteum infiltrated with lidocaine. For aspiration a large-bore needle with a stylus is slowly advanced into the marrow and the stylus removed. Bone marrow is aspirated and smeared on slides, allowed to air-dry (no fixative or other preservative is required), and then taken to the pathology laboratory. In the biopsy procedure an incision is made and a core biopsy instrument used.

VALUE OF THE TEST

- Evaluates the manufacture of red cells, white cells, and platelet precursors (megakaryocytes) in their developmental stages
- Useful in the differential diagnosis of thrombocytopenia, leukemia, granulomatous disease, and aplastic, hypoplastic, or megaloblastic anemias
- Useful in the diagnosis of multiple myeloma
- Documents a deficiency in body iron stores in certain cases of suspected iron deficiency anemia
- Demonstrates metastatic neoplasm and some types of infectious disease
- Differentiates between chronic iron deficiency anemia and anemia of chronic disease, in which case the test shows stainable storage iron

NURSING ACTION

1. Inform the patient that there are no dietary restrictions before this test.
2. Explain the procedure to the patient and avoid creating anxiety. Patient cooperation is essential. The area will be anesthetized and the initial sensation will be that of pressure; as the needle enters the bone some pain will occur. A sedative may be necessary.
3. Obtain signed informed consent.
4. Assess coagulation studies before the procedure.
5. Prepare the aspiration site for sterile procedure. Aspiration sites in adults are the sternum and iliac crests. The aspiration site for very young children is the proximal tibia. Observe meticulous aseptic technique throughout the procedure.
6. Aspiration of bone marrow is performed in the patient's room by a physician with the assistance of the nurse.
7. After withdrawing the needle apply firm pressure to prevent hemorrhage.
8. Observe the dressing site for bleeding and inflammation.
9. Check the patient for vital signs reflecting hemorrhage and infection.

INTERFERING FACTORS

Blood transfusion within the preceding few weeks
Iron, vitamin B_{12}, folic acid, or cytotoxic agents may alter cells.

CLINICAL IMPLICATIONS

Acute leukemia. In acute leukemia, the bone marrow is saturated with blast forms of cells that are almost always present in the peripheral blood.

Chronic iron deficiency anemia. When the bone marrow aspiration or biopsy specimen is stained with Prussian blue, the absence of a stainable iron is confirmatory of chronic iron deficiency.

In the early stage of iron deficiency anemia, bone marrow examination reveals normoblastic hyperplasia but this dissipates with severe iron deficiency. The normoblasts are small, with frayed edges and poor hemoglobinization.

In the absence of inflammation, serum ferritin levels correlate well with total iron stores and fairly well with bone marrow stores of iron and can be obtained easily and in a noninvasive manner. Thus, in most cases ferritin level determinations obviate the need for bone marrow examination in the diagnosis of iron deficiency anemia.

Macrocytic anemias. Although the levels of vitamin B_{12} and folic acid in the blood are diagnostic or megaloblastic anemia, bone marrow aspiration may reveal various hematologic conditions resulting in vitamin B_{12} and folic acid deficiencies.

Multiple myeloma. On occasion, bone marrow aspiration can be diagnostic in multiple myeloma if larger collections of plasma cells occupying most of the marrow elements are seen. The plasma cells may vary considerably in their cellularity (10% to 90%) within the marrow. The degree of involvement may be focal within the red marrow.

Hemolytic anemias. A bone marrow examination may be useful in determining whether hemolysis is complicated by a lack of compensatory erythropoietic response, although it does not help a physician differentiate between the various causes of hemolytic anemias.

Idiopathic thrombocytopenic purpura. In bleeding disorders that result from a decrease in the number of platelets, a bone marrow examination is helpful in differentiating between idiopathic thrombocytopenic purpura (in which there are normal or increased numbers of megakaryocytes) and numerous other hematologic disorders that result in thrombocytopenia owing to depletion of megakaryocytes. A normal or increased number of megakaryocytes indicates that platelets are being destroyed in the patient's circulation, while the depletion of megakaryocytes indicates a defect in platelet production.

NURSING ALERT

Note that bone marrow biopsy is contraindicated in uncooperative patients and in those with severe bleeding disorders.

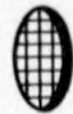

TRANSFERRIN SATURATION

Reference range

30%-50%

EXPLANATION OF THE TEST

Transferrin saturation is the percentage of the total iron-binding protein that is saturated with iron. It is derived by dividing the serum iron value by the total iron-binding capacity (TIBC) and is a good index for evaluating protein malnutrition.

VALUE OF THE TEST

A sensitive screening test for chronic iron deficiency
Differentiates iron-limited erythropoiesis (transferrin saturation less than 30%) from the microcytosis associated with thalassemia and sideroblastic anemia (transferrin saturation greater than 30%).

NURSING ACTION

1. Inform the patient that there are no dietary restrictions before this test.
2. Collect venous blood in a 7-ml red-top tube.
3. Handle the specimen with care to prevent hemolysis, which will cause a falsely elevated level.

CLINICAL IMPLICATIONS
Increased level

Hemolytic or megaloblastic anemia
Sideroblastic anemia
Iron overload
Hemochromatosis

Decreased level (<30%)

Chronic iron deficiency anemia
Anemia of chronic disease
Anemia of chronic renal failure

SERUM FERRITIN

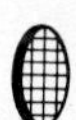

Adult reference range

Borderline iron deficiency: 13-20 ng/ml (SI units: 5.21-8 nmol/L)
Iron deficiency: 0-12 ng/ml (SI units: 0-4.8 nmol/L)

EXPLANATION OF THE TEST

Serum ferritin can be measured by radioimmunoassay or enzyme-linked immunoassay. The level is directly related to the amount of stored iron.

VALUE AND LIMITATIONS OF THE TEST

This is currently the most sensitive test available for detecting iron deficiency.

It is used to monitor iron status in chronic renal failure.

A markedly elevated level is a "tumor marker" for hepatoma.

In the case of iron-limited erythropoiesis, levels will help to distinguish between a true iron deficiency (iron ferritin < 15 ng/ml) and block preventing release of iron from storage (iron ferritin $>$ 15 ng/ml).

Clinically it is difficult to evaluate ferritin levels in an inflammatory state.

NURSING ACTION

1. Inform patient that there are no dietary restrictions before test.
2. Withdraw venous blood into a 10-ml red-top tube.

INTERFERING FACTORS

A recent transfusion may cause elevated levels.

Ferritin values vary by 10% to 15% daily in the same individual.

CLINICAL IMPLICATIONS

A decrease in serum ferritin is diagnostic of iron deficiency.

An increase is seen in various chronic diseases, including those that affect serum iron and TIBC (as described above) and in some patients with leukemia and aplastic anemia, with blood transfusions, megaloblastic anemia, hemolytic anemia, iron overload (i.e., hemochromatosis and acute iron poisoning), and pregnancy.

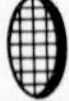

VITAMIN B_{12} ASSAY

Reference range

205-876 pg/ml (SI units: 150-674 pmol/L)

EXPLANATION OF THE TEST

Vitamin B_{12} determinations are usually performed along with serum folic acid, since deficiencies in both are the most common causes of megaloblastic anemia. Vitamin B_{12} has a role in folic acid metabolism and is therefore necessary for DNA synthesis, hematopoiesis, growth, myelin synthesis, and nervous system integrity. Vitamin B_{12} forms a complex with intrinsic factor before being absorbed from the ileum and stored in the liver. When being transported in the serum, it is bound to serum proteins termed as *transcobalamin*. Megaloblastic anemia results from a deficiency of either vitamin B_{12} or folic acid.

VALUE OF THE TEST

Useful in the differential diagnosis of megaloblastic anemia (vitamin B_{12} or folic acid deficiency), and in the differential diagnosis of CNS disorders affecting the peripheral and spinal myelinated nerves

NURSING ACTION

1. Inform the patient that there are no dietary restrictions before the test.
2. Collect venous blood in a 7-ml red-top tube.
3. Handle the specimen gently to prevent hemolysis and immediately transport to the laboratory.

CLINICAL IMPLICATIONS

Increased levels

Hepatic disease (i.e., cirrhosis, acute or chronic hepatitis)
Increase in vitamin B_{12}-binding protein
Myeloproliferative disorders (chronic myelocytic leukemia)

Decreased levels

Inadequate dietary intake
Malabsorption syndromes
Isolated malabsorption of vitamin B_{12}
Hypermetabolic states
Pregnancy

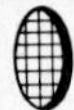

SERUM FOLIC ACID

Reference range

>3.3 ng/ml (radioimmunoassay) (SI units: > 7.3 nmol/L)
Borderline low: 2.5-3.2 ng/ml (SI units: 5.75-7.39 nmol/L)

EXPLANATION OF THE TEST

This test is easiest done by radioimmunoassay. Folic acid (folate) is a water-soluble vitamin like vitamin B_{12}, that is necessary for hematopoiesis, DNA synthesis, and overall body growth.

VALUE OF THE TEST

Aids in the differential diagnosis of megaloblastic anemia
Assesses folate stores in pregnancy

NURSING ACTION

1. Inform the patient not to eat or drink from the night before the test.
2. Collect venous blood in a 7-ml red-top tube.
3. Handle the specimen gently to prevent hemolysis and immediately transport it to the laboratory.

CLINICAL IMPLICATIONS

Increased levels

Excessive dietary intake
Hepatic disease (i.e., cirrhosis, acute or chronic hepatitis)
Myeloproliferative disorders (chronic myelocytic leukemia)

Decreased levels

Megaloblastic anemia
Inadequate dietary intake
Malabsorption syndromes (primary small bowel disease)
Pregnancy
Hyperthyroidism
Estrogens
Oral contraceptives
Dyrenium (Dyzide, Maxide)
Trimetoprim

Phenytoin (Dilantin)
Alcohol

SERUM IRON

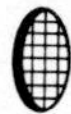

Adult reference range

50-150 μg/dl (SI units: 10-27 umol/L)

Pediatric reference range

Newborns: 100-200 μg/dl
6 months-2 years: 40-100 μg/dl

EXPLANATION OF THE TEST

Serum iron measurements reflect iron bound to the transport protein, transferrin. Thus serum iron values depend on the amount of iron and the amount of transferrin present. Such measurements are made in the absence of blood loss.

LIMITATIONS OF THE TEST

Although, theoretically, serum iron levels should be sensitive to iron deficiency in anemic patients, they at times only reflect low-normal values in such patients.

Diurnal variations occur with peak values having been found at 8 AM in some patients and 4 PM in others.

Day-to-day variations (20% to 25%) have been noted among individuals.

NURSING ACTION

1. Usually the patient may not eat or drink for 8 hours before the test.
2. Collect 5 to 10 ml of venous blood in a red-top tube.
3. Handle the specimen with care to prevent hemolysis, which will cause a falsely elevated level.

INTERFERING FACTORS

Increased levels may be caused by chloramphenicol, oral contraceptives, and excessive use of iron supplements.

CLINICAL IMPLICATIONS
Increased levels

Hemolytic anemia
Iron overload conditions (hemochromatosis)
Progesteronal birth control pills
Acute hepatitis
Thalassemia minor (usually)

Decreased levels

Iron deficiency anemia
Rheumatoid-collagen diseases
Anemia of chronic disease
Pregnancy
Defective absorption (sprue)

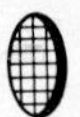

SERUM TOTAL IRON-BINDING CAPACITY (TIBC)

Adult reference range

300-400 μg/dl (20%-50% saturation)

Pediatric reference range

Newborns: 60-175 μg/dl
Infant (6 months-2 years): 100-350 μg/dl

EXPLANATION OF THE TEST

This test estimates the amount of iron that would be present if all the binding sites on transferrin were occupied. Normally they are only 30% occupied. The percentage of saturation is obtained by dividing the serum iron value by the TIBC.

VALUE AND LIMITATIONS OF THE TEST

Since iron is bound by other proteins besides transferrin, the TIBC is not an exact measurement.
In a substantial number of patients with chronic iron deficiency anemia the TIBC remains normal or elevated.

NURSING ACTION

1. Inform the patient that there are no dietary restrictions before this test.

2. Collect venous blood in a 7-ml red-top tube.
3. Handle the specimen with care to prevent hemolysis, which will cause a falsely elevated level.

INTERFERING FACTORS

Chloramphenicol and excessive use of iron supplements (decreased levels)
Oral contraceptives (increased levels)

CLINICAL IMPLICATIONS

Increased levels

Chronic iron deficiency anemia (however, a substantial number of patients do not show elevation)
Other conditions increasing the transferrin level (pregnancy, estrogen therapy, alcoholism, and acute hepatitis)

Decreased levels

Various chronic diseases (that also decrease the serum iron levels)
Hypoproteinemia
Iron overload conditions

BLEEDING DISORDERS

Mechanism of coagulation

Each of the substances involved in coagulation has been assigned a Roman numeral (I to XIII, with VI having been dropped because it was identical to activated factor V).

The activation of the coagulation process involves two sequential pathways, intrinsic and extrinsic, each of which is sometimes described as a "waterfall" or a "cascade" because it involves step-by-step interactions and the dependency of one reaction upon another. The two pathways of coagulation eventually interact to form a common pathway (Fig. 10-1).

The origination of the extrinsic pathway with the initial injury may be due to blood vessel endothelium as well as a variety of other tissue. The released tissue factor (factor III, tissue thromboplastin) activates factor VII in the presence of calcium ion. In turn, factor VII activates factors IX and X.

The intrinsic pathway involves protein-protein interactions and is slower than the extrinsic system in vitro. As the name implies, the intrinsic factors are within the blood itself.

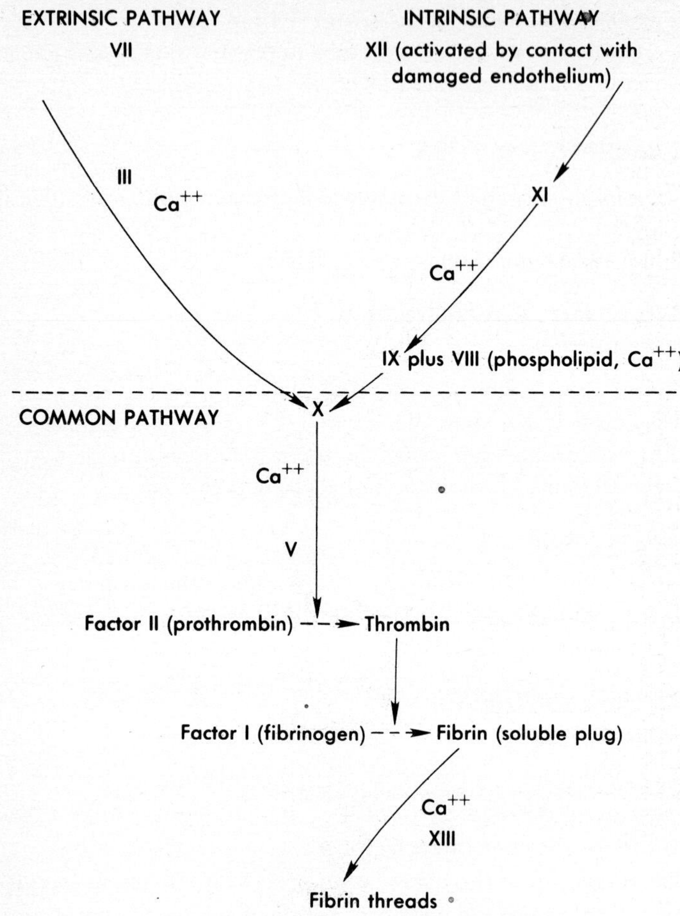

Fig. 10-1. *Mechanism of coagulation.*

Factor XII is the plasma component that is apparently activated by endothelial injury with exposure of negatively charged surface. Once activated, factor XII activates factor XI, which in turn, in the presence of calcium ion, activates factor IX ("Christmas factor"), which is synthesized in the liver in a vitamin K–dependent process.

The factor VIII molecule is composed of two portions: (1) the von Willebrand portion, with high molecular weight, which is made in endothelium and megakaryocytes, and (2) a coagulant portion, with low molecular weight, which is of unknown origin but considered probably to be produced by sinusoidal endothelium of the liver. In terms of function, factor VIII forms a complex with activated factor IX, with phospholipid and calcium ion, and greatly enhances activation of factor X by factor IX. Factor VIII is also involved in promoting platelet adhesiveness.

Prothrombin is converted into thrombin by factor X (Stuart-Prower factor), in the presence of calcium ion and factor V. Factor X may be activated by the products of either the intrinsic pathway or the extrinsic pathway, and thus begins the *common pathway* of coagulation (see Fig. 10-1).

Factor V, a glycoprotein, acts as a catalyst in the activation of factor II. It thus participates in prothrombin activation.

Thrombin acts as an enzyme to convert fibrinogen into fibrin threads to form a soluble plug, the first visible sign of coagulation. Finally, the clot structure is strengthened by factor XIII, the fibrin-stabilizing factor.

Coagulation tests

Laboratory evaluation of coagulation, combined with a complete history taking and physical examination, with emphasis on family history, can greatly facilitate the definitive diagnosis of coagulation disorders. If there is no family history of bleeding problems, presurgery screening tests include platelet count, bleeding time, partial thromboplastin time, and prothrombin time. Bleeding time is the screening test for platelet function in the presence of a normal platelet count; partial thromboplastin time and prothrombin time are the screening tests for intrinsic, extrinsic, and common pathway abnormalities. If an abnormality is found, or if there is a family history of a bleeding problem, then more specific tests are required, such as specific factor assays and tests for qualitative platelet abnormalities.

Table 10-2 lists defects of coagulation factors and the abnormal laboratory tests that result.

Pathophysiology of bleeding disorders

Bleeding disorders usually result from one of the following:

1. A clotting problem, which is exemplified by hemophilia. Such a problem involves bleeding in joints and soft tissue or extended bleeding as a result of trauma or surgery.
2. A hemostatic plug problem, which usually is the result of a platelet or factor VIII (von Willebrand factor) abnormality and is char-

Table 10-2 Coagulation factors

Factor	Synonyms	Deficiency state	Inheritance pattern	Abnormal tests
I	Fibrinogen	Afibrinogenemia	Autosomal recessive	PT, PTT, TCT
		Dysfibrinogenemia	Autosomal dominant	PT, PTT, TCT
II	Prothrombin	Hypoprothrombinemia	Autosomal recessive	PT, PTT
		Dysprothrombinemia	? Autosomal recessive	PT, PTT
III	Tissue thromboplastin	None		
IV	Calcium	None		
V	Accelerator globulin (proaccelerin)	Factor V deficiency†	Autosomal recessive	PT, PTT, BT (prolonged in ⅓)
VII	Proconvertin	Factor VII deficiency*	Autosomal recessive	PT
VIII	Antihemophilic factor	Classic hemophilia* (hemophilia A)	X-linked recessive	PTT
		von Willebrand's disease	Autosomal dominant or recessive	BT, PTT
IX	Plasma thromboplastin component	Hemophilia B* (Christmas disease)	X-linked recessive	PTT

Adapted from Blatt, P.M., Zietler, K.D., and Roberts, H.R.: Hemophilia and other hereditary defects of coagulation. In Conn, H.F., and Conn, R.B., Jr., editors: Current diagnosis, Philadelphia, 1980, W.B. Saunders Co.

Key: BT = bleeding time; PT = prothrombin time; PTT = partial thromboplastin time; TCT = thrombin clotting time.

*Genetic heterogeneity identified with some patients showing "true" deficiency of factor synthesis while other patients have abnormal molecules incapable of supporting procoagulant activity yet present in antigenically normal quantity.

†Genetic heterogeneity suggested by variable levels of factor V activity.

Table 10-2 Coagulation factors—cont'd

Factor	Synonyms	Deficiency state	Inheritance pattern	Abnormal tests
X	Stuart factor	Factor X deficiency*	Autosomal recessive	PT, PTT
XI	Plasma thromboplastin antecedent	Factor XI deficiency*	Autosomal recessive	PTT
XII	Hageman factor	Factor XII deficiency*	Autosomal recessive (most)	PTT
Fletcher	—	Fletcher factor deficiency	Autosomal recessive and dominant	PTT
Fitzgerald	—	Fitzgerald factor deficiency	Autosomal recessive	PTT
Passavoy	—	Passavoy factor deficiency	Autosomal dominant	PTT
XIII	Fibrin stabilizing factor	Factor XIII deficiency*	Autosomal recessive	Clot solubility increased in 5 M urea

acterized by small vessel bleeding, petechiae, and mucous membrane bleeding.

Hemostasis (prevention of blood loss) is achieved through vascular spasm, formation of a platelet plug, and blood coagulation, forming fibrin threads to strengthen the blood clot. Immediately after a blood vessel is cut or ruptures, the wall of the vessel contracts locally, permitting platelet plugging and the process of coagulation. When a vessel wall is injured, factor III (thromboplastin) is released from the damaged cells. The platelets exposed to the recently disrupted endothelial surface of the vessel come into contact with collagen fibers and connective tissue, whereupon they change their characteristics. There follows a complicated process, which is greatly oversimplified here.

The sequence of platelet plug formation is shown in Fig. 10-2. When the platelets are exposed to the collagen of the injured vessel

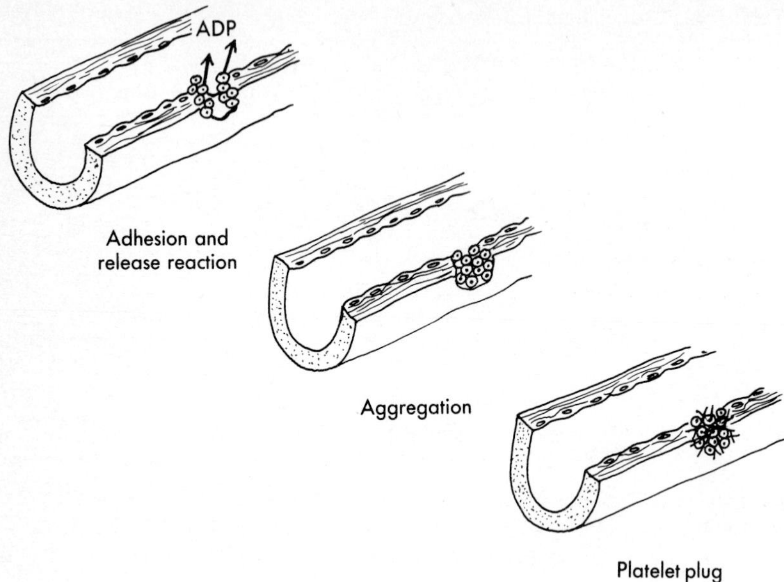

Fig. 10-2. *Sequence of platelet plug formation.*

wall they begin to adhere to the vessel wall and to clump together. Adhesion to the vessel wall (Fig. 10-2, *A*) and exposure to thrombin, which is being generated from the clotting systems, stimulates the platelets to release their intracellular pool of adenosine diphosphate (ADP), adenosine triphosphate (ATP), serotonin, and calcium. Platelet aggregation (Fig. 10-2, *B*) results from the exposure of the platelets to the extracellular pool of ADP and to thrombin. The platelets secrete substances that maintain vasoconstriction and thus participate in blood coagulation. The vasoconstriction and the platelet aggregation result in the formation of the platelet plug (Fig. 10-2, *C*), the maintenance of which is achieved through the interaction of platelets, thrombin, and fibrin.

Clinical application of laboratory tests when there is bleeding

When purpura is encountered clinically, the diagnostic process begins with a *platelet count* and a *CBC*, with emphasis on the *peripheral smear*. These tests have been described in Chapter 2.

If there is thrombocytopenia, a *bone marrow aspiration* (both clot section and smear technique) is usually in order.

If thrombocytopenia is *not* found, a *bleeding time* test is performed to evaluate platelet function. *Platelet function tests* may also be ordered. Other abnormalities would already have been ruled out by the other tests for hemorrhagic disease.

If there is active bleeding, the following tests are in order: *bleeding time* to evaluate platelet formation; *peripheral blood smear* to look for abnormal platelet morphology and estimated number, and evaluate RBC morphology; *activated partial thromboplastin time* (APTT) to assess for intrinsic pathway abnormalities and *prothrombin time* (PT), for extrinsic pathway abnormalities; and a test for *fibrinogen degradation products* (FDP) to assess for disseminated intravascular coagulation (DIC). If the bleeding time is abnormal do a *platelet count;* if the prothrombin and partial thromboplastin times are abnormal, do a *fibrinogen level* test. If there is active bleeding, a platelet count should be performed whether the bleeding time is abnormal or not. Idiopathic thrombocytopenic purpura (ITP) is notable for ecchymoses and severe thrombocytopenia, but a normal bleeding time.

Thrombin time is not as widely used a test as the other coagulation procedures. If thrombin time is prolonged, quantitation of fibrinogen levels is required and in suspected DIC, the test for FDP is also done.

Thrombocytopenias

Thrombocytopenia is the most common bleeding disorder involving platelets. It may be the result of defects in platelet production (infiltrative disease of the bone marrow, drug-induced or the result of chemotherapy), increased destruction of platelets (idiopathic thrombocytopenic purpura, DIC), or a redistribution of platelets with splenic pooling.

Hemophilias

Hemophilia is a group of congenital bleeding disorders that involves a defect of a single coagulation protein. It is possible to divide the disorder into hemophilia A (classic hemophilia; factor VIII deficiency) and hemophilia B (Christmas disease; factor IX deficiency) by laboratory tests; however, the two types are clinically indistinguishable. In the routine screening test the *partial thromboplastin (PTT)* or activated partial thromboplastin time is prolonged; *pro-*

thrombin time, *bleeding time*, and *thrombin time* are all normal. The definitive diagnosis is made by specific assay or, less specifically, by means of the PTT. If the PTT is corrected with barium sulfate–absorbed plasma but not with aged serum, the deficiency is in factor VIII; if the opposite is the case, the deficiency is in factor IX.

von Willebrand's disease

This is a congenital bleeding disorder characterized by prolonged bleeding time, impaired platelet adhesiveness, impaired ristocetin, induced platelet aggregation, and often a concordant decrease in the levels of antihemophilic factor VIII and von Willebrand factor. Note that pregnancy and the use of birth control pills can normalize many of the test results that are usually abnormal in von Willebrand's disease. Also test results can vary from day to day or month to month in the same patient.

Disseminated intravascular coagulation (DIC)

DIC is an acquired clotting disorder that is usually secondary to serious systemic disease. It is characterized by intravascular formation of fibrin thrombi, along with reductions in the consumption of clotting factors, platelets, and fibrinogen, resulting in the activation of the fibrinolytic system. The fibrinolytic process produces potent circulating anticoagulants. The levels of factors I, II, V, and VIII are frequently decreased. *Prothrombin time* and *partial thromboplastin time* are increased; the *platelet count* and the *fibrinogen* level are decreased. Definitive tests are an assay for *fibrinogen degradation products*, which will have a positive titer, and *thrombin time*, which will be increased. The *peripheral blood smear* will show fragmented red cells (schistocytes) and decreased platelets.

LABORATORY TESTS FOR BLEEDING DISORDERS

The platelet count has already been covered in Chapter 2.

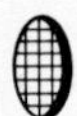

BLEEDING TIME

Reference range

3-9.5 minutes (Simplate method)
(SI units: 180-570 seconds)

EXPLANATION OF THE TEST

This test measures the duration of bleeding after a standardized skin incision. The template (Meilke) modification of the Ivy technique is the standard test.

VALUE AND LIMITATIONS OF THE TEST

Evaluates platelet number and function
Roughly correlates with the degree of thrombocytopenia in the presence of functionally normal platelets
Used for preoperative screening
The normal range may vary if the puncture is not standard size.
Elevated bleeding times do not necessarily predict the possibility of hemorrhage.

NURSING ACTION

1. Inform the patient that there are no food or fluid restrictions before the test.
2. Explain the procedure to the patient and advise him or her that the incisions will leave a small hairline scar.
3. Notify the laboratory if the patient has been taking drugs that prolong bleeding time.
4. The standard procedure is the template method. Some laboratories use the Simplate method, in which a small spring-driven lancet makes a uniform incision 5 mm long and 1 mm deep.
5. The blood pressure cuff is wrapped around the upper arm and inflated to 40 mm Hg.
6. An area on the forearm that is free of superficial veins is cleansed with antiseptic.
7. After the skin has dried the incision is made and the stopwatch started. The blood is gently blotted with filter paper every 30 seconds until bleeding stops. The bleeding time is then recorded.

INTERFERING FACTORS

Bleeding time may be prolonged by aspirin and other nonsteroidal antiinflammatory drugs, and by antihistamines and various antibiotics.

CLINICAL IMPLICATIONS

Bleeding time is normal in disorders of coagulation, but is abnormal in severe thrombocytopenia, defects of platelet function, von Willebrand's disease (usually), or when there is afibrinoginemia.

NURSING ALERT

If bleeding continues beyond 15 minutes, apply pressure and notify the physician.

When bleeding time is 1½ times the upper limit of the reference range, there is a possibility of excessive bleeding during surgery.

When the bleeding time is more than 2 times the upper reference range, there is a definite risk of excessive bleeding during surgery.

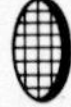

PLATELET AGGREGATION

Reference range

Full response to ADP, epinephrine, and collagen (SI units: 1.0)

EXPLANATION OF THE TEST

Normal platelet aggregation refers to the clumping of platelets at vascular injury sites. This in vitro test measures the rate of platelet aggregation in a sample of citrated platelet-rich plasma after the addition of an aggregating reagent (ADP, epinephrine thrombin, collagen, or ristocetin).

VALUE OF THE TEST

Detection of von Willebrand's disease and other inherited syndromes of platelet dysfunction

NURSING ACTION

1. Instruct the patient to fast for 8 hours before the test to ensure a fat-free diet. Water may be taken.

2. The patient should be as free of medications as possible before the test. In particular, he or she should abstain from aspirin or aspirin compounds for 14 days, and phenylbutazone, sulfinpyrazone, phenothiazines, antihistamines, antiinflammatory drugs, and tricyclic antidepressants for 48 hours before the test.
3. Venous blood is collected in a 7-ml blue-top siliconized tube.
4. Completely fill the collection tube and invert it gently to mix the anticoagulant.
5. Handle the specimen gently and maintain between 71.6° F (22° C) and 98.6° F (37° C) to prevent aggregation.

INTERFERING FACTORS

Platelet aggregation is inhibited by aspirin, phenylbutazone, sulfinpyrazone, phenothiazines, antihistamines, antiinflammatory drugs, and tricyclic antidepressants.

CLINICAL IMPLICATIONS

Uremia, severe liver disease, and advanced alcohol-related conditions depress the release-inducing effect of collagen, epinephrine, or exogenous ADP. This may also be the case in myeloproliferative disorders and dysproteinemias.

In von Willebrand's disease it is not the platelet that is abnormal, but there is a factor missing in the plasma so that the platelets do not adhere with the addition of ristocetin, although they respond normally to the other additives.

NURSING ALERT

Do not excessively probe the venipuncture site or leave the tourniquet on too long. If a coagulation defect is present this will cause excessive bleeding and bruising.

Apply pressure to the venipuncture site for 5 minutes following needle withdrawal.

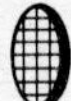

ACTIVATED PARTIAL THROMBOPLASTIN TIME (APTT)

Normal result

A fibrin clot forms 25-38 seconds after the reagent is added to the specimen.

EXPLANATION OF THE TEST

This test is a modification of the partial thromboplastin time (PTT), which does not contain added contact activator and is relatively insensitive to the effects of heparin. A contact activator is added to the PTT reagent, activating factor XII (contact factor) and shortening clotting time. The APTT test is sensitive to heparin and evaluates all the clotting factors of the intrinsic and common pathways (that is, all factors except factor VII and factor XIII).

The partial thromboplastin time (PTT) is less sensitive and less frequently performed. It relies on contact with the glass surface of the test tube to activate the blood clotting process.

VALUE AND LIMITATIONS OF THE TEST

The APTT test is fast, reproducible, easy to perform, and can be automated.

Monitors heparin therapy

Not as sensitive to prothrombin abnormalities as is the prothrombin time (PT)

Not influenced by platelet abnormalities

Blood levels of heparin that are above the anticoagulant range cause the test to be nonlinear, prolonged, and unreliable.

The test is prolonged by Coumadin.

It may be impossible to compare values from different laboratories since different techniques and equipment produce different results on the same specimen.

NURSING ACTION

1. Inform the patient that there are no food or fluid restrictions before the test.
2. Collect venous blood in a 7-ml blue-top tube; fill the tube completely and gently invert it to mix the anticoagulant.
3. If a vacuum tube is used to collect the specimen and not opened, the plasma remains stable for a longer period of time.

4. If the specimen cannot be sent immediately to the laboratory, pack it in ice.
5. Prevent hemolysis: handle the specimen gently and avoid excessive probing at the venipuncture site.

INTERFERING FACTORS

If the collection tube is not filled there will be too much anticoagulant relative to the amount of plasma and the test may be falsely prolonged.

Use of heparin flushes to keep intravenous lines open will prolong test results.

CLINICAL IMPLICATIONS

In the clinical setting of active bleeding, if the APTT is the only abnormality, it is repeated with the patient's plasma being diluted 1:1 with fresh normal plasma. A normal result implies that there is an intrinsic pathway factor deficiency; an abnormal result implies the existence of a circulating anticoagulant or an inhibitor.

PROTHROMBIN TIME (PT)

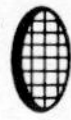

Reference range

Less than 2 seconds deviation from control

EXPLANATION OF THE TEST

This test measures the time required for a fibrin clot to form following the addition of a source of tissue extract and calcium ions to citrated plasma; it is used for preoperative screening.

VALUE OF THE TEST

Identifies defects of the vitamin K–dependent coagulation factors in the extrinsic and common pathways (factors VII, X, and II), as well as factors V and I.

NURSING ACTION

1. Inform the patient that there are no food or fluid restrictions before the test.

2. Collect venous blood in a 7-ml blue-top tube.
3. Completely fill the collection tube and gently invert it to mix the contents.
4. Send the sample to the laboratory immediately. More than 4 hours at room temperature causes a deterioration of factor V, prolonging the PT; however, if the specimen is refrigerated, factor VII may be activated, shortening the PT.

INTERFERING FACTORS

Excessive probing during venipuncture or rough handling of the specimen

Failure to fill the tube, mix the sample, or deliver to the laboratory promptly

Plasma fibrinogen levels of less than 100 mg/dl prolongs PT (reference range 200 to 400 mg/dl)

Most of the drugs listed for their effect on prothrombin time act through their interference with or promotion of coumarin effects.

Some drugs that thus shorten PT are

- Barbiturates, diuretics, diphenhydramine (Benadryl), oral contraceptives, rifampin, metaproterenol (Metaprel), vitamin K

Drugs that prolong PT include

- Penicillin, streptomycin, carbenicillin, chloramphenicol (Chloromycetin), kanamycin (Kantrex), neomycin, tetracyclines, chlordiazepoxide (Librium), phenytoin (Dilantin), heparin, methyldopa (Aldomet), mithramycin, reserpine (Serpasil), phenylbutazone (Butazolidin), quinidine, salicylates, sulfonamides

CLINICAL IMPLICATIONS

Prolonged PT may indicate parenchymal liver disease, vitamin K deficiency, or deficiencies in factor V, VII, or X.

If the APTT and the PT are both abnormal, the diagnostic possibilities are disseminated intravascular coagulation syndrome, coumarin therapy or heparin (i.e., heparin flushes), hepatic disease, or circulating antithrombins or fibrinolysins.

NURSING ALERT

If the patient has received a subcutaneous heparin injection, it is necessary to wait 6 hours for the effects to disappear before performing a PT or inform the laboratory so that the heparin may be absorbed before performance of the test.

FIBRINOGEN DEGRADATION PRODUCTS (FDP) (FIBRIN SPLIT PRODUCTS)

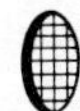

Reference range

Negative reaction at <1:4 dilution (SI units: 0 at 1:4 dilution)

EXPLANATION OF THE TEST

The normal process for dissolving a clot is accomplished by the fibrinolytic system. The fibrin (and fibrinogen) molecules are broken down by the enzyme plasmin, causing fibrin degradation products to be released. Many laboratories are using a new 2-minute latex agglutination slide procedure, the Thrombo-Wellcotest (Burroughs-Wellcome).

VALUE AND LIMITATIONS OF THE TEST

Assessment of disseminated intravascular coagulation (DIC) syndrome

Determination of the degree of fibrinolysis during coagulation

There is an overlap in results between normal and mild DIC syndrome.

NURSING ACTION

1. Inform the patient that there are no food or fluid restrictions before the test.
2. Draw the sample before administering heparin.
3. Completely fill the collection tube and gently invert it to mix the contents.

INTERFERING FACTORS

Pretest administration of heparin

Fibrinolytic drugs

CLINICAL IMPLICATIONS

Thrombo-Wellcotest titer over 1:40: classic DIC syndrome
Thrombo-Wellcotest between 1:10 and 1:40: mild DIC syndrome and occasionally a clinically normal individual
Venous thrombosis can produce an elevated value.

> **NURSING ALERT**
>
> In the event of the development of a hematoma at the venipuncture site, apply warm packs.

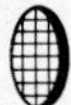

FIBRINOGEN LEVEL

Reference range

200-400 mg/dl (SI units: 2.00 to 4.99 g/L)

EXPLANATION OF THE TEST

This test measures the plasma concentration of fibrinogen available for coagulation. It is usually measured by the thrombin time technique although there are newer immunologic methods.

VALUE OF THE TEST

Aids in the diagnosis of suspected bleeding disorders
Most methods are not reliable when there are high titers of plasmin or heparin present.

NURSING ACTION

1. Inform the patient that there are no food or fluid restrictions before the test.
2. Collect venous blood in a 7-ml blue-top tube.
3. Completely fill the collection tube and gently invert it to mix the contents.
4. If the specimen cannot be immediately transported to the laboratory, it should be placed on ice.

INTERFERING FACTORS

Elevated levels may occur in the third trimester of pregnancy and in postoperative patients.

CLINICAL IMPLICATIONS

The most common cause of depressed levels is DIC syndrome. Another cause is high titer of plasmin.

> **NURSING ALERT**
>
> If the patient is receiving heparin, notify the laboratory because this necessitates the use of a different reagent.

PROTHROMBIN CONSUMPTION TIME (PCT)

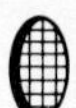

(SERUM PROTHROMBIN TIME; TWO-STAGE PROTHROMBIN TIME)

Reference range

Complete after 20 seconds

EXPLANATION OF THE TEST

Prothrombin consumption time is the rate and amount of prothrombin activation in the clotting process. This test is performed on the serum remaining after clotting in the standard prothrombin time test.

VALUE AND LIMITATIONS OF THE TEST

Detects abnormalities in platelets or intrinsic pathway clotting factors essential to thromboplastin formation (factors VIII, IX, XI, XII) prior to the prothrombin stage

This test is not influenced by prothrombin or fibrinogen defects unless there is a circulating anticoagulant.

NURSING ACTION

1. Inform the patient that there are no food or fluid restrictions before the test.

2. Collect venous blood in a 7-ml red-top tube.
3. Handle the specimen gently; if it cannot be immediately transported to the laboratory, it should be placed on ice.

INTERFERING FACTORS

Anticoagulant therapy

CLINICAL IMPLICATIONS

Normal

Normal utilization of prothrombin during the clotting process leaves a very small amount of prothrombin in the serum and the PT is prolonged.

Shortened PCT

Defect in platelet quantity or function or defect of factors VII, IX, X, XI, or XII of the intrinsic pathway. In such cases the utilization of prothrombin in the clotting process is decreased and more remains in the serum, shortening the serum PT.

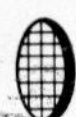

THROMBIN TIME

Reference range

Control ± 5 seconds

EXPLANATION OF THE TEST

Thrombin time is the time required for plasma to clot after the addition of commercially supplied thrombin. Two strengths of thrombin are used. The time required for clot formation is used to estimate the rate of fibrin formation.

VALUE AND LIMITATIONS OF THE TEST

Detection of abnormalities in the fibrinogen/fibrin stage of coagulation

Evaluation of the effectiveness of treatment with heparin, streptokinase, or urokinase

The test is influenced by the amount of patient fibrinogen available and the presence of inhibitors such as fibrin split products, antithrombins, or fibrinolysins.

NURSING ACTION

1. Inform the patient that there are no food or fluid restrictions before the test.
2. Collect venous blood in a 7-ml blue-top tube. Completely fill the collection tube and invert it gently to mix the anticoagulant.
3. Handle the specimen gently; if it cannot be immediately transported to the laboratory, it should be placed on ice.

INTERFERING FACTORS

Improper and rough collecting techniques
Heparin
Plasmin

CLINICAL IMPLICATIONS

Prolonged thrombin time may indicate hepatic disease, DIC, hypofibrinogenemia, or dysfibrinogenemia. It is also prolonged in the newborn and in patients with macroglobulinemia and multiple myeloma.

HEMOLYTIC DISORDERS

Pathophysiology and clinical application of laboratory tests

Hemolysis is the premature destruction of red blood cells, which, if intravascular, would result in the release of hemoglobin into the blood. In the hemolytic anemias this process is the ability of the bone marrow to compensate. Recognition of its presence and determination of its degree are based on the identification of compensatory red blood cell production (erythropoiesis) and increased red blood cell destruction. Red blood cells are usually destroyed in the reticuloendothelial cells, where the hemoglobin is degraded and converted into bilirubin, then released into the plasma and conjugated by the liver. The resulting bilirubin glucuronide is excreted through the biliary system and is measured in the blood as *direct-reacting bilirubin*. If the rate of bilirubin formation exceeds the liver's capacity to conjugate and excrete, there will be an increase in the amount of *indirect bilirubin* in the serum. The unconjugated bilirubin is not found in the urine, because it is not water soluble and not cleared by the kidney.

Routine screening tests for hemolysis are tests for compensatory red blood cell production (reticulocyte count and peripheral smear) and tests for increased red blood cell destruction, reflected by an increase in the level of *indirect-reacting bilirubinemia* and a reduction in the level of *haptoglobins*. If the hemolysis is severe, one sees *hemoglobinuria* (p. 84), which indicates that the amount of plasma hemoglobin exceeds the amount of haptoglobin available to bind it; *hemosiderinuria*, which indicates chronic hemoglobinuria (iron from the reabsorbed hemoglobin is present in shed renal tubular cells from the kidneys and produces this condition); and increased amounts of plasma *lactic dehydrogenase (LD)* (p. 33). Hemosiderinuria may also occur without severe states and elevated LD with extravascular as well as intravascular hemolysis.

Hemolysis can usually be documented with the screening tests just mentioned unless, in addition to hemolysis, there is bone marrow depression (caused by infection, drugs), in which case there would not be reticulocytosis. Other tests that may be used to document the hemolysis and to suggest diagnostic possibilities include *osmotic fragility, autohemolysis, direct and indirect Coombs' test, RBC enzyme assay,* and *hemoglobin electrophoresis*.

Hemolytic anemias

Red blood cells must travel approximately 180 miles in their 10 to 120 days of life. They must pass through micropores smaller than one fifth their resting diameter and therefore must be able to assume different forms. When this quality of "deformability" is lost, it becomes impossible to negotiate the microcirculation and the red blood cell is entrapped and destroyed in the spleen. In the hemolytic anemias there is a premature destruction of red blood cells. This process exceeds the capacity of the bone marrow to produce red blood cells in sufficient numbers to compensate for the premature loss.

The *peripheral smear* provides a rough index of the degree of reticulocytosis, but a *reticulocyte count* is more specific by measuring the number of red cells recently delivered to the blood from the marrow per 100 erythrocytes. The degree of reticulocytosis has some correlation (inverse) with the degree of anemia. If compensatory red blood cell production is occurring, examination of the *bone marrow* reveals erythroid hyperplasia and early megaloblastic changes resulting from folic acid deficiency. RBC hemolysis also causes an elevation of LDH_1 as well as the *total LD* and *potassium* (see Chapter 1). A normal total LD helps to rule out severe hemolytic anemia. It may also cause an increase in *uric acid, AST, ALT*, and *serum iron* to varying degrees.

Laboratory test results for various hemolytic anemias

Reticulocyte count: more than 2.5%
Peripheral blood smear: polychromatophilia, spherocytes, poikilocytes, sickle cells, and so forth
Indirect bilirubin: elevated levels
Lactic dehydrogenase: elevated levels
Haptoglobin: decreased levels
Plasma free hemoglobin: increased levels
Folic acid (serum and red blood cell): decreased levels
Urine analysis: free hemoglobin or hemosiderin
Bone marrow: erythroid hyperplasia

The hemolytic anemias may be divided into 5 classes according to their pathophysiology: (1) hemoglobinopathies, (2) membrane defects, (3) metabolic defects, (4) autoimmune defects, and (5) physical defects.

1. *Hemoglobinopathies* are genetic abnormalities resulting in clinical syndromes such as the thalassemias, sickle cell anemia, and anemias associated with unstable hemoglobins. Technically, hemoglobinopathies refer to production of an abnormal globin (a qualitative defect), whereas thalassemia refers to diminished production (quantitative defect).

The patient's personal and family history suggests the diagnosis and *hemoglobin electrophoresis* usually confirms it (α-thalassemia minor is associated with normal hemoglobin electrophoresis in adults). The *peripheral blood smear* in thalassemias reveals hypochromic, microcytic red cells with frequent target cells; in sickle cell anemia, characteristic sickle forms; and in unstable hemoglobin disease, spherocytes are present and Heinz body preparations are positive. *Gene mapping* is available to definitively diagnose the thalassemias and hemoglobin variants.

2. *RBC membrane defects* may be either inherited or acquired and may be associated with liver disease (especially alcohol-induced cirrhosis) and uremia. Inherited defects are those of membrane cytoskeletal protein constituents, the most common of which are hereditary spherocytosis, hereditary elliptocytosis, and hereditary sto-

matocytosis. Laboratory tests in hereditary spherocytosis reveal spherocytes dominating the peripheral smear, increased osmotic fragility, and mild to moderate anemia; in hereditary elliptocytosis there are elliptic RBCs seen on the peripheral smears and anemia is absent or there is a modest decrease in hematocrit; in hereditary stomatocytosis there are large numbers of stomatocytes seen on the peripheral smear; in anemia of liver disease the peripheral smear reveals acanthocytes (RBCs with irregular membrane spicules, diminished deformability, and decreased survival); in acute alcoholic hepatitis or Zieve's syndrome there is hyperlipemia, hemolysis, and the peripheral smear shows target cells and acanthocytes; in profound hypophosphatemia (<0.25 mg/dl) the RBC adenosine triphosphate is 25% below normal and the peripheral smear shows RBC rigidity, spherocytosis, and hemolytic anemia.

3. *Metabolic defects* constitute a glycolytic enzyme abnormality in which the RBC is less able to adapt to microcirculations and is prematurely destroyed. Metabolic defects include pyruvate kinase (PK) deficiency, glucose-6-phosphate dehydrogenase (G6PD) deficiency, and Wilson's disease.

4. *Autoimmune defects* result from the presence of autoantibodies (warm-reacting IgG or cold-reacting IgM) to RBC antigens, or is an acquired stem cell disorder known as paroxysmal nocturnal hemoglobinuria that is characterized by the production of an RBC clone that has a marked sensitivity to the lytic action of complement. In autoimmune hemolytic anemia the direct Coombs' antiglobulin test is positive, there is reticulocytosis, spherocytosis, and complement components on the RBC surface (50% of patients). In paroxysmal nocturnal hemoglobinuria there is iron deficiency, and the acid hemolysis and sugar water lysis tests are positive.

5. *Physical defects* result when RBCs are driven at high flow rates across fibrin strands causing hemolysis. This can occur with intravascular processes such as disseminated intravascular coagulation, cavernous hemangiomas, hemolytic-uremic syndrome, thrombotic thrombocytopenic purpura, and renal homograft rejection. Physical hemolysis may also occur because of metastatic mucinous adenocarcinoma, cardiac valvular disease, and prosthetic cardiac valves or patches; it also occurs in soldiers who march, joggers, and congo drummers.

LABORATORY TESTS FOR HEMOLYTIC DISORDERS

PERIPHERAL BLOOD FILM

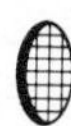

See also p. 69.

CLINICAL IMPLICATIONS IN HEMOLYTIC DISORDERS

Examination of the peripheral blood film may reveal anisocytosis, macrocytosis, and poikilocytosis. Also the following may be suggested from a careful examination of the blood smear:

1. Marked spherocytosis suggests hereditary spherocytosis.
2. Mild spherocytosis suggests hemoglobin C disease.
3. Mild spherocytosis plus a positive reaction to Coombs' test suggests autoimmune hemolysis.
4. The presence of schistocytes in significant numbers or of helmet cells suggests microangiopathic hemolytic anemia (for example, anemia associated with an aortic valve prosthesis).
5. The presence of Heinz bodies during a hemolytic crisis strongly suggests hemolysis caused by red cell enzyme deficiency or unstable hemoglobins.

SERUM HAPTOGLOBIN

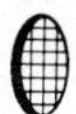

Reference range

60-270 mg/dl (SI units: 0.6-2.7 g/L)

EXPLANATION OF THE TEST

Haptoglobins are produced by the liver to act as transport proteins for hemoglobin. They bind free hemoglobin that has been released as a result of RBC destruction, thus preventing it from being lost in the urine and conserving body iron. Haptoglobin levels decrease 8 hours following hemolysis, suggesting that the available haptoglobin has been bound to free hemoglobin.

VALUE OF THE TEST

Considered to have a sensitivity equal to the reticulocyte count for hemolytic anemia

Combined with reticulocytosis, used to differentiate hemolytic anemia from acute bleeding and from the treatment phase of iron deficiency anemia

CLINICAL IMPLICATIONS

Increased levels

Severe infection, tissue destruction, burns, and in some cases of cancer

Decreased levels

Megaloblastic anemia
Severe liver disease, hematomas
Congenital absence of haptoglobin (3% of blacks)

> **NURSING ALERT**
>
> If the serum haptoglobin level is found to be low, observe the patient for symptoms of hemolysis (chills, fever, back pain, flushing, distended neck veins, tachycardia, tachypnea, and hypotension).

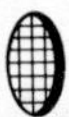

HEMOGLOBIN ELECTROPHORESIS

Reference range

Adults: Hgb A, 95%; Hgb A_2, 2%-3%; Hgb F, <1%. Hgb S and Hgb C are absent.
Neonates: Hgb F is about half the total

EXPLANATION OF THE TEST

This test separates normal from certain abnormal hemoglobins. However, note that there are different methods used for this test, with different patterns depending on the medium used.

VALUE OF THE TEST

Detection of and differential diagnosis among the abnormal hemoglobins

NURSING ACTION

1. Inform the patient that there are no food or fluid restrictions before this test.

2. Collect venous blood in a 7-ml lavender-top tube; completely fill the collection tube and gently invert it to mix the anticoagulant.

CLINICAL IMPLICATIONS

The most common abnormal hemoglobins are Hgb S (sickle cell disease) and Hgb C (mild hemolytic anemia).

Measurement of the Hgb A_2 level is important in the diagnosis of the thalassemias and is commonly ordered in conjunction with tests for the level of Hgb F, since both may be increased in thalassemia.

OSMOTIC FRAGILITY

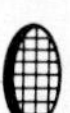

EXPLANATION OF THE TEST

This is a measurement of the ability of a cell to hold extra water. A normal red blood cell is biconcave; in a hypotonic medium, it will fill with water until the osmotic pressure is the same inside and outside of the cell. At a certain critical volume (about 1.8 times the resting volume), a normal cell becomes a perfect sphere and further entry of water produces lysis. A cell that is already spherical can admit less water before it lyses. In this test, RBCs are placed in bottles containing sodium chloride of decreasing concentrations. At a certain concentration RBCs hemolyze.

VALUE OF THE TEST

Useful in the diagnosis of hemolytic anemia
Most useful diagnostic test in congenital spherocytosis

NURSING ACTION

1. Inform the patient that there are no dietary restrictions before this test.
2. Notify the laboratory since this is not a routine test.
3. Withdraw venous blood in a 7-ml green-top tube or a special heparinized tube for collecting defibrinated blood.
4. Completely fill the tube and invert it gently to mix the anticoagulant. Handle the specimen gently to prevent hemolysis.

CLINICAL IMPLICATIONS

Since spherocytes hemolyze at concentrations of sodium chloride above normal range, an increased osmotic fragility strongly suggests hereditary spherocytosis.

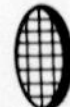

RBC ENZYME ASSAYS

EXPLANATION OF THE TEST

Numerous forms of hemolytic anemia are associated with a deficiency of erythrocyte enzymes. Although quantitative assays are necessary for the identification of most of these anemias, simple screening tests are available for the more common deficiencies in glucose-6-phosphate dehydrogenase (favism), pyruvate kinase, triosephosphate isomerase, and glutathione reductase.

VALUE OF THE TEST

Aids in the differential diagnosis of hemolytic anemia

NURSING ACTION

1. Inform the patient that there are no food or fluid restrictions before this test.
2. Collect venous blood in a 7 ml red-top tube.
3. Handle the specimen gently to avoid hemolysis and transport it immediately to the laboratory.

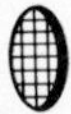

RBC SURVIVAL TIME

Reference range

A normal RBC survives about 120 days, with a half-life of 60 days. The ^{51}Cr-labeled RBCs have a half-life of 25 to 30 days.

EXPLANATION OF THE TEST

A radioactive isotope that will tag the patient's RBCs is given in vitro, the tagged cells are reinjected, and blood samples drawn periodically for isotope counting. The time taken for the tagged cells to disappear is then noted.

VALUE AND LIMITATIONS OF THE TEST

Demonstrates low-grade hemolytic anemias
Not useful in the case of chronic occult extravascular blood loss
Data on the survival of the RBC are not accurate (only approximate)
An expensive and inconvenient test, requiring blood sampling for a few weeks

NURSING ACTION

1. Inform the patient that there are no food or fluid restrictions before this test.
2. Instruct the patient regarding the details of the test.
3. Draw a blood sample and label it with ^{51}Cr.
4. Collect venous blood in a 7-ml lavender-top tube at 24 hours and then at 2 to 3 day intervals for 30 days.

CLINICAL IMPLICATIONS

Demonstrates decreased RBC survival, which defines hemolysis

ACIDIFIED SERUM LYSIS TEST (HAM TESTS)

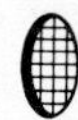

Normal findings

No hemolysis

EXPLANATION OF THE TEST

In paroxysmal nocturnal hemoglobinuria (PNH) the RBCs are more susceptible to hemolysis in acid pH. Therefore, serum is acidified to a point that will not affect normal RBCs, but will hemolyze the RBCs of paroxysmal nocturnal hemoglobinuria.

VALUE OF THE TEST

Determines the cause of undiagnosed hemolytic anemia, hemoglobinuria, and bone marrow aplasia as PNH
A much more specific test than is the urine hemosiderin examination for PNH

NURSING ACTION

1. Inform the patient that there are no dietary restrictions before this test.
2. Laboratory personnel will collect the venous sample since the blood sample must be defibrinated immediately.

INTERFERING FACTORS

False-positive test results from blood containing large numbers of spherocytes and from patients with congenital dyserythropoietic anemia or *hereditary erythrocytic multinuclearity with positive acidified serum* (HEMPAS) (a rare hematologic disorder).

CLINICAL IMPLICATIONS

Hemolysis of the red blood cells indicates paroxysmal nocturnal hemoglobinuria.

FREE HEMOGLOBIN IN PLASMA

Normal findings

Absent

EXPLANATION OF THE TEST

A small amount of free hemoglobin is usually present in plasma because of the technique of drawing the blood and processing (less in plasma than in serum). However, true free plasma hemoglobin occurs when the hemoglobin in the blood has exhausted binding sites on the plasma proteins.

VALUE OF THE TEST

Diagnostic of severe intravascular hemolysis

NURSING ACTION

1. Inform the patient that there are no food or fluid restrictions before the test.
2. Collect venous blood in a 7-ml blue-top tube. Completely fill the collection tube and invert it gently to mix the anticoagulant.

INTERFERING FACTORS

Excessive probing with the needle during venous puncture and rough handling of the specimen

CLINICAL IMPLICATIONS

Severe intravascular hemolysis (after ruling out laboratory artifact)

FREE HEMOGLOBIN IN URINE

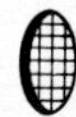

Normal findings

Absent

EXPLANATION OF THE TEST

Normally hemoglobin is not found in the urine. However, if the plasma level of hemoglobin is greater than that of haptoglobin (a plasma α_2-globulin to which free hemoglobin binds), the excess hemoglobin is excreted in the urine. This test utilizes the effect of heme proteins on organic substances to oxidize them and produce a blue color in the specimen.

VALUE OF THE TEST

Aids in the diagnosis of hemolytic anemia or transfusion reaction

NURSING ACTION

1. Inform the patient that there are no food or fluid restrictions before this test.
2. Instruct the patient in the collection of a random urine specimen.
3. The test should be rescheduled if there is menstruation.
4. Send the specimen to the laboratory immediately.

CLINICAL IMPLICATIONS

Severe intravascular hemolysis caused by blood transfusion reaction, burns, or a crush injury

Acquired hemolytic anemias resulting from chemical or drug intoxication or malaria

Hemolytic anemia (paroxysmal nocturnal hemoglobinuria)

Congenital hemolytic anemias (hemoglobinopathies or enzyme defects)

Less commonly, cystitis, ureteral calculi, urethritis
Glomerulonephritis or pyelonephritis (from renal epithelial damage)
Renal tumor or infarction

GAMMOPATHIES

The gammopathies are a group of immunologic disorders in which neoplastic cells synthesize and secrete immunoglobulins, which may be monoclonal or polyclonal.

Monoclonal gammopathy results in increased plasma levels of a monoclonal immunoglobulin (IgG, IgM, IgA, IgG, IgE) and includes diseases such as multiple myeloma, Waldenström's macroglobulinemia, amyloidosis, heavy-chain disease, and chronic lymphocytic leukemia.

Polyclonal gammopathy results in a heterogeneous increase in immunoglobulins involving more than one clonal line and includes diseases such as cirrhosis of the liver, Hodgkin's disease, rheumatoid arthritis, lupus erythematosus, tuberculosis, leishmaniasis, certain lymphomas, and metastatic carcinoma.

The two major gammopathies are multiple myeloma and Waldenström's macroglobulinemia. Monoclonal gammopathies are usually detected because *clinical symptoms* suggest myeloma and *serum protein electrophoresis* is then ordered. *Bone marrow aspiration* is required to support the diagnosis by demonstration of atypical plasmocytosis. If the only protein abnormality is urinary excretion of Bence Jones protein, there may be no monoclonal-type serum peak and it is necessary to perform *urine protein electrophoresis* on a concentrated specimen. In some cases, when the diagnosis is not evident, *serum and urine immunoelectrophoresis* is necessary and many authorities advocate this for all patients being screened for gammopathies.

Nonspecific tests are markedly elevated sedimentation rate, rouleaux formation in the blood smear, hyperuricemia (reflecting abnormal cell turnover or renal failure), and increased alkaline phosphatase level.

LABORATORY TESTS FOR THE GAMMOPATHIES

Protein electrophoresis (p. 44) and bone marrow aspiration have already been discussed.

IMMUNOELECTROPHORESIS

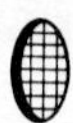

EXPLANATION OF THE TEST

Immunoelectrophoresis is a sensitive, relatively uncomplicated procedure useful in detecting the specific monoclonal proteins. In this test, after ordinary protein electrophoresis is performed, antiserum against a specific type of human globulin is added, and the areas of reaction within a gel between the patient's immunoglobulin fractions and corresponding antibodies form visual lines.

VALUE OF THE TEST

An important diagnostic test in patients with symptoms of myeloma or pathologic findings in the peripheral blood, bone marrow, or lymph node

Useful in differentiating macroglobulinemia from other types of monoclonal gammopathy

Level of IgE helpful in assessing allergic states.

NURSING ACTION

1. Inform patient that he or she should take nothing by mouth except for water and medications 8 hours before collection of specimen.
2. Collect venous blood in 7-ml red-top tube. Handle specimen gently to prevent hemolysis.

DIRECT COOMBS' TEST (DIRECT ANTIGLOBULIN TEST)

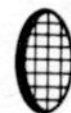

Normal results

Negative in adults and children (no agglutination)

Positive results

1+-4+

EXPLANATION OF THE TEST

This test detects autoantibodies against RBCs. Coombs' serum is anti–human globulin developed from rabbit serum. The patient's serum and the red cells are mixed and incubated with the Coombs' serum. The antibodies in this serum will attach to any antibody coating the RBC and cause agglutination (a positive result). Lack of agglutination is a normal response and indicates that there are no circulating antibodies against RBC antigens in the patient's serum.

VALUE AND LIMITATIONS OF THE TEST

Differentiates acquired immunologic hemolytic anemias (globulin on the RBCs) from nonimmunologically mediated hemolytic anemias

Useful in the early diagnosis of hemolytic disease of the newborn (erythroblastosis fetalis), idiopathic autoimmune hemolytic anemia, drug-induced hemolytic anemia, and hemolytic transfusion reactions

Detects immunoglobulin (IgG) and/or complement coating the erythrocytes of patients with warm-antibody autoimmune hemolytic anemia

Detects antibodies to red cell antigens before transfusion

Detects anti $Rh_0(D)$ antibody in maternal blood

Assists in the diagnosis of acquired hemolytic anemia

A positive result does not identify the antibody responsible.

NURSING ACTION

1. Inform the patient that there are no food or fluid restrictions before this test.
2. Collect venous blood in a purple-top tube. The Coombs' serum is added directly to the fresh blood either in the test tube or on a slide.
3. Send the specimen to the laboratory immediately.

NURSING ALERT

Watch for the development of a hematoma at the venipuncture site. Apply warm soaks in this event.

INTERFERING FACTORS

Presence of reticulocytosis, which may result in a weakly positive reaction owing to the binding of transferrin (a globulin) to the reticulocyte membranes

A prior transfusion that resulted in minor blood group incompatibility

The most common drugs that, although they do not actually interfere with the test, are possible causes of immune-mediated hemolysis are:

cephaloridine (Loridine)	cephalothin (Keflin)
penicillin	streptomycin
tetracycline	aminopyrine (Pyradone)
chlorpromazine (Thorazine)	phenytoin (Dilantin)
ethosuximide (Zarontin)	hydralazine (Apresoline)
isoniazid (INH)	levodopa
methyldopa (Aldomet)	procainamide (Pronestyl)
quinidine	rifampin (Rifadin)
sulfonamides	

Heparin may produce a false-negative test in individuals with acquired hemolytic anemia.

CLINICAL IMPLICATIONS

The direct Coombs' test may be positive in

Autoimmune hemolytic anemia (idiopathic, drug-induced, associated with disease such as lymphomas and lupus erythematosus).

Laboratory artifact associated with sepsis, cephalothin, penicillin.

Umbilical cord blood indicates hemolytic disease caused by maternal antibodies crossing the placenta. A transfusion of Rh-negative blood may be necessary.

ABO BLOOD TYPING

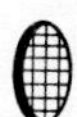

EXPLANATION OF THE TEST

Before blood transfusions are given, the blood group of the recipient and of the donor must be determined to ensure the similarity of the antigenic properties of the blood of the two individuals. If the necessary precautions are not taken, red blood cell agglutination and hemolysis may result. This situation (transfusion reaction) can lead to the death of the recipient.

The surfaces of the red blood cells contain antigens, which determine the blood type of the individual. Normally, people do not form antibodies against the antigens of their own red cells, but if a person receives a transfusion with blood containing different antigens, antibodies may be formed against all of the foreign antigens. Among the antigens, two groups, the ABO and Rh groups, are highly antigenic and can cause a transfusion reaction if they are transfused into persons with incompatible blood types.

VALUE OF THE TEST

Assures the transfusion of compatible blood

NURSING ACTION

1. Inform the patient that there are no dietary restrictions before this test.
2. Check the patient's history for recent transfusion, or administration of intravenous dextran or contrast media.
3. Withdraw venous blood in a 10-ml lavender-top tube or a red-top tube if cross-matching is also to be done.
4. Handle the specimen gently to avoid hemolysis and send it to the laboratory immediately.

RESULTS OF THE TEST

Forward typing

Type A: agglutination occurs when the patient's red cells are mixed with anti-A serum.

Type B: agglutination occurs when the patient's red cells are mixed with anti-B serum.

Type AB: agglutination occurs with both anti-A and anti-B serum.

Type O: agglutination does not occur with either anti-A or anti-B serum.

Reverse typing

Type A: agglutination occurs when B cells are mixed with the patient's serum.

Type B: agglutination occurs when A cells are mixed with the patient's serum.

Type AB: agglutination does not occur when A and B cells are mixed with the patient's serum.

Type O: agglutination occurs when A and B cells are mixed with the patient's serum.

Rh Typing:

Rh Positive: agglutination occurs when serum containing anti-D antibodies is added to the patient's blood.

Rh Negative: agglutination does not occur when serum containing anti-D antibodies is added to the patient's blood.

CROSS-MATCHING

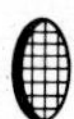

EXPLANATION OF THE TEST

Cross-matching avoids transfusion reactions by establishing compatibility or incompatibility between the blood of the recipient and the donor. A complete cross-match takes from 45 minutes to 2 hours and tests for compatibility between the donor's red cells and the recipient's serum.

VALUE OF THE TEST

Makes the final compatibility check before a transfusion is initiated

NURSING ACTION

1. Inform the patient that there are no dietary restrictions before this test.
2. Check the patient's history for recent transfusion, or administration of intravenous dextran or contrast media.
3. Withdraw venous blood in a 10-ml red-top tube if cross-matching is also to be done.
4. Handle the specimen gently to avoid hemolysis and send it to the laboratory immediately.

RESULTS OF THE TEST

Positive: indicates incompatibility between the donor and the patient's blood: agglutination when the donor's red cells and the recipient's serum are mixed and incubated

Negative: indicates probable compatibility between donor and patient blood: absence of agglutination

11

Diagnostic tests for neurologic disorders

ANATOMY AND PHYSIOLOGY OF THE BRAIN

The brain consists of three major parts: the cerebrum, the cerebellum, and the brain stem. The cerebrum is the largest division and is divided into two hemispheres, each of which has four lobes—frontal, temporal, parietal, and occipital. The *cerebrum* is the highest integrative center of the nervous system; it is responsible for sensation, perception, memory, consciousness, judgment, and will. The *cerebellum,* located just below the posterior portion of the cerebrum, functions in the control of skeletal muscles. The *brain stem* is composed of the midbrain, the pons, and the medulla oblongata, which connects the brain with the spinal cord and controls breathing, heart rate, and blood pressure. (See Fig. 11-1.)

The three meninges or membranes that envelop the brain and spinal cord are the *dura mater,* the *arachnoid mater,* and the *pia mater* (Fig. 11-2). Their names imply their qualities: the dura is the strong, tough outer layer; the arachnoid is a delicate layer between the dura mater and the pia mater; and the pia adheres to the brain surface like a delicate skin. The pia, which could also be compared to a delicate, transparent layer of cellophane, contains numerous capillaries and arterioles. It is the pia and arachnoid membranes that become inflamed and thickened as a result of infection or hemorrhage and that account for the headache and neck stiffness occurring in those conditions.

A potential space, called the *subdural space,* lies between the dura mater and the arachnoid mater. Between the arachnoid mater and the pia mater lies an actual space, called the *subarachnoid space,* which is filled with cerebrospinal fluid (CSF).

Cerebrospinal fluid is produced by filtration from blood circulating through the richly vascular tissue of the choroid plexuses, which

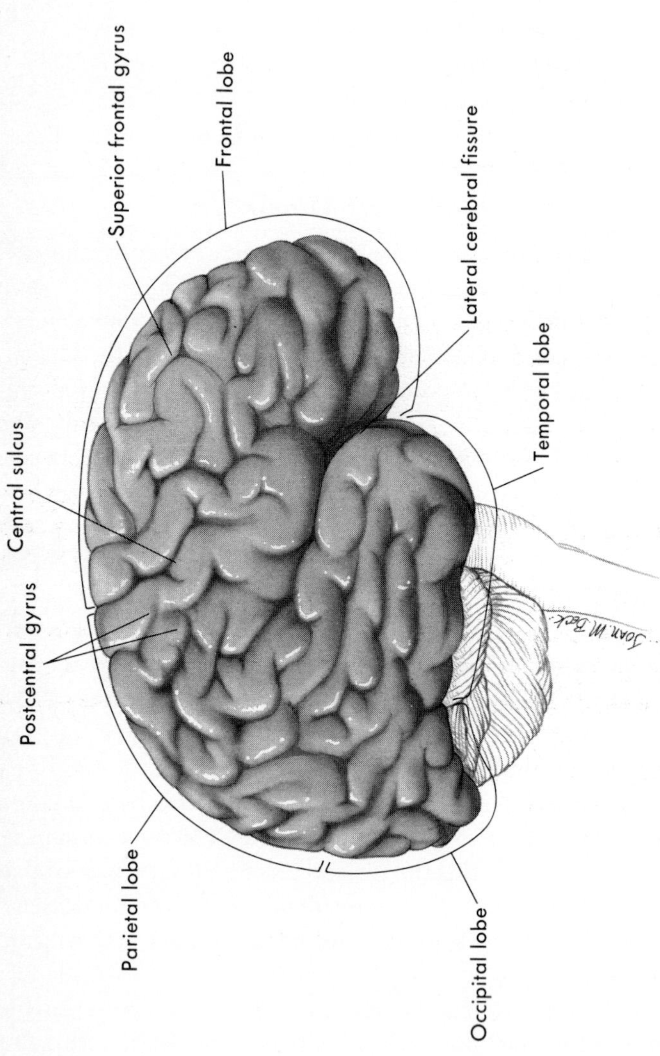

Fig. 11-1. *Right hemisphere of Cerebrum, lateral surface.* (*From Thibodeau, G.A.: Textbook of anatomy and physiology, ed. 12, St. Louis, 1987, Times Mirror/Mosby College Publishing.*)

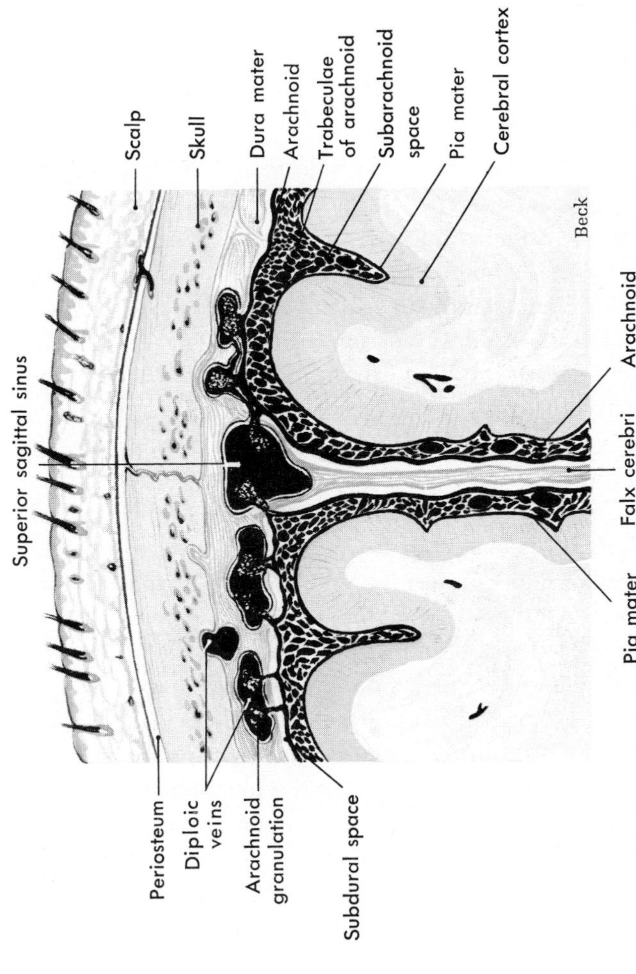

Fig. 11-2. *The meninges of the brain as seen in coronal section through the skull. (From Thibodeau, G.A.: Textbook of anatomy and physiology, ed. 12, St. Louis, 1987, Times Mirror/Mosby College Publishing.)*

are secretory modifications of the pia mater that project into the ventricles of the brain. The continuously formed, fresh cerebrospinal fluid must drain out of the ventricles through the apertures in the fourth ventricle, in the brain stem. It must freely circulate through the subarachnoid spaces and over all the surfaces of the brain and spinal cord. It is then mostly reabsorbed into the venous system by specially modified arachnoid tissue, called arachnoid granulations (see Fig. 11-2).

PATHOPHYSIOLOGY

The skull can expand in response to increasing intracranial pressure resulting from hydrocephalus or tumor, until skull sutures ossify at age 12 or 13. After that age, increasing pressure inside the then rigid skull pushes the brain downward and backward into the foramen magnum. This foramen is the largest opening in the skull; it surrounds the lower brain stem and its junction with the spinal cord. Increasing intracranial pressure resulting from trauma, hemorrhage, tumor, infection, or hypoxia can force the cone-shaped brain stem ever lower into the bony foramen magnum until the brain stem and the adjacent cerebellar tonsils become tightly wedged or impacted in the foramen magnum. This situation is invariably accompanied by rapid clinical deterioration, as evidenced by decreased responsiveness to stimuli, coma, dilated and/or nonreactive pupils, and Cheyne-Stokes respiration, apnea, or other abnormal respiratory patterns.

Another special area of brain vulnerability is the midbrain. Here the cerebral peduncles, which connect each hemisphere with the brain stem, must pass through a small, semicircular, sharp-edged opening, the incisura in the tentorium, a strong dural structure on each side of the brain stem that forms the roof of the posterior fossa. Any substantial increase in the volume of one cerebral hemisphere, whether from head injury, hemorrhage, tumor, abscess, or large infarction, can wedge the inferior and medial portion of the temporal lobe (the uncus) down into this semicircular opening in the tentorium. This forces the midbrain laterally into the opposite knifelike dural edge of the tentorium and usually results in multiple hemorrhages in the midbrain and compression of either the ipsilateral or the contralateral third nerves as they sweep around the lateral margins of the midbrain en route to the orbits.

Despite the remarkable versatility of the brain, it reacts to most clinical insults by either localized or generalized swelling. Thus the following conditions can all cause serious problems in clinical management of increased intracranial pressure: traumatic head injury; hypertensive or idiopathic intracerebral hemorrhage; subarachnoid hemorrhage caused by ruptured aneurysms; large infarcts resulting from thrombosis or cerebral embolus; hypoxia resulting from cardiac arrest, drowning, or neonatal asphyxia; bacterial meningitis or viral encephalitis; brain abscess; electrolyte depletion; and poisoning with lead or mercury.

The most critical practical considerations in regard to brain anatomy and physiology are the fact that the size of the skull is fixed, allowing no room for expansion of an injured and swollen brain, and the fact that brain swelling is the end result of most metabolic insults. Continuous monitoring of intracranial pressure is therefore becoming widely used in large intensive care units; a manometer is placed in a skull burr hole by a neurosurgeon. Continuous monitoring is of considerable advantage in assessing the need for:

1. Medical decompression by means of dexamethasone (Decadron), mannitol, or urea
2. Controlled hyperventilation to lower PCO_2
3. Intravenous administration of barbiturates to further lower intracranial pressure in certain head injuries
4. Surgical decompression of the brain by ventricular drainage, by evacuation of intracerebral blood clots or necrotic brain tissue, or by ventricular shunts. Surgical decompression is used when medical decompression is inadequate or not the method of choice.

CLINICAL APPLICATION OF LABORATORY TESTS

Cerebral thrombosis

Usually there is an onset over a period of minutes to a few hours of a neurologic deficit such as limb weakness or numbness or speech impairment, which slowly improves or even resolves over the next few days, weeks, or months.

When history, physical findings, and hospital course are all well documented and consistent with the clinical impression of cerebral thrombosis, extensive laboratory evaluations are usually not required.

Patients who fell at the onset of their neurologic symptoms, or who were found on the floor, and/or have scalp contusions or other evidence of recent injury should have *skull films* taken.

Patients who develop headaches, vomiting, seizures, neck stiffness, decreasing alertness, or decreasing speech or limb function after hospital admission should have *computed tomographic (CT) brain scans* to rule out intracranial hemorrhage, hematoma, or brain swelling secondary to infarction. A *spinal tap* is usually not required in an ordinary case of cerebral thrombosis, but it is of value in ruling out hemorrhage when a patient's condition deteriorates in the hospital and CT scans are not available. *Electroencephalograms* are not routine when the history and physical examination are fairly characteristic of cerebral infarction, unless there is a clinical suspicion of seizure activity.

Stroke in progress

An occasional patient who shows progressive or stepwise deterioration after admission to the hospital will have a normal CT scan but will have an isotope perfusion scan that shows a focal perfusion defect. Many such patients have progressive strokes; if these patients are normotensive, they may be candidates for intravenous heparin treatment, after clear spinal fluid has first been demonstrated.

Cerebral embolus

Because there is not time for development of a collateral source of blood flow in a case of cerebral embolus, unlike the situation in an instance of a slowly enlarging atheroma in a cerebral thrombosis case, the onset of embolic stroke is often more dramatic and rapid than the onset of cerebral thrombosis and the neurologic deficits can peak in a few minutes.

The following are common predisposing conditions: recent myocardial infarction, with formation of a mural thrombus; atrial fibrillation; ulcerated plaque in the aortic arch or in the common or internal carotid artery; fibrin or platelet emboli resulting from prosthetic heart valves; mitral stenosis, with enlarged left atrium; mitral valve prolapse syndrome; and subacute bacterial endocarditis.

If cholesterol crystals or fibrin emboli are seen on *funduscopic examination*, or if an *echocardiogram* and other cardiac evaluations suggest a source for an embolus, the risk posed by the possibility that additional cerebral emboli will occur is usually greater than the risks involved in anticoagulation therapy (in normotensive patients). There is, however, a controversy over whether to begin anticoagulation therapy immediately or to wait a few days or a week.

The indications for *EEG, spinal tap*, and *CT or isotope scans* are similar to those described for cerebral thrombosis patients. In some patients no cardiac source for a suspected embolus is present, and careful funduscopic examination may show small quantities of cholesterol or fibrin debris lodged in retinal artery branch points. In such a case, if the residual neurologic deficit is not severe and the patient is otherwise a surgical candidate, *arch angiograms* should be done to look for ulcerated atheromatous plaques in the common and internal carotid arteries.

Intracerebral hemorrhage

Long-standing and poorly controlled hypertension is the most significant risk factor for an intracerebral hemorrhage. Such hemorrhages usually occur deep in the hemispheres—in the basal ganglia and the internal capsule—but they also occur in the pons and the cerebellum. The onset is often announced by a sudden headache in a previously well patient, usually followed quickly by nausea, vomiting, and disturbed speech (if the hemorrhage is in the dominant hemisphere or the brain stem), and by hemiparesis.

A *spinal tap* can be hazardous in such a patient if intracranial pressure is elevated; it is not ordinarily necessary for diagnosis when CT scans can be quickly obtained. Emergency surgical drainage of hemorrhages is often done when they occur in cerebellar hemispheres or in nondominant cerebral hemispheres and the patient is still thought to have a chance to recover.

Subarachnoid hemorrhage

A subarachnoid hemorrhage is most commonly the result of the rupture of an aneurysm on the circle of Willis, which is located at the base of the brain. A subarachnoid hemorrhage typically causes sudden headache, followed within 1 or 2 hours by neck stiffness and pain caused by blood free in the basal cisterns diffusing down into the cervical subarachnoid space. A leaking aneurysm of the anterior communicating artery usually causes no physical findings except for neck stiffness; a leaking aneurysm of the posterior communicating artery frequently causes diplopia and third-nerve weakness; a leaking aneurysm of the middle cerebral artery often causes varying degrees of contralateral hemiparesis and may cause dysphasic speech if it is in the dominant hemisphere.

Since small amounts of subarachnoid bleeding can be missed on a *CT scan*, a *spinal fluid examination* is still necessary in cases in which a CT scan is normal but clinical suspicion of a subarachnoid hemorrhage remains strong.

Transient ischemic attack (TIA)

Transient ischemic attacks are caused by brief but critical periods of blood flow reduction distal to an atherosclerotic narrowing of an internal carotid, vertebral, or basilar artery, or by small emboli that lodge temporarily at cerebral artery branch points and then break up and move on into small, more distal arteries. Such attacks last from 1 or 2 minutes to several hours, with the average being 15 minutes. Carotid system TIAs most often produce transient monocular blindness (amaurosis fugax) or transient hemiparesis and hemisensory loss with or without dysphasic speech. Vertebral basilar transient attacks are suggested by the presence of one or more of the following transient symptoms: diplopia, numbness of the lips and tongue, slurred speech, drop attacks, ataxia, or hemiparetic episodes that alternate from one side of the body to the other.

One third to one half of all patients who have cerebral thrombosis have a warning TIA hours, days, or weeks before the completed stroke, and 10% to 15% of all untreated patients who have a TIA develop a completed stroke within 1 year. Most of these strokes occur in the first 5 or 6 months after the TIA.

When the history is typical and reliable, a patient is usually referred for *arch angiography* or *selective cerebral angiograms*. When a history of TIA is doubtful or less reliable, *noninvasive cerebral flow studies* can be most helpful in identifying internal carotid flow restriction.

Patients who are found to have significant atheromatous stenosis at the internal carotid artery origin or ulcerated plaques at that location are ordinarily advised to have a carotid endarterectomy. This procedure has been shown to reduce the incidence of subsequent TIAs and of strokes, and it has had a combined operative mortality and morbidity of less than 3% in many hospitals. In cases in which internal carotid stenosis is not severe and no ulcerated plaques are present, anticoagulants or antiplatelet drugs may reduce the incidence of further TIAs and of strokes.

Acute head injury

Skull films should be obtained after any acute head injury that leads to a period of unconsciousness or that is followed by vomiting or confusion. A nondepressed skull fracture is not in itself of much clinical significance, but it could indicate that a blow has been strong enough to cause injury to the brain or meningeal arteries. Fractures through the base of the skull into the ear or sinuses should be suspected when trauma is followed by clear or serous drainage from an ear or the nose. Such patients often are given broad-spectrum antibiotics to reduce the risk of intracranial infection.

Anterior-posterior and lateral cervical spinal films should be made, along with skull films, in any case of acute head injury in which the patient does not move all limbs well, is confused, or has depressed consciousness.

An *emergency CT brain scan* is invaluable in the case of a head-injured patient who has a depressed state of consciousness or whose neurologic status deteriorates (as reported by relatives, if the patient has been at home, or by hospital personnel). Such deterioration in a previously awake and talking patient suggests acute epidural or subdural hematoma. Such findings on a CT scan or, if a CT scanner is not available, on an angiogram ordinarily call for prompt neurosurgical intervention.

An *electroencephalogram* is usually not very helpful in evaluating acute head injuries, but it can be of prognostic help in subacute and recovery stages.

A *spinal tap* is usually unnecessary and can be hazardous. It is performed only if a head injury is suspected of being complicated by intracranial infection.

Intracranial pressure monitoring by means of an epidural, subdural, or intraventricular manometer placed through a skull burr hole is being used in large hospitals. The procedure is being used in certain cases of severe head injury in which high intracranial pressure is life threatening.

Spinal cord injury or tumor

Plain spine films are indicated whenever spinal injuries or spinal cord tumors are suspected.

Myelography, performed promptly, is in order when clinical suspicion is increased because of the history and the physical findings of progressive limb weakness and numbness, with or without back pain or impaired bladder control. This procedure should generally not be delayed for performance of a spinal tap, a Queckenstedt test, or electromyography (EMG). Myelographic findings of partial or complete spinal canal block resulting from fracture-dislocation or from a tumor usually call for prompt neurosurgical and/or orthopedic consultation. Some cases of cord compression resulting from metastatic cancer may be treated with dexamethasone (Decadron) and irradiation as an alternative to surgery.

Myopathic disorders

The most common cause of generalized muscle weakness in hospital patients is hypokalemia; serum potassium levels should therefore be checked in such patients. High doses of steroids, alcoholism, myxedema, and occult carcinoma are examples of other causes of generalized myopathy, which often appears first in the hip girdle muscles. Such patients must use their arms to push themselves up out of low chairs. Muscular dystrophies typically are characterized by very slowly progressive and painless weakness of the limbs and limb girdles without any sensory impairment. Careful inquiry into a patient's family history will usually reveal that other family members are also affected. Duchenne dystrophy is unique in that the weakened leg muscles of affected young boys usually appear larger than normal and both the boys and their asymptomatic carrier mothers have elevated serum levels of creatine kinase (CK).

Special histochemical stains and electron microscopic studies of muscle biopsy specimens are the most useful laboratory examinations in muscle disease; they have resulted in the classification of many subtypes of muscular dystrophy in recent years. The identification of a carnitine enzyme deficiency in some forms of limb-girdle dystrophy has enabled affected patients to be treated with carnitine supplements.

Seizure disorders

In seizure disorders the workup varies according to individual circumstances, but a few general principles can be stated.

Focal seizures have a higher correlation with structural brain lesions such as tumors, hemorrhages, and abscesses than do generalized seizures.

Seizures in pediatric patients are less likely to be caused by structural brain lesions than are seizures in adults.

Seizures that first appear in patients who are hospitalized for other conditions are often of metabolic origin. Among the occasional inciting causes are the following: hyponatremia; excessive use of, or withdrawal from the use of, alcohol or hypnotic or tranquilizing drugs before hospital admission; high serum levels of aminophylline or lidocaine; and cerebral hypoxia.

Laboratory tests usually include electroencephalography, skull x-ray films, and, in adults, a CT scan as well. An electroencephalogram (EEG) is abnormal in about 75% of patients with seizures. Sleep EEGs may be useful in patients who have normal routine EEGs but who have primarily nocturnal seizures or temporal lobe seizures.

When seizures are suspected to be of metabolic origin, the following tests are usually done: serum electrolytes levels, calcium levels, magnesium levels, blood glucose levels, and, in selected patients, arterial blood gas determinations and serum lidocaine and aminophylline levels.

If a patient has a history of seizures and has been prescribed anticonvulsants, determinations of serum anticonvulsant drug levels are helpful in assessing the patient's compliance with the physician's instructions. Such determinations also help a physician to adjust an anticonvulsant drug regimen.

Headaches

Since headaches can have dozens of causes, the extent of laboratory investigation depends heavily on the history and the physical examination. In general, headaches that are constant or progressive in intensity or frequency, awaken a patient from sleep, or are accompanied by stiff neck, anorexia, nausea, or vomiting require fairly extensive laboratory investigation. Headaches that are episodic, with interim periods of good health, begin during the day in fairly regular relation to job or other stresses, remit during vacations, and are relieved by simple analgesics are usually less extensively investigated. The most common headaches seen in outpatient practice are migraine and tension headaches.

Migraine headaches are typically periodic temporal-frontal-orbital headaches that occur in persons who are otherwise well; these headaches often are accompanied by photophobia or bright scotomas in the visual fields and by nausea or vomiting. They often are severe enough to prevent a person from continuing daily activity. Migraine headaches are frequently alleviated by ergotamine-containing medications and by sleep. A family history of migraines is common.

Tension headaches are usually occipital, cervical, or generalized. They begin during the day, they are often associated with environmental stresses, and they do not awaken a person at night. Such a headache often remits on holidays or during vacations, and it frequently clears as a result of simple analgesics, reassurance, and rearrangement of daily schedules to minimize frustrations and stresses.

A rare cause of headaches in persons over 55 years of age is temporal arteritis. Any patient over that age presenting with headaches should have a *Westergren sedimentation rate test* done, which is an excellent screening tool. It is important to identify this disease because, although rare, it carries with it a significant risk of blindness if undiagnosed and untreated. Treatment consists of the administration of steroids.

A frequent cause of headaches that regularly begin on *awakening* in the morning is undiagnosed or inadequately controlled hypertension. Blood pressure control usually results in prompt headache relief.

If the history and the physical examination lead a clinician to order laboratory investigation of the cause of a patient's headaches, one generally starts with *skull films*, *sinus films*, and an *electroencephalogram*. If the suspicion of an intracranial mass persists, the clinician goes on to a *CT brain scan*, if it is available, or to an *isotope brain scan*. Most patients who have unremitting headaches accompanied by unexplained fever or persistent neck stiffness and who have negative brain scans should also have *cerebrospinal fluid examinations* to rule out minimal subarachnoid hemorrhage or central nervous system infections.

Coma

The causes of coma are legion. A clinician's first task is to determine whether a patient's coma is of primary (central nervous system) origin or of metabolic origin. This determination is complex and beyond the purposes of this book. However, a few generalizations can be made. Localized abnormalities, as shown by neurologic examination or an electroencephalogram, suggest a central nervous system cause; generalized or symmetrical abnormalities usually correlate with metabolic causes.

Laboratory tests for metabolic causes of coma might include most or all of the following: *serum hypnotic screening panel, blood alcohol level, electrolyte levels, and levels of calcium, phosphorus, magnesium, blood urea nitrogen (BUN), creatinine, triiodothyronine, thyroxine, blood glucose, arterial blood gases, aspartate aminotransferase (AST), alanine aminotransferase (ALT), alkaline phosphatase,* and *serum ammonia*.

Suspected central nervous system causes of coma ideally would be investigated by *EEG* and by *CT* or *isotope brain scans* before a physician proceeds to *cerebrospinal fluid examination*. However, when a comatose patient has an unexplained fever and petechiae, or there is other reason to suspect acute meningitis, time is of critical importance; in most such instances the physician should do a spinal fluid examination promptly, without waiting for an EEG or scans.

NEUROLOGIC LABORATORY TESTS

CEREBROSPINAL FLUID (CSF) EXAMINATION

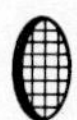

EXPLANATION OF THE TEST

A lumbar spinal tap is a relatively harmless procedure; it can be quickly and easily done on cooperative patients by physicians with some experience. Cisternal puncture, however, is very hazardous unless done by experienced physicians; patients must be cooperative or sedated. Fortunately, a cisternal tap is only rarely necessary–for example, in the treatment of fungal meningitis, when it is indicated for instillation of a small amount of amphotericin into the cisternal cerebrospinal fluid.

VALUE OF THE TEST

Essential in the diagnosis and management of herpes simplex encephalitis, bacterial or fungal meningitis, or meningeal leukemia or carcinoma

May be necessary when cerebral hemorrhage is suspected. Although clear evidence of hemorrhage on a CT scan of the brain usually eliminates the need for a spinal tap, a normal CT scan does not always eliminate the possibility of a small subarachnoid hemorrhage and a spinal tap may be indicated.

NURSING ACTION

1. Inform the patient that there are no dietary restrictions before this test.
2. Describe the procedure to the patient and explain that this test enables the physician to evaluate the fluid within the spinal column. Stress the importance of full cooperation during the test.
3. Obtain a signed consent.
4. Evaluate the patient for signs of anxiety, assess vital signs, and notify the physician if warranted.
5. The patient is usually placed in the lateral decubitus position, with the back even with the edge of the mattress and knees folded up against the chest to the extent consistent with comfort. Drapes obscure landmarks and are best avoided. If the patient is obese or apprehensive or has scoliosis, the procedure is best accomplished with the patient sitting across the bed with legs extended and trunk flexed forward to the extent consistent with comfort.
6. Following the test advise the patient to lie flat, although he or she may turn from side to side, for 8 hours or as ordered. There is a high risk of spinal headache if even a 30-degree elevation of the head of the bed is permitted.
7. Observe the puncture site for redness and swelling.

THE QUECKENSTEDT MANEUVER

The Queckenstedt maneuver involves temporary compression of both jugular veins to see if the cerebrospinal fluid level promptly rises in a manometer and then promptly falls with jugular release. This maneuver is dangerous when intracranial pressure is elevated; it *should not be done* under the following circumstances:

1. When opening pressure on the spinal tap is elevated
2. When the diagnosis is uncertain
3. When an intracranial mass, hemorrhage, or edema is suspected

The maneuver is only justified when compression of the spinal cord as a result of tumor, blood clot, or acute vertebral fracture is suspected.

Normal opening pressure is 180 mm of water in relaxed patients who are in the lateral decubitus position. The cerebrospinal fluid level is at or below the level of the foramen magnum in patients who are in the sitting position.

CLINICAL IMPLICATIONS OF CSF

Grossly clear

Routine cerebrospinal fluid tests on grossly clear specimens include red cell and white cell counts, determination of glucose and protein levels, and the Venereal Disease Research Laboratories (VDRL) test.

Blood

The presence of blood could result from recent intracranial or intraspinal bleeding, or it could result from the needle striking a small vein or capillary as it penetrates the arachnoid membrane to enter the lumbar subarachnoid space, a fairly common occurrence that causes diagnostic confusion. The most reliable method of distinguishing this mere "bloody tap" from preexisting and critically important recent intracranial or intraspinal hemorrhage is to take the tubes of cerebrospinal fluid *immediately* to the laboratory and have one tube centrifuged *at once*. If the blood in the cerebrospinal fluid has been freshly released as a result of needle puncture of the arachnoid membrane, the spun supernatant cerebrospinal fluid will be crystal clear because red cells will not yet have hemolyzed and caused staining of the supernatant fluid.

Intracranial or intraspinal hemorrhage that has occurred an hour or more before the tap usually has resulted in enough hemolysis of red cells so that supernatant cerebrospinal fluid is slightly pink or straw colored, or yields a positive *Hematest* result. This centrifuge test is much more reliable than determining the percentage of crenated red cells in the cerebrospinal fluid or the degree of clearing of blood in serial tubes of cerebrospinal fluid.

Important: Since red cells in tubes of cerebrospinal fluid can hemolyze in 20 to 30 minutes while sitting at nursing stations or in laboratory receiving areas, all cerebrospinal fluid specimens should be sent to the laboratory *at once* and processed *immediately* upon arrival. This promptness is also crucial to accurate red cell and white cell counts, accurate glucose level determinations, and valid cerebrospinal fluid cytological or cell button examinations.

Cloudy

Cloudy fluid requires an immediate Gram stain and usually acid-fast stains as well as cultures for aerobic, anaerobic, and acid-fast bacteria. It is a good policy for hospital laboratories to telephone all results of Gram and acid-fast stains and all abnormal cell counts and low glucose values to the physician promptly so that he or she may initiate additional bacterial or other studies while the remaining cerebrospinal fluid specimen is still fresh.

The findings of 100 or fewer lymphocytes, a normal or modestly increased protein level, a negative Gram stain, and a normal glucose level are characteristic of viral meningoencephalitis. The same spinal fluid, except for the substitution of a low glucose level, suggests tuberculous or fungal meningitis, meningeal leukemia, meningeal carcinoma, or incompletely treated bacterial meningitis.

Acute bacterial meningitis usually produces cloudy or turbid cerebrospinal fluid containing many hundreds or thousands of white cells per cubic millimeter, predominantly polymorphonuclear cells. Protein levels in such cases often are greater than 250 mg/dl and can reach 800 to 1000 mg/dl.

Tuberculous (TB) meningitis usually produces several hundred white cells, predominantly mononuclear cells, along with low glucose levels and high protein levels (more than 200 mg/dl). The low cerebrospinal fluid chloride level long reported to be associated with TB meningitis is thought by some to be correlated with systemic chloride depletion as a result of repeated vomiting rather than with any intrinsic disturbance of chloride metabolism in the spinal fluid.

An acid-fast stain is sometimes diagnostic; acid-fast cultures are often not positive for 4 to 6 weeks.

The differential diagnosis of TB meningitis often includes fungal meningitis, in which case india ink preparations and cerebrospinal fluid tests for cryptococcal antigen and for antibodies to *Coccidioides immitis* are helpful.

Glucose

Normally the glucose level in the cerebrospinal fluid is two thirds the blood glucose level, or about 45 to 70 mg/dl in the fasting adult. Because of the filtration of glucose into the cerebrospinal fluid from blood, the glucose level of the cerebrospinal fluid bears a direct relationship to the current blood level. Therefore, the lower limit of the normal cerebrospinal fluid glucose concentration for a particular patient can be reliably determined only by means of a simultaneous blood glucose determination. Thus, whenever a central nervous system infection is suspected, a blood glucose determination should also be performed at the time of spinal puncture.

CYTOLOGICAL CSF EXAMINATION

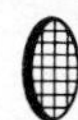

In cases of suspected neoplasm—particularly meningeal leukemia or lymphoma, meningeal carcinoma, or medulloblastoma, but also other neoplasms—cytological examination of cerebrospinal fluid may be of diagnostic help.

The laboratory should be alerted beforehand so that it can expedite the handling of the specimen on receipt. Expeditious processing is important to the validity of the results of cytological cerebrospinal fluid examinations.

VENEREAL DISEASE RESEARCH LABORATORIES (VDRL) TEST

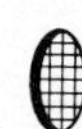

The VDRL test on cerebrospinal fluid should be performed in cases of suspected central nervous system (CNS) syphilis, particularly when there is no history of syphilis and there is a question as to whether a positive result of a blood serological test is false-positive. VDRL or other similar serologic tests are now routine on all cerebrospinal fluid specimens sent to hospital laboratories.

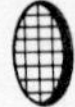

SKULL FILMS

VALUE OF THE TEST

Provides clues to the existence of chronic increased intracranial pressure

If there is chronic increased intracranial pressure skull films show erosion of the dorsum sellae and the clinoid processes in adults and suture separation in children.

Superior to routine CT scans in the diagnosis of pituitary tumors

In older patients who are likely to have physiological calcification in the pineal gland, the skull film raises suspicion of the presence of a tumor in a hemisphere or a subdural hematoma when there is lateral displacement of the normally midline pineal gland, as best seen in the Towne projection.

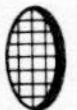

FILMS OF THE LUMBOSACRAL SPINE

VALUE OF THE TEST

Invaluable in the evaluation of low back pain, especially when the pain radiates down the back of one or both legs, a situation that suggests the presence of degenerated disks at lower lumbar levels. In such cases, x-ray findings of narrowed intervertebral disk spaces in lateral views and of calcified spurs in intervertebral foramina in oblique views are quite common.

Occasionally may reveal the collapse of vertebral bodies as a result of osteoporosis, trauma, or metastases

Aids in the evaluation of patients with unexplained bladder or bowel incontinence accompanied by leg weakness or numbness with or without back or leg pain (usually includes dorsal and lumbar spinal x-ray films and often cervical films)

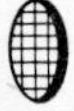

CT SCAN

CT is covered on pp. 161-166.

VALUE AND LIMITATIONS OF CT SCAN OF THE SPINE

Increasingly useful in the diagnosis of herniated disks, intraspinal tumors, and spinal stenosis (sometimes used with an injection of a few milliliters of soluble contrast agent)

Is more time consuming than CT brain scan and requires cooperative or sedated patients

The cross-sectional anatomy of the spinal cord and spinal canal that is visualized is very complementary to the anteroposterior (AP), lateral, and oblique views seen with myelography.

VALUE AND LIMITATIONS OF CT BRAIN SCAN

Provides an outline of the cerebral sulci and gyri, ventricles, and subarachnoid cisterns, as well as pathologic conditions

Certain tumors are seen better when contrast media are given intravenously just before or during scanning.

Occasionally renal shutdown may result from large amounts of contrast media being injected into elderly, dehydrated, or diabetic patients.

Pathologic conditions such as tumors, hemorrhages, hematomas, hydrocephalus, or atrophy can be visualized with CT scanning of the brain.

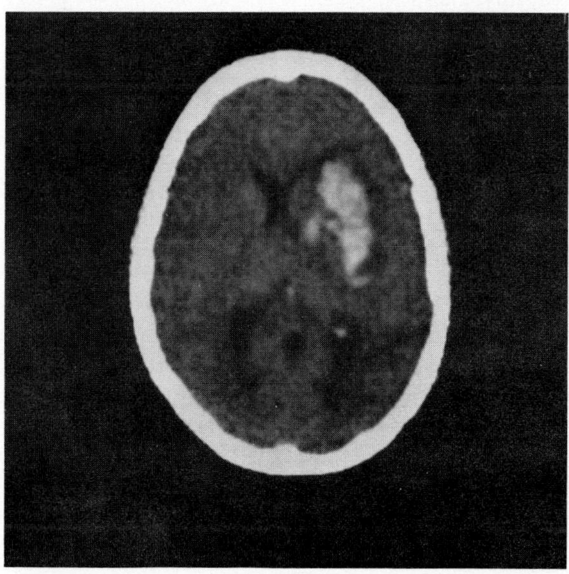

Fig. 11-3. *CT scan of brain, showing large hemorrhage into the left basal ganglia. This 40-year-old man developed sudden loss of speech and weakness of the right limbs, followed by seizures. (Courtesy Valley Presbyterian Hospital Radiology Department, Van Nuys, Calif.)*

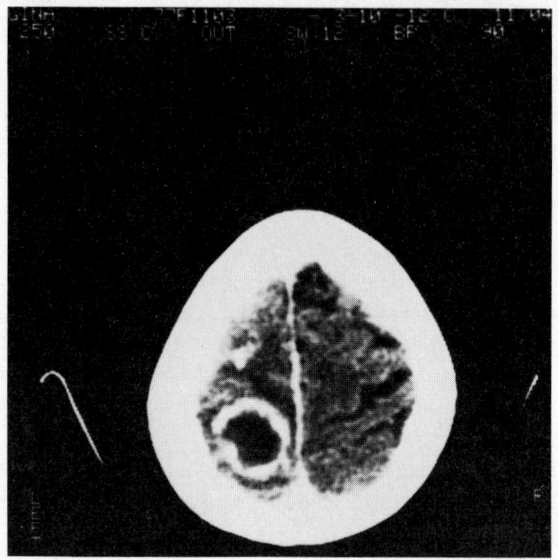

Fig. 11-4. *CT scan of brain, showing circular mass in the upper left parietal-occipital area, surrounded by a dense rim. During surgery the mass proved to be an abscess and was evacuated. This 77-year-old patient was well until 3 days before admission to the hospital, when the onset of right-sided seizures and a minimal right-sided limb weakness occurred. (Courtesy Valley Presbyterian Hospital Radiology Department, Van Nuys, Calif.)*

CLINICAL IMPLICATIONS OF CT BRAIN SCANNING

Fig. 11-3 is a CT brain scan showing a large hemorrhage into the left basal ganglia. Fig. 11-4 shows a circular mass in the upper left parietal-occipital area; the mass is surrounded by a dense rim. Subsequent surgery revealed the mass to be an abscess, which was evacuated.

MYELOGRAPHY

Normal findings

The contrast medium flows freely through the subarachnoid space, revealing no obstructions.

EXPLANATION OF THE TEST

Myelography evaluates the subarachnoid space using fluoroscopy and radiography, following an injection of contrast medium into the lumbar subarachnoid space. The contrast medium is heavier than CSF and will flow to the dependent area of the subarachnoid space. Thus, the patient can be tilted allowing fluoroscopic visualization of the outline of the subarachnoid space as the contrast medium flows through it. AP, lateral, and oblique films of the area of interest are made.

Oil-based (Pantopaque) and water-soluble (Amipaque) dyes are in common use. A new contrast agent, Omnipaque, is now becoming widely used and has a significantly lower risk of CNS toxicity than does Amipaque.

Pantopaque is usually used when a pathologic condition is suspected in the cervical or upper dorsal spine, since a fluoroscopist can more readily prevent this material from going up into the cerebral subarachnoid spaces.

VALUE OF THE TEST

Performed when the physician suspects that the nerve roots or spinal cord are being compressed by degenerated disks or tumors, or as a result of fracture dislocations of the spine.

NURSING ACTION

1. Inform the patient that he or she is to fast for 3 to 4 hours before the procedure.
2. The task of explaining this procedure to the patient belongs to the physician.
3. Obtain informed consent.
4. Check the patient's history for epilepsy or hypersensitivity to iodine and iodine-containing substances (e.g., shellfish) and radiographic contrast medium.
5. The patient is placed in the lateral decubitus position, with the back even with the edge of the mattress and knees folded up against the chest to the extent consistent with comfort. Drapes obscure landmarks and are best avoided. If the patient is obese

or apprehensive or has scoliosis, the procedure is best accomplished with the patient sitting across the bed with legs extended and trunk flexed forward to the extent consistent with comfort.

6. When Pantopaque has been used as the contrast medium, the patient is kept flat in bed for 4 hours or more after the procedure. However 10% to 15% of patients still develop a postspinal headache and must be kept flat for an additional 12 to 24 hours.
7. When Amipaque contrast material has been used, keep the patient semirecumbent with the head elevated at 20 to 30 degrees for the next 8 hours to minimize the diffusion of the water-soluble dye into cerebral subarachnoid spaces.
8. Since high concentrations of Amipaque in cerebral subarachnoid fluid can cause confusion and even seizures, observe the patient frequently for 8 to 12 hours after the myelogram has been obtained.

CLINICAL IMPLICATIONS

Myelography identifies extradural lesions such as herniated intervertebral disks and metastatic tumors, lesions within the subarachnoid space such as neurofibromas and meningiomas, and lesions within the spinal cord such as ependymomas and astrocytomas. Fig. 11-5 illustrates the lateral view of the lumbar area revealing a disk protrusion or a tumor causing a filling defect in the column of contrast material.

NURSING ALERT

When contrast medium is to be administered

Watch the patient for adverse reactions to the radiocontrast material such as anaphylactic reaction, volume overload and congestive heart failure, acute right ventricular failure, and acute renal failure.

In order to recognize a nephrotoxic response to the contrast medium should it occur, closely monitor urinary output, renal function (BUN and creatinine), and electrolytes for 24 to 48 hours following the use of radiocontrast material.

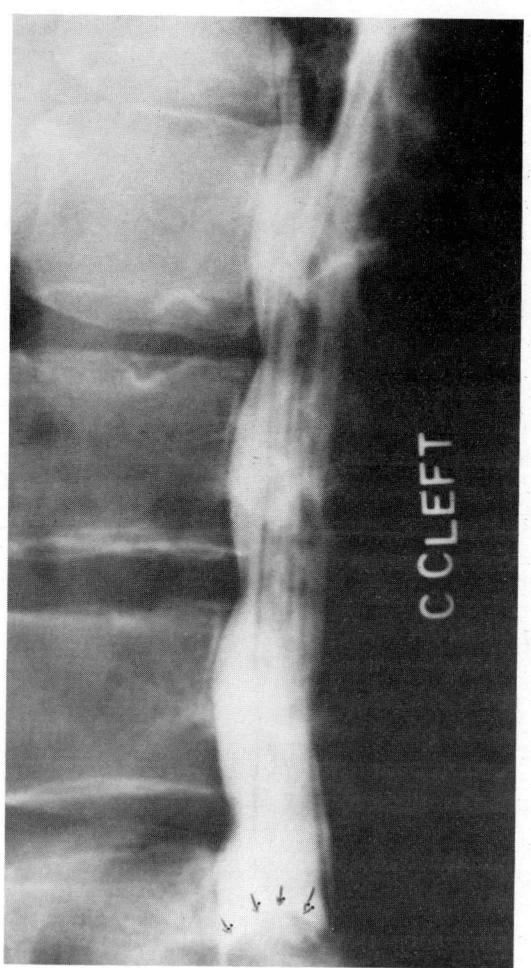

Fig. 11-5. *Myelogram. Lateral view of lumbar area. Arrows outline a filling defect in dye column that, during surgery, proved to be a neurofibroma attached to the right S1 nerve root. For 3 years this 21-year-old man had complained of low back pain radiating down the back of the right leg. (Courtesy Valley Presbyterian Hospital Radiology Department, Van Nuys, Calif.)*

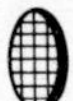

RADIONUCLIDE BRAIN SCAN

Normal findings

When the blood-brain barrier is maintained, only a small amount of isotope activity is recorded from gray and white matter. Greater vascularity causes choroid plexi and other vascular structures such as venous sinuses to be well outlined. Most injuries to the blood-brain barrier cause "leaks" in capillary membranes, which result in increased escape of isotope, outlining the injured area.

EXPLANATION OF THE TEST

This test uses a gamma scintillation camera to produce images of the brain following intravenous injection of a radionuclide.

VALUE AND LIMITATIONS OF THE TEST

Essentially a risk-free test

Reveals cerebral perfusion defects immediately after the onset of cerebral thrombosis or embolism and fully 2 or 3 days before infarcts can be seen in CT scans

Accurate in identifying chronic subdural hematomas, including the 5% or 10% of subdural hematomas that are not seen on CT scans because the x-ray density of the encapsulated mix of blood breakdown products and spinal fluid is equal to the x-ray density of the underlying brain

Requires that the patient be either cooperative or sedated, so that the head can be immobilized under the gamma camera

NURSING ACTION

1. Inform the patient that there are no dietary restrictions before this test.
2. Explain that this test helps the physician to visualize the brain.
3. Reassure the patient that there is no pain involved in the test and that the exposure to radiation is minimal.

CLINICAL IMPLICATIONS

Usually the radionuclide accumulates in lesions such as malignant gliomas, meningiomas, metastases, and abscesses, which can then be detected. However, there is less accumulation in benign tumors.

MAGNETIC RESONANCE IMAGING (MRI) OF THE BRAIN

EXPLANATION OF THE TEST

MRI uses static and changing magnetic fields in the body and radio frequency pulses from the resulting alignment of hydrogen protons in the magnetic field to generate tomographic images of the body with high contrast of soft tissue. This noninvasive technique provides excellent tissue characterization without the use of injected contrast.

VALUE AND LIMITATIONS OF THE TEST

Permits visualization of tissues without exposure to ionizing radiation and without administration of contrast media

Soft tissue adjacent to bone is easily viewed since MRI does not visualize bone.

Permits visualization of cerebral lesions not evident on CT scans, especially early brain abscess, encephalitis, and brain stem tumors

Is able to delineate white matter from gray matter and has a potential application for localizing lesions in the white matter, such as in multiple sclerosis

Imaging of the brain and spinal cord is already in widespread use and of great clinical utility, but imaging of other organ systems is still being developed.

Requires a metal-free environment, and therefore patients on life support equipment or with implanted metal objects such as pacemakers or intracranial aneurysm clips are not suitable candidates

NURSING ACTION

1. Inform the patient that there are no dietary restrictions before this test.
2. Explain the procedure to the patient and assure him or her that it is painless and involves no exposure to radiation.
3. Describe the MRI cylinder that houses the magnets.
4. Ask the patient to remove all metal objects because they may be damaged by the strong magnetic field.
5. Warn the patient that excessive movement while the test is in progress could blur the images.

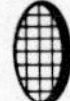

ELECTROENCEPHALOGRAPHY

EXPLANATION OF THE TEST

In electroencephalography electrodes are attached to standard areas of the patient's scalp for the purpose of recording a portion of the electrical activity of the brain ("brain waves"). The electroencephalograph magnifies the electrical impulses 1 million times; the resultant recording is called an electroencephalogram (EEG).

Sleep EEG. Some patients with seizures, particularly those who have temporal lobe seizures or seizures only during sleep, may not have EEG abnormalities when they are awake. Such abnormalities may be revealed by EEGs taken during either natural or sedative-induced sleep. In infants and small children, natural sleep is preferable and safer; the test can best be performed at the child's usual nap time or after feeding.

VALUE AND LIMITATIONS OF THE TEST

A very useful and economical screening test for brain tumors and subdural hematomas, in which case the EEG is abnormal in over 80% of cases

Provides the most complete information when the patient is cooperative and can provide valuable information on an uncooperative patient who can be sedated

Indicated in almost all patients with unexplained episodes of confusion or unconsciousness, and in all patients presenting with first seizures

May provide supporting evidence for the clinical determination of brain death; of itself the EEG does not establish brain death

CT scanning usually takes precedence over an EEG in the evaluation of head injuries that have produced stupor or coma.

NURSING ACTION

1. Inform the patient that there are no dietary restrictions before this test.
2. Ask the patient to void before going to the EEG laboratory to avoid this necessity after 21 scalp and ECG electrodes are in place.
3. Inform the patient who is taking anticonvulsive medications that he or she may continue to do so.

CLINICAL IMPLICATIONS

The two cerebral hemispheres normally produce electrical rhythms that are quite symmetrical in older children and adults. Thus, focal slowing or disorganization of background alpha activity, or the appearance of focal spike or sharp waves, usually correlates with the presence of underlying brain lesions.

Spikes that recur with characteristic location or rhythmicity are clues to petit mal epilepsy, Jakob-Creutzfeldt disease, herpes encephalitis, or, in some instances, recent temporal lobe infarction.

The finding of generalized slow activity in an EEG of a patient with coma of unknown origin is more suggestive of hypoxia or other metabolic disorders than of a focal structural brain lesion.

EVOKED BRAIN POTENTIALS

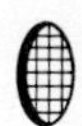

EXPLANATION OF THE TEST

These tests use four or more EEG amplifier channels linked to a stimulus signal generator and a computer to evaluate nerve conduction through the central nervous system. The extremely small stimulus-linked cerebral potentials resulting from repetitive visual, auditory, or peripheral sensory nerve stimuli can be stored and amplified by the computer. A smooth, flat baseline is achieved as a background for the desired evoked potentials because the computer averages out unwanted background resulting from random EEG and artifactitious waves.

VALUE OF THE TEST

Used in adults with suspected tumors of the brain stem or of the eighth cranial nerve, or with suspected multiple sclerosis

Auditory brain stem evoked potentials in infants who have sustained a large variety of serious perinatal insults can provide evidence of abnormal conduction through the brain stem structures and of hearing impairment

NURSING ACTION

Nursing action for evoked brain potentials is the same as for electroencephalography, discussed opposite.

CLINICAL IMPLICATIONS

In a patient known to have normal hearing before suspected brain death, the absence of brain stem auditory evoked potentials constitutes additional or confirmatory evidence of brain death when EEGs are equivocal because of an unusual artifact, or when they are suboptimal for other technical reasons.

Fig. 11-6 shows brain stem auditory evoked responses to click stimuli of 80 dB HL in an infant born without a right ear canal and external earlobe. The responses prove the presence of an underlying functioning right cochlea and auditory nerve.

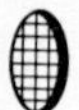

ECHOENCEPHALOGRAPHY

EXPLANATION OF THE TEST

In echoencephalography a sound transducer-receiver placed against the scalp beams sound waves of very high frequency through the brain. Whenever the sound waves pass through an interface

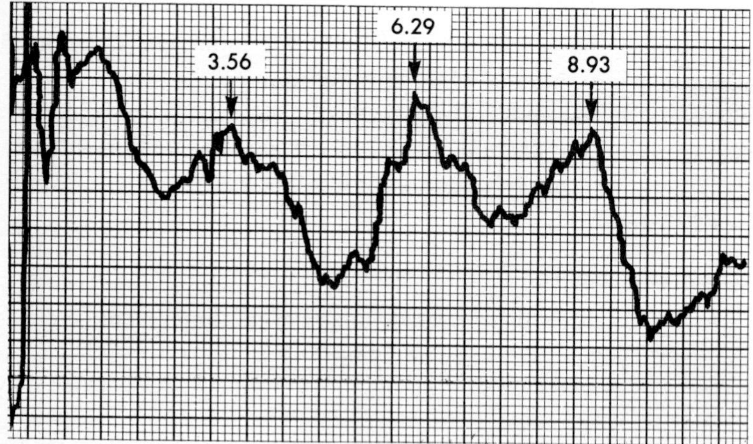

Fig. 11-6. *Brain stem auditory evoked responses to click stimuli in an infant born without a right ear canal and external earlobe. Responses prove the presence of an underlying functioning right cochlea and auditory nerve. Stimulus intensity was 80 dB HL, with white noise masking on the normal left side. (Courtesy Valley Presbyterian Hospital Neurology Department, Van Nuys, Calif.)*

between brain tissue and a substance of different sound transmission properties, such as cerebrospinal fluid in the ventricles or blood from an intracerebral hemorrhage, echoes are reflected back to the receiver, thus outlining the structures encountered by the sound waves. This test has been superseded by the widespread availability of CT scans.

VALUE OF THE TEST

May be done on agitated patients
Inexpensive

NURSING ACTION

1. Inform the patient that there are no dietary restrictions before this test.
2. Explain the test to the patient.

ELECTROMYOGRAPHY

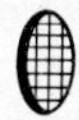

EXPLANATION OF THE TEST

An electromyogram (EMG) facilitates an analysis of voluntary and spontaneous muscle action potentials in selected muscles of one or more limbs or limb girdles and in paraspinal muscles. These potentials are examined (1) on needle insertion, (2) with complete muscle relaxation, (3) with minimal voluntary muscle contraction, and (4) with maximal contraction.

VALUE OF THE TEST

Useful in cases of suspected cervical or lumbar disk disease, polymyositis, muscular dystrophy, motor neuron disease, myasthenia gravis, and a myasthenia-like disease (Eaton-Lambert syndrome), which occurs with certain cancers.

NURSING ACTION

1. Inform the patient that there are no dietary restrictions before this test unless the physician has ordered restrictions on cigarettes or caffeine.

2. Explain the test to the patient and tell him or her that a needle will be inserted into selected muscles to assess their activity.
3. Obtain a signed consent.

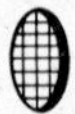

NERVE CONDUCTION VELOCITIES

EXPLANATION OF THE TEST

This test measures the velocity of electrical impulse conduction along motor or sensory nerves, frequently in conjunction with an EMG. The measurement of nerve conduction times involves the electrical stimulation of a nerve through the overlying skin. A recording electrode placed over a supplied muscle, or further along the nerve at a measured distance from the point of stimulus, records the response from the stimulated nerve. The time between stimulation and response is measured on an oscilloscope and the speed of conduction is calculated by dividing the distance between the point of stimulus and the recording electrode by the time between stimulus and response.

VALUE OF THE TEST

Aid in the diagnosis of peripheral nerve injuries and diseases affecting the peripheral nervous system, such as peripheral neuropathies

NURSING ACTION

1. Inform the patient that there are no dietary restrictions before the test.
2. Explain the procedure to the patient.

CLINICAL IMPLICATIONS

Velocities are generally low in persons with poorly controlled diabetes, in long-term renal dialysis patients, and in patients who have polyneuritis resulting from any of a variety of other causes. Focal slowing of median nerve velocity across the wrist or of ulnar velocity across the elbow is good evidence of entrapment neuropathy at those locations.

ANGIOGRAPHY

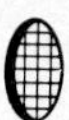

EXPLANATION OF THE TEST

Angiography is performed by cannulation of a femoral artery, through which a catheter is advanced to the aortic arch or into the orifices of carotid or vertebral arteries for injection of contrast media.

DIGITAL-SUBTRACTION ANGIOGRAPHY provides arterial imaging of good quality by means of an x-ray image intensifier linked to a computer, which enables small differences in x-ray absorption between an artery and surrounding tissues to be converted to digital information and stored. A "mask" exposure of the area of interest is made a few seconds before the injection of intravenous contrast medium. Four or more exposures are then made while the contrast medium is circulating through the arteries. The computer then subtracts the preinjection mask image from the postinjection images, thus removing all undesired tissue images (such as bone) and leaving arterial images of high contrast and high quality.

VALUE AND LIMITATIONS OF THE TEST

Important in the identification and localization of rupture aneurysms or of arteriovenous malformations

Provides the surgeon with accurate preoperative information about the blood supply of certain tumors

Although arch injections do not permit optimal evaluation of intracerebral arteries, they often suffice when there is a strong suspicion of atherosclerotic stenosis of the internal carotid artery in the neck.

NURSING ACTION

1. Instruct the patient to take nothing by mouth for at least 3 hours before angiography.
2. Explain the procedure to the patient and obtain an informed consent.
3. Ensure that dentures are removed before the patient leaves the hospital room for the catheterization laboratory.
4. Before administering premedication ensure that a baseline neurologic assessment has been done. This includes state of alertness, fluency of speech, and estimates of symmetry of limb strength or tone and the symmetry of pedal pulses.

5. After the procedure keep the patient flat and instruct him or her to avoid flexing the thigh that was cannulated for at least 2 or 3 hours. This will reduce the risk of late bleeding at the site of femoral artery puncture.
6. Encourage elderly or diabetic patients to increase fluid inake for 14 hours following the test.

NURSING ALERT

Immediately report to the physician complaints of groin pain, coldness of the leg, or observations of loss of pedal pulse distal to the arterial puncture site.

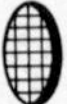

PNEUMOENCEPHALOGRAPHY

EXPLANATION OF THE TEST

This test requires a lumbar spinal tap so that air can be injected into the lumbar subarachnoid space.

VALUE OF THE TEST

Almost obsolete because of CT scanning
An adjunct to CT scanning

CLINICAL IMPLICATIONS

Small injections of air (5 to 10 cc) or small amounts of water-soluble contrast medium are occasionally introduced into the lumbar subarachnoid space to provide better contrast in CT scanning for suspected posterior fossa tumors.

NURSING ACTION

1. Inform the patient that there are no dietary restrictions before this test.
2. Describe the procedure to the patient and stress the importance of full cooperation during the test.
3. Obtain informed consent.
4. Evaluate the patient for signs of anxiety, assess vital signs, and notify the physician if warranted.

5. The patient must be in a sitting position so that the air rises to the head and outlines the cerebral cisterns and the ventricles.
6. Following the test advise the patient to lie flat, although he or she may turn from side to side, for 8 hours or as ordered. There is a high risk of spinal headache if even a 30° elevation of the head of the bed is permitted.
7. Observe the puncture site for redness and swelling.

NONINVASIVE CEREBROVASCULAR FLOW TESTS

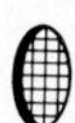

EXPLANATION OF THE TESTS

A commonly available battery of noninvasive cerebrovascular flow tests are:

1. Oculoplethysmography, which involves evaluation of retinal artery pressures and/or pulse waves (see also p. 182).
2. Doppler evaluation of arterial pulses in periorbital arteries connecting the internal and external carotid arterial systems
3. Phonoangiographic recording of bruits over the cervical portion of the carotid arteries

The larger hospital laboratories often offer Doppler evaluation of flow velocity at the carotid bifurcation and ultrasound imaging of the carotid bifurcation.

VALUE OF THE TESTS

Useful in the identification of patients who may be at risk of stroke because of embolic or thromboembolic lesions in the internal carotid system

CLINICAL IMPLICATIONS

Although a patient with a history of transient ischemic attacks of the internal carotid system ordinarily proceeds directly to angiography if he or she is otherwise a surgical candidate, many histories are less clear and the physical examination may not reveal carotid bruits. By the same token, a patient who has had no cerebral symptoms but who needs major surgery may have a carotid bruit on physical examination. Hearing this bruit should remind the physician to order noninvasive cerebral flow tests *before* the operation. A seriously obstructed carotid artery should ideally be identified and rendered patent *before* the contemplated major surgery is performed.

12

Diagnostic tests for rheumatologic disorders

PATHOPHYSIOLOGY AND CLINICAL APPLICATION OF LABORATORY TESTS

Rheumatoid arthritis (RA)

Rheumatoid arthritis is a chronic systemic disease of unknown origin. The primary manifestation is inflammation of the peripheral joints. Rheumatoid factors (antiglobulin antibodies) combine with immunoglobulin (usually IgG or IgM) in the synovial fluid to form immune complexes. Polymorphonuclear leukocytes are thus attracted to the joint space, causing destruction of joint structures.

The diagnosis is made because of the clinical features after ruling out other inflammatory arthritides. Laboratory findings may include *anemia,* low *serum iron* level and *iron-binding capacity,* mild *leukocytosis,* elevated *erythrocyte sedimentation rate* (ESR), reduced albumin on *protein electrophoresis,* and increased levels of *rheumatoid factors* (not diagnostic). *Synovial fluid* is turbid in appearance with neutrophils 10,000 to 75,000/mm^3.

Juvenile rheumatoid arthritis (JRA)

Juvenile rheumatoid arthritis is divided into three groups: systemic-onset, polyarticular, and pauciarticular disease. The diagnosis is made because of the clinical symptoms and the following laboratory tests.

Systemic-onset JRA: Anemia, leukocytosis, negative rheumatoid factors, and antinuclear antibodies (ANA)

Polyarticular JRA: ANA in 25% of cases; rheumatoid factors negative by standard method, but positive for IgG and IgA with special techniques

Pauciarticular JRA: ANA in 50% of cases; rheumatoid factors absent

Systemic lupus erythematosus (SLE)

SLE is a disorder of unknown origin associated with immunologic mechanisms of tissue injury and occurring most frequently in women of childbearing age. The diagnosis is suspected because of clinical features and a positive test for antinuclear antibodies, the most characteristic laboratory abnormality. Other laboratory findings may be mild *anemia* (normochromic, normocytic), *leukopenia* (over 50%), abnormal *urinalysis* and *renal function tests* (over 50%), reversed serum *albumin-globulin ratio,* and gamma globulin elevation on *serum electrophoresis.*

Rheumatic fever

Rheumatic fever is an inflammatory disease related to previous infection with group A β-hemolytic streptococci and involving mainly the heart, joints, central nervous system, skin, and subcutaneous tissues.

Although laboratory tests do not indicate the presence of rheumatic fever per se, they may indicate continued rheumatic inflammation. Of the streptococcal antibody tests, the *antistreptolysin O tests* are the most widely used and provide evidence of recent infection; another such test is the *anti-deoxyribonucleotidase B test.*

Progressive systemic sclerosis (diffuse scleroderma)

Progressive systemic sclerosis is a multisystem disorder characterized by alterations in connective tissue, leading to fibrosis of the skin and internal organs.

The diagnosis is strictly clinical, but *antinuclear antibodies* in high titer is very suggestive. There may be elevated *ESR, anemia,* elevated *IgG* (50%), *rheumatoid factor* in low titer (15%), and *antinuclear antibodies* (70%).

Mixed connective tissue disease

Affected patients have clinically overlapping features of scleroderma, SLE, and polyarthritis. High titers of antibody to *nuclear ribonucleoprotein* are found even during clinical remissions. However, this is also true of SLE, discoid lupus, rheumatoid arthritis, and progressive systemic sclerosis.

Spondyloarthropathies

In these conditions inflammation affects the spine and lumbosacral joints (ankylosing spondylitis), the urethra (Reiter's syndrome), and the skin (psoriatic arthritis). Ankylosing spondylitis has typical radiologic changes at early, progressive, and advanced stages. Although the *HLA-B27* antigen is present in more than 90% of cases, most persons who have a positive test do not have the disease. The absence of HLA-B27 antigen in whites is some evidence against the presence of ankylosing spondylitis. Other laboratory findings may be *anemia* (25%) and elevated *ESR* (80% to 90%).

Reiter's syndrome is associated with an increased white blood cell (WBC) count on *synovial fluid examination*. Often present are mild *leukocytosis* and elevated *erythrocyte sedimentation rate* and *HLA-B27* antigen; *rheumatoid factor* is negative. In psoriatic arthritis the level of HLA-B27 antigen is elevated in 40% of cases.

Gouty arthritis

Gouty arthritis is an acute clinical manifestation of gout, usually appearing abruptly, with the initial attack involving the metatarsal-phalangeal joint of the great toe in 50% to 70% of cases. There is usually an elevation of the *uric acid* level, but the diagnosis is made by observing monosodium urate crystals in white cells of *synovial fluid*.

Septic arthritis

Septic arthritis is usually monoarticular and is considered a medical emergency. *Radiologic examination* shows soft tissue swelling. *Synovial fluid* is purulent with the leukocyte count between 50,000 and 100,000/mm^3, with 90% or more being neutrophils, and decreased glucose concentration. A Gram stain and culture should be performed on the synovial fluid immediately to establish the definitive diagnosis and treatment.

Degenerative arthritis or osteoarthritis

This condition is found in 85% of persons over the age of 70. The results of serologic tests are normal and the radiologic examination is quite characteristic. *Synovial fluid* has decreased viscosity, good mucin clotting ability, and a WBC count of less than 200/mm^3. The glucose level is normal.

Sjögren's syndrome

Sjögren's syndrome may be either primary or secondary. The primary syndrome is associated with destruction of the parenchymal cells of the salivary glands, lacrimal glands, and labial glands. Secondary Sjögren's syndrome coexists with another disease such as rheumatoid arthritis and systemic lupus erythematosus. The diagnosis is made because of the symptoms. *Biopsy* of the salivary or labial glands, or the presence of SS-A or B autoantibodies in high titer substantiates the diagnosis.

LABORATORY TESTS FOR RHEUMATOLOGIC DISORDERS

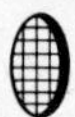

ANTI-DEOXYRIBONUCLEIC ACID (ANTI-DNA) ANTIBODIES

Reference range

Negative at a 1:10 dilution of serum

EXPLANATION OF THE TEST

The anti-DNA assay detects antibodies against native, double-stranded DNA, important in the diagnosis of systemic lupus erythematosus (SLE).

VALUE OF THE TEST

Strongly supports a diagnosis of SLE when the antinuclear antibody test has been positive

Monitors the patient's response to therapy

NURSING ACTION

1. Inform the patient that there are no dietary restrictions before this test.
2. Withdraw venous blood in a 7-ml red-top tube (some laboratories may use gray-top or lavender-top tubes).
3. Handle the specimen gently to prevent hemolysis.

INTERFERING FACTORS

Radioactive scan within 1 week before the test.

CLINICAL IMPLICATIONS

Increased levels (10 to 15 μg/ml)

Active SLE

Decreased levels (1 to 2.5 μg/ml)

Remission phase of SLE or the presence of other autoimmune disorders

Depressed levels following immunosuppressive therapy are diagnostic of effective treatment of SLE.

ANTI-DEOXYRIBONUCLEOTIDASE B TEST

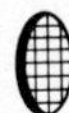

(ANTI-DNase B)

Adult reference range

<85 Todd units/ml

Pediatric reference range

Preschool child: <60 Todd units/ml
Child: <170 Todd units/ml

EXPLANATION OF THE TEST

DNase B is a potent enzyme produced by all group A streptococci. The anti-DNase B test detects antibodies to DNase B.

VALUE OF THE TEST

Detects reactions to group A streptococcal pyoderma when ASO titers have false-negative results

NURSING ACTION

1. Inform the patient that there are no food or fluid restrictions before the test.
2. Explain the test to the patient.
3. Collect venous blood in a 7-ml red-top tube.
4. Handle the specimen gently to prevent hemolysis.

CLINICAL IMPLICATIONS

Elevated levels

Acute rheumatic fever (80%)

Poststreptococcal glomerulonephritis following streptococcal pharyngitis (75%)

Glomerulonephritis following group A streptococcal pyoderma (60%)

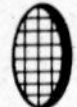

ANTINUCLEAR ANTIBODIES (ANA)

Reference range

Negative at a 1:87 dilution of serum
Varies with the laboratory

EXPLANATION OF THE TEST

The antinuclear antibodies are immunoglobulins (IgM, IgG, or IgA) that are produced in response to the nuclear DNA component of leukocytes perceived to be abnormal. If the ANA forms antigen-antibody complexes, there is tissue damage such as is observed in systemic lupus erythematosus. They are detected by fluorescent methods that measure the relative concentration of ANA. Serial dilutions of the patient's serum are mixed with cell nuclei from a rat. If there is ANA present in the patient's serum, it forms antigen-antibody complexes with the normal cell nuclei. Fluorescein-labeled antihuman serum is added and examined under ultraviolet microscope. The nuclei will be fluorescent if ANA is present. The titer is the greatest dilution to still show fluorescence.

VALUE AND LIMITATIONS OF THE TEST

Screens for systemic lupus erythematosus (SLE); if negative the chances of the disease being present is low; if positive further tests are indicated

Monitors effectiveness of immunosuppressive treatment for SLE

Is more frequently abnormal than is the lupus erythematosus cell test in conditions other than SLE

False-negative results have been reported.

Different sources for cell nuclei used in the test do not have equal sensitivity.

The fluorescent patterns are not specific for any one autoantibody or one disease.

There is disagreement among the experts as to which fluorescent pattern is found more often in a particular disease.

NURSING ACTION

1. Inform the patient that there are no food or fluid restrictions before the test.
2. Explain the test to the patient.

3. Collect venous blood in a 7-ml red-top tube.
4. Apply warm packs in the event of a hematoma at the site.

INTERFERING FACTORS

The most common drug to cause a false-positive result is procainamide; others are isoniazid, hydralazine, para-aminosalicylic acid, chlorpromazine, clofibrate, phenytoin, griseofulvin, ethosuximide, gold salts, methyldopa, oral contraceptives, penicillin, propylthiouracil, phenylbutazone, methysergide, streptomycin, sulfonamides, tetracyclines, mephenytoin, quinidine, primidone, reserpine, and trimethadione.

CLINICAL IMPLICATIONS

ANA results are reports both by titer and distribution of fluorescence. Patterns seen are illustrated in Fig. 12-1.

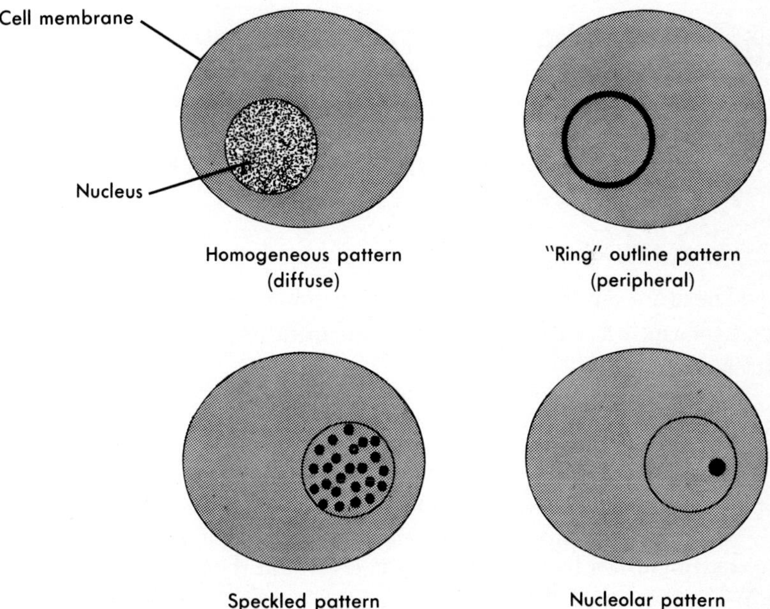

Fig. 12-1. *Fluorescence patterns of ANA antibodies.* **A,** *Rim or outline pattern (fluorescence only of the nuclear border).* **B,** *Homogeneous or solid pattern (the entire nucleus is fluorescent).* **C,** *Speckled pattern (fluorescence is distributed in dots throughout the nucleus).* **D,** *Nucleolar pattern (fluorescence only of the nucleolar area of the nucleus). See text for discussion.*

1. Rim or outline pattern (fluorescence only of the nuclear border). This along with an ANA titer of 1:160 or more is strongly characteristic of SLE. In other rheumatoid collagen diseases or in drug-induced SLE there is not usually a rim pattern. However, with lower ANA titers there is overlap with other diseases.
2. Homogeneous or solid pattern (the entire nucleus is fluorescent). Most frequent pattern in SLE and is especially diagnostic if the ANA titer is high as well. In noncollagen diseases the titer is usually less than 1:160.
3. Speckled pattern (fluorescence is distributed in dots throughout the nucleus). This pattern is characteristic of mixed connective tissue syndrome, especially if the ANA titer is high. The pattern has been reported in some cases of SLE (25%) and rheumatoid arthritis, progressive systemic sclerosis, and Sjögren's syndrome and in some elderly individuals.
4. Nucleolar pattern (fluorescence only of the nucleolar area of the nucleus). This suggests progressive systemic sclerosis if the ANA titer is high.

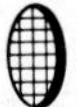

ANTISTREPTOLYSIN O (ASO) TESTS

Reference range

Less than 166 Todd units depending on the prevalence of group A β-hemolytic streptococcal infections

EXPLANATION OF THE TEST

These are serological tests (neutralization or particle agglutination) that measure the relative serum concentrations of the antibody to streptolysin O.

VALUE AND LIMITATIONS OF THE TEST

Confirms a recent or ongoing infection with β-hemolytic streptococci

Aids in the diagnosis of rheumatic fever and poststreptococcal glomerulonephritis in the presence of clinical symptoms

Distinguishes between rheumatic fever and rheumatoid arthritis in the presence of joint pain

It takes 7 to 10 days for antibody elevation. Therefore a throat culture is done when the patient presents with acute onset of a sore throat to identify or rule out the group A β-hemolytic streptococci.

Commercial tests vary in reliability.

A positive test does not prove the existence of acute rheumatic fever or that the present symptoms are the cause of the antibodies.

NURSING ACTION

1. Inform the patient that there are no food or fluid restrictions before the test.
2. Explain the test to the patient.
3. Collect venous blood in a 7-ml red-top tube.

INTERFERING FACTORS

Antibiotic or corticosteroid therapy (may suppress the streptococcal antibody response)

CLINICAL IMPLICATIONS

Elevated levels

Streptococcal pharyngitis patients (approximately 80%) who develop rheumatic fever or glomerular nephritis

Uncomplicated streptococcal disease (60%), except for streptococcal pyoderma, in which only 25% of patients have an elevated ASO titer even though acute glomerular nephritis may also be present

HLA-B27 ANTIGEN TEST

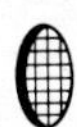

Reference range

Usually absent but may be a normal finding in 6% to 8% of white and 3% to 4% of black Americans

EXPLANATION OF THE TEST

The HLA complex has to do with antigenic differences among humans. These genes, designated HLA-A, HLA-B, HLA-C, and HLA-D, produce antigenic glycoproteins that determine whether or not a foreign graft will be accepted or rejected. The glycoproteins span the cell membrane and remain unchanged throughout an individual's life. By international agreement the letters HLA are the human counterpart for the major histocompatibility complex (MHC) antigens first studied in the animal model. HLA-B refers to the loci on the chromosome (each individual has six serologically defined

HLA-A, HLA-B, and HLA-C antigens, three from each parent). HLA-B27 refers to a certain antigen group. A number of disease processes are positively associated with HLA-B27 antigens.

VALUE OF THE TEST

Absence of the HLA-B27 antigen in whites helps to rule out the diagnosis of ankylosing spondylitis when the case is clinically borderline.

Aids in the diagnosis of ankylosing spondylitis, Reiter's syndrome, and some cases of psoriatic arthritis

NURSING ACTION

1. Inform the patient that there are no food or fluid restrictions before the test.
2. Explain the test to the patient.
3. Collect venous blood in a 7-ml red-top tube.

CLINICAL IMPLICATIONS

HLA-B27 is present in
Ankylosing spondylitis (90% of cases)
Reiter's syndrome (85% of cases)
Psoriatic arthritis (35% of cases)

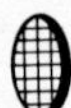

LUPUS ERYTHEMATOSUS (LE) CELL PREPARATION

Normal results

No LE cells present

EXPLANATION OF THE TEST

The LE cell preparation is only rarely performed and has been replaced by the anti-DNA titer. The LE cell preparation is an in vitro test that is based on the fact that antibodies against certain nuclear constituents produced in systemic lupus erythematosus react with the nuclei of damaged cells. Thus, the LE cell phenomenon can be visualized. This consists of the complexing of the LE factor (an autoantibody) with the nuclei of the damaged cells (the antigen). This material becomes an amorphous mass that is stained and is then phagocytized by polymorphonuclear neutrophils. The phagocytes with the engulfed material are the so-called LE cells. The presence of LE cells is strongly suggestive of SLE except in patients taking certain drugs (see interfering factors).

VALUE AND LIMITATIONS OF THE TEST

Aids in the diagnosis of SLE

Monitors the treatment of SLE

Many drugs cause a positive test.

Some patients with rheumatoid arthritis, other collagen diseases besides SLE, or some individuals with chronic active hepatitis or cirrhosis may have a positive LE preparation.

Neutrophils with ingested red blood cells (RBCs) can be misdiagnosed as LE cells by the inexperienced.

Artifacts may cause false-positive determinations. For example, the nuclear structure that is phagocytized must have no remaining nuclear structure at all. If the phagocytized nuclear material still has some features of a nucleus ("tart cell") it has no diagnostic significance.

NURSING ACTION

1. Inform the patient that there are no food or fluid restrictions before the test.
2. Explain the test to the patient.
3. Collect venous blood in a 7-ml red-top tube.
4. Handle the specimen gently to prevent hemolysis.

INTERFERING FACTORS

Hypersensitivity to hydralazine (Apresoline)

Procainamide: 50% of patients taking more than 1.5 g of procainamide per day develop positive LE preparations and 75% develop antinuclear antibodies.

Other such drugs include para-aminosalicylic acid, chlorpromazine, clofibrate, phenytoin, griseofulvin, ethosuximide, gold salts, methyldopa, oral contraceptives, penicillin, propylthiouracil, phenylbutazone, methysergide, streptomycin, sulfonamides, tetracyclines, mephenytoin, quinidine, primidone, reserpine, and trimethadione.

CLINICAL IMPLICATIONS

A positive LE preparation is strongly suggestive of systemic lupus erythematosus.

> **NURSING ALERT**
>
> Be sure to establish what drugs the patient has been taking and compare them to the list of drugs responsible for positive LE preparations.

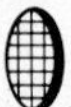

RHEUMATOID FACTORS

Normal findings

Negative

EXPLANATION OF THE TEST

Rheumatoid arthritis (RA) and related diseases cause a production of globulins known as rheumatoid factors (IgG and IgM antibodies). The most important is the IgM macroglobulin. These are produced by lymphocytes in the synovial joints and react with other IgG or IgM antibodies to produce immune complexes, complement activation, and tissue destruction. The IgM globulin can combine in vitro with normal gamma globulin and complement is fixed during the reaction. There are many newly developed methods that are either tube tests or rapid slide tests. The slide tests have a slightly greater sensitivity than tube tests but are less specific and should be used mainly for screening. The latex fixation tube test, known as the *Plotz-Singer latex test,* is considered the standard diagnostic method with a sensitivity in adult RA of 75%.

VALUE AND LIMITATIONS OF THE TEST

Useful in establishing the diagnosis of rheumatoid arthritis

It takes several weeks to 6 months for RA serologic tests to become abnormal.

Titers between 1:20 and 1:80 occur in many diseases.

Five percent of the general population and 25% of the elderly have positive RF titers.

A negative titer does not rule out RA.

NURSING ACTION

1. Inform the patient that there are no food or fluid restrictions before the test.
2. Explain the test to the patient.
3. Collect venous blood in a 7-ml red-top tube.

INTERFERING FACTORS

Inadequately activated complement (false-positive results)
High lipid or cryoglobulin levels in the patient's serum (false-positive results)
High IgG levels in the patient's serum (false-negative results)

CLINICAL IMPLICATIONS

A positive test (>1:80) is only considered diagnostic of RA when evaluated along with the total clinical picture.

SYNOVIAL FLUID EXAMINATION

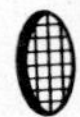

Normal results

Normal synovial fluid is straw colored and clear. A normal mucin clot is compact, the WBC/mm^3 is less than 200 with fewer than 25% polymorphonuclear cells. Normal synovial fluid strings out for more than 3 cm (viscosity) as it slowly drips from the end of a needle. The normal glucose content is 10 mg/dl of the serum glucose value.

EXPLANATION OF THE TEST

In synovial fluid aspiration (arthrocentesis) a fluid specimen is aspirated from a joint space under strict aseptic technique.

VALUE AND LIMITATIONS OF THE TEST

Aids in the differential diagnosis of arthritis
Essential in the diagnosis of gout and in the differential diagnosis of pseudogout
Identifies the cause of joint effusion
Relieves pain and distention
Gram stain for microbiologic studies is sometimes difficult to interpret because of joint debris in the specimen.

Previous antibiotic therapy decreases the possibility of diagnoses by culture.

There is an overlap in the WBC count between noninflammatory conditions and noninfectious inflammatory diseases, and between infectious disease and noninfectious inflammatory disease, rendering only a very high or a very low count diagnostically useful of itself.

NURSING ACTION

1. Explain the procedure to the patient and obtain a signed consent.
2. Obtain a blood specimen for blood glucose evaluation as close in time as possible to the joint aspiration.
3. Inform the patient that he or she should fast at least 6 to 8 hours before the procedure if the specimen is to be tested for glucose; otherwise there are no restrictions.
4. The skin is prepared and anesthetized as for a surgical procedure. A 20-ml syringe will be needed for the aspiration of fluid.
5. Tubes will be needed for culture, cytologic, clot, and glucose analysis: an anticoagulated tube (heparin is preferred, but liquid EDTA can be used) for cell count, WBC differential, and examination for crystals; a sterile tube for fluid to be cultured with heparin. A tube without anticoagulant is necessary for the mucin, complement assay, and glucose assay.
6. A minimum of 10 ml of synovial fluid is aspirated; 20 ml is preferred. The heparinized tube for cell count also contains 1 ml or more. Invert the tube to mix the anticoagulant. If the complement assay is not to be performed within 1 to 2 hours, this specimen should be frozen immediately.
7. The culture tubes are clearly labeled "synovial fluid" and sent immediately to the laboratory.
8. Apply pressure for 2 minutes to prevent bleeding. Apply a sterile dressing.
9. Cold packs may be used to decrease swelling. Apply an elastic bandage to stabilize the joint.

NURSING ALERT

Observe strict aseptic technique during the procedure.

Table 12-1 Characteristics of synovial fluid in major joint disease

Disease	Appearance	Fibrin clot	Mucin clot	Crystals	WBC/mm³	Polymorphonuclear cells	Glucose (approx. % of blood level)
Degenerative joint disease	Turbid	Small	Good	None	< 2000	< 25	100
Acute gout	Turbid	Large	Fair to poor	Monosodium urate	5000-50,000	> 75	90
Pseudogout	Turbid	Large	Fair to poor	Calcium pyrophosphate	5000-50,000	> 75	90
Traumatic arthritis	Straw colored, bloody, or xanthochromic	Small	Good	None	2000	< 25	100
Tuberculous arthritis	Turbid	Large	Poor	None	25,000	Varies	< 50
Septic arthritis	Turbid or purulent	Large	Poor	None	10,000->100,000	> 80	< 50
Rheumatoid arthritis	Turbid	Large	Fair to poor	None	5000-50,000	> 65	75
Other inflammatory arthritis	Turbid	Large	Fair to poor	None	5000-50,000	> 50	75

Adapted from Gilliland, B.C., and Mannik, M.: Disorders of the joints and connective tissues. In Petersdorf, R.G., et al., eds. Harrison's principles of internal medicine, ed. 10, New York, 1983, McGraw-Hill Book Co., p. 1976.

CLINICAL IMPLICATIONS (see also Table 12-1)

Acute bacterial infection: poor clot
Noninflammatory arthritides: good clot
Noninfectious inflammation: good to poor clot
Gout: strongly negative birefringent urate crystals
Pseudogout: positive birefringent calcium pyrophosphate crystals

Viscosity (string sign)

Acute inflammatory conditions: little or no stringing
Noninflammatory arthritides: normal stringing

Glucose content

Acute inflammatory noninfectious arthritis (e.g., LE, RA, gout): mild to moderate decrease
Acute bacterial arthritis: marked decrease in 50% of cases

13

Diagnostic tests for infectious diseases

The definitive diagnosis of infectious diseases is made by (1) the traditional staining and culture of the agent responsible for the disease, (2) the nontraditional methods for detection of the product of the infectious agent in material obtained from the patient, and (3) detection of the immune response specific for that particular organism. In this chapter a description of the laboratory tests for each category of infectious disease follows a brief description of the diseases themselves.

Since infections involve multiorgans, it is important to correlate the laboratory testing in infectious disease with the clinical state and clinical information; close communication with the pathology department is needed. Some of the new developments in bacteriology and virology are already in clinical use or will be introduced into clinical medicine in the near future; some will remain research tools. There are five reasons for the accelerated research and new laboratory tests.

1. It has been recognized that certain infectious agents, besides causing a transient infection, may cause latent and/or persistent infections (e.g., herpes simplex virus, cytomegalovirus, Epstein-Barr virus, rubella virus, measles virus, hepatitis B virus).
2. It is necessary to arrive more rapidly at a diagnosis for effective clinical management.
3. The cost of lengthy hospitalization for diagnostic purposes is prohibitive.
4. New technology is available, such as monoclonal techniques and computers assisting in the diagnostic laboratory.
5. Some infectious diseases have changed their clinical features, for example, a significant decrease in rheumatic fever and streptococcal pharyngeal infection, and new infections have emerged, for example, there is an AIDS epidemic with all of its secondary viral and bacterial infections, which are classified as opportunistic infections and have no consequences when immunity is intact but cause mortality and significant morbidity in immune-compromised patients.

CLINICAL APPLICATION OF LABORATORY TESTS

PNEUMONIAS

Bacterial pneumonia

In the diagnosis of bacterial pneumonias, a *chest x-ray* study is nearly always essential. In addition to substantiating the existence of an inflammatory infectious condition, the consolidation pattern may indicate the cause. For example, a lobar distribution usually indicates that the cause is a pneumococcus organism, while a bronchial distribution suggests other gram-positive organisms. *Klebsiella* and staphylococci also have some unique radiological characteristics. An untreated or inadequately treated bacterial pneumonia may resolve into a lung abscess. All of the diagnostic tests helpful in pneumonia are employed in the diagnosis of lung abscess. Occasionally, surgical evacuation is needed for specific bacteriological diagnosis.

A *Gram stain of the sputum* may be suggestive enough to indicate therapy before a culture is available. Occasionally transtracheal aspiration of sputum is necessary, especially with anaerobic infections. *Blood cultures* are useful both in substantiating the sputum culture result and in indicating bacteremia, thus raising the possibility of distant metastatic infection and the need for modification of therapy. *Arterial blood gas determinations* are helpful in documenting the degree of hypoxemia. A *pleural tap* may yield the offending organism if there is associated pleural fluid. *Bronchoscopy* is performed to exclude obstruction in the tracheobronchial tree when the pneumonia is recurrent or slowly resolving.

Mycoplasmal pneumonia

This disease occurs primarily in children and young adults, spreading by means of respiratory tract secretions. It is important to arrive at the specific diagnosis rapidly because mycoplasmal pneumonia does not respond to penicillin but rather to tetracycline and erythromycin. *Chest x-ray* studies and the clinical picture aid in the diagnosis. Serologic tests are the usual means of diagnosis, the most widely used being *complement fixation*. A fourfold rise in titer between the acute serum and the convalescent serum drawn 2 to 4 weeks later is diagnostic. Titers in single serum specimens greater than or equal to 1:128 suggest recent infection. *Enzyme-linked immunosorbent assay (ELISA)* and *indirect immunofluorescence* methods should soon be clinically available.

Viral pneumonias

Viral infections are a common cause of upper respiratory tract infections, last 2 to 3 days, and are usually of no clinical consequence. The usual viruses involved are influenza, adenovirus, varicella, rubeola, or respiratory syncytial virus. Secondary bacterial infection may occur in some patients, usually in the form of bronchitis. In such a case there will be purulent sputum and a normal chest x-ray film. The infecting organism is usually β-hemolytic streptococci, pneumococci, *Staphylococcus aureus*, *Branhamella catarrhalis*, *Hemophilus influenzae*, and *Neisseria meningitidis*.

Psittacosis (ornithosis)

The causative organism, *Chlamydia psittaci*, is transmitted from birds to humans by inhalation, deposited in the alveoli where some are ingested by macrophages, and carried to the lymph nodes. They are then disseminated and begin to grow in the reticuloendothelial system. Pneumonia results along with hepatosplenomegaly, headache, and changes in mentation. Although *C. psittaci* is endemic in all birds, psittacine birds such as parrots and parakeets are the usual contacts for the human disease. Psittacosis has also been diagnosed in individuals who process turkeys or who have frequent contact with pigeons.

Diagnosis is by *serological methods*. *Sputum culture* is safe only if performed by laboratories with type III biohazard containment facilities. *Microindirect immunofluorescence* is a new and sensitive test, but it is difficult to perform. *Chest x-ray* study shows patchy pneumonitis resembling *Mycoplasma* infection.

Legionnaires' disease

A gram-negative bacillus *(Legionella pneumophila)* causes what is known as Legionnaires' disease, producing severe, consolidated pneumonia as the main symptom, although multiple organs are involved. Cell-mediated immune responses are required to overcome the disease. The organism is distributed in soil, mud, lakes, and streams and can be found in air-conditioning cooling-tower water, air-conditioning condensate, reservoir water, shower heads, whirlpool baths, and institutional potable water systems. The disease is acquired through aerosols and not by person-to-person transmission. Those at increased risk are immunosuppressed individuals and smokers.

The organism can be isolated from respiratory tract secretions (sputum, pleural fluid), blood, and biopsy material from the lung or transbronchi. A biological safety cabinet is necessary for handling of the specimen, which is immediately smeared on slides for *direct fluorescent antibody testing* and inoculated to agar plates for *culture*.

Recently developed, but commercially unavailable, immunological tests are detection of antigen in urine by radioimmunoassay (RIA) or ELISA methods, nucleic acid probe, and a radiolabeled ribonucleic acid (RNA) probe. ELISA has also been used to detect circulating antigens in serum. The nucleic acid probe specifically detects genetic material of *L. pneumophila*, and the radiolabeled RNA probe recognizes the oganism. All of these new testing methods are under study. Details on the laboratory diagnosis of Legionnaires' disease can be found in the works by Edelstein and co-workers listed in the Bibliography at the end of the book.

TULAREMIA

Tularemia (rabbit fever, deer fly fever, Ohara's disease) is transmitted to humans from animals by direct contact or through an insect host. The causative organism is *Francisella tularensis*, a gram-negative bacillus. This highly invasive organism has intracellular parasites, which survive in the cells of the reticuloendothelial system after the bacteremic phase. Pneumonia is a common complication of the disease.

The diagnosis is usually made with the *febrile agglutination test* (whole cell agglutination) or by ELISA techniques.

Note: Tularemia is one of the most common laboratory-acquired infections and special precautions are necessary when handling specimens. It is advisable to send the specimen to state or reference laboratories where fluorescent antibody stains are available for direct detection of the organism from lesion smears.

MENINGITIS

Acute meningitis

In acute meningitis it is extremely important to make an etiological diagnosis. Common bacterial infections are those caused by *Meningococcus*, *Hemophilus influenzae* (especially in children), *Pneumococcus*, and *Mycobacterium tuberculosis*. Less common causative agents are *Escherichia coli*, *Streptococcus*, and *Staphylococcus*. *Listeria monocytogenes* may be found in immunosuppressed and terminally ill patients.

The *spinal tap* is the most important test in the diagnosis of bacterial meningitis. The usual measurements are polymorphonuclear neutrophils greater than 1000/mm^3; glucose level decreased (corresponding to the serum glucose level; the normal ratio of cerebrospinal fluid [CSF] to serum glucose is about 0.6); and serum protein increased. Further details of the spinal tap are discussed on p. 459.

Blood cultures may be important, especially if the CSF contains no bacteria. *Skull x-ray* studies may show osteomyelitis and mastoiditis. These results may help in determining where to obtain cultures and in establishing a specific diagnosis and a possible causative agent. *Chest x-ray* study is necessary, since bacterial meningitis may be secondary to underlying pneumonitis.

Tuberculous meningitis

In tuberculous meningitis the *white blood cell (WBC) count in the CSF* is not as high as in bacterial meningitis and consists mainly of monocytes and lymphocytes. In the differential diagnosis between tuberculous meningitis and viral meningitis, the *glucose level* is important. It is decreased in tuberculous meningitis and normal in viral or aseptic meningitis.

Viral meningitis

In viral meningitis the serum protein level in the *spinal tap* is usually elevated, the WBC count slightly elevated (mainly lymphocytes), and the glucose level normal. CSF lactate levels are not elevated.

BRAIN ABSCESS

Changes in the CSF may occur that mimic meningitis. The CSF pressure is elevated and the WBC count between 50 and 300/μl (mainly lymphocytes). If the abscess communicates with the ventricular system, the WBC count will increase in the CSF, with an increase in the number of polymorphonuclear leukocytes, and the infecting organism can be cultured from spinal fluid. If there is no such communication, the findings will indicate a space-occupying lesion of the brain. Magnetic resonance imaging (MRI) and CT scanning may help in the differential diagnosis.

URINARY TRACT INFECTIONS

Since lower urinary tract infection is common in females, the usual practice is to assume that cystitis is the result of this without elaborate laboratory workups. However, in repeated urinary tract infections, urinalysis should be performed with a Gram stain and a culture (p. 521). The necessary test for urinary tract obstruction should also be ordered (p. 255). In asymptomatic bacteriuria a colony count of 100,000/ml or more of gram-negative rods is diagnostic of infection. A colony count of only 10,000/ml of enterococci is diagnostic.

In genitourinary tuberculosis, the most common finding is asymptomatic pyuria and hematuria. In the elderly such a combination should alert the clinician to order the proper cultures to rule out tuberculous involvement of the urinary tract.

PHARYNGITIS AND TONSILLITIS

The differential diagnosis in acute tonsillitis and pharyngitis is between bacterial infection, mainly with β-hemolytic streptococci, and viral infection. Unless one is already committed to the use of penicillin, it is essential to identify the organism by throat culture. For an unknown reason, the epidemiology of β-hemolytic streptococci is changing and its dreaded complications are significantly diminished in the United States. Thus we would like to emphasize the need for specific diagnosis so that unnecessary and potentially harmful use of antibiotics for a nonspecific diagnosis of sore throat can be avoided. There is no need for sensitivity testing once the culture identifies the organism. If the result of the culture is negative, a viral infection is usually indicated. *Antistreptolysin O (ASO) titers* will help in diagnosing β-hemolytic streptococcal infection and its complications.

DIPHTHERIA

Diphtheria is an infection of the mucous membranes of the pharynx by *Corynebacterium diphtheriae,* with toxin production causing widespread inflammation, trauma, and destruction. If the disease is suspected, antitoxin should be administered immediately, even before any specific diagnosis is attempted. However, antibiotics should be withheld until *cultures* have been taken. For best results, swabs from both throat and nasopharynx should be cultured. A *Gram stain* will show gram-positive rods. Testing for toxigenicity is done either by animal inoculation or by in vitro testing. The purpose is to demonstrate that the suspected bacteria are capable of producing toxin. Testing for immunity is accomplished through the *Schick skin test*. Diphtheria toxin is given intradermally. A positive reaction indicates that the patient does not have circulating antibodies.

PERTUSSIS

Pertussis (whooping cough) is an acute infection of the mucous membranes of the respiratory tract. The organism responsible for this condition, *Bordetella pertussis,* is isolated from the upper respiratory tract. It can be cultured only on special media. Serologic tests are not practical, since the antibodies are in low titer and appear only after 2 weeks. The *blood count* reveals leukocytosis, from 15,000 to 40,000 cells/mm^3, with 90% being lymphocytes.

SALMONELLA TYPHOSA

Salmonella typhosa causes typhoid fever. The organisms are ingested, enter the bloodstream, and are sequestered in the liver, spleen, and bone marrow, multiplying within the reticuloendothelial system to be discharged from the bile into the intestine. Three percent of patients will become carriers, with subclinical infections of the gallbladder and the biliary tract.

Blood cultures will have positive results in 70% to 90% of patients during the first week. By the third week only 30% to 40% of patients will have positive results. *Bone marrow cultures* may be positive in partially treated patients when blood culture results are negative. *Throat cultures* will be positive in 10% to 15% of patients the first week, increasing to 75% by the third week. *Serological tests* show an increase in agglutinins against the typhoid bacillus antigens after the first week of illness, rising to a peak by the fifth or sixth week. Such a rise is highly supportive of the presence of infection with the typhoid bacillus, but is not specific since other organisms also produce such a rise. The *blood count* reveals leukopenia during the acute febrile phase. A sudden appearance of leukocytosis suggests a complication, such as rupture of the bowel.

SALMONELLA *GASTROENTERITIS*

Salmonella gastroenteritis usually causes severe nausea, vomiting, and diarrhea. The organism can be isolated from suspected food and from the feces. Blood cultures are usually negative.

SHIGELLOSIS

The *Shigella* organism causes acute enterocolitis with fever, abdominal pain, and diarrhea. A *stool culture* confirms the diagnosis. The *WBC count* ranges from 5000 to 15,000/mm^3. Usually there are electrolyte abnormalities, depending on the severity of the symptoms.

TUBERCULOSIS

The causative organism of tuberculosis, *Mycobacterium tuberculosis*, enters the lungs by aerosol particle. Macrophages phagocytize it and carry it to the lymph nodes, where the organism multiplies, destroys the macrophages, and spills into the bloodstream. Thus the tubercle bacilli arrive in many parts of the body and most of them are eradicated by the immune system. The bacilli that remain are usually in the apex of the lung. If the patient has immune defects the bacilli are not eradicated when they enter the bloodstream and *miliary tuberculosis* results.

An *acid-fast stain* from sputum and gastric washings is sufficient for a tentative diagnosis and initiation of therapy. However, a *culture* of the organism is the only absolute proof of existing infection. For this, multiple sputum specimens and gastric washings are needed for a sufficient positive yield. A positive acid-fast stain of spinal fluid is fairly diagnostic and indicates the need for immediate initiation of therapy.

Radiological methods give valuable information and provide a tentative diagnosis, but never a definitive one. They are also useful in follow-up and evaluation of treatment.

The *tuberculin skin test* (purified protein derivative, PPD) does not differentiate between present active infection and dormant and subclinical infections, nor does a negative result rule out active tuberculosis, since anergic states such as Hodgkin's disease, sarcoidosis, massive infection, and pleural effusion cause false-negative results.

When the result of a routine urine culture is negative in the presence of hematuria with pyuria, one should suspect tuberculous infection of the kidney and perform a culture of the urine for the tubercle bacilli.

A *biopsy* of the liver, bone marrow, or lymph nodes may be diagnostic of miliary tuberculosis. A pleural biopsy may be very helpful in the presence of pleural effusion, which is usually an exudate. Bacteriological study and fluid analysis should also be performed. The needle pleural biopsy usually reveals the typical granuloma of tuberculosis, with giant cells showing caseous necrosis. Such findings are sufficiently diagnostic to initiate therapy.

The biopsy specimen or gastric washings should be processed promptly, since the bacillus dies quickly in such specimens.

RICKETTSIAL DISEASES

The rickettsiae are intracellular parasites maintained by a cycle involving an insect vector and an animal reservoir host, with man being an incidental victim. The organism typically invades the endothelial cells of small blood vessels, with perivascular infiltration and thrombosis. Diagnosis is important because treatment is specific.

The *Weil-Felix tests* evaluate for cross-reacting antibodies. Some microorganisms can be agglutinated by antibodies produced by another organism. Rickettsiae produce antibodies that agglutinate *Proteus* bacteria. Thus, this test gives positive results in patients with Rocky Mountain spotted fever or murine typhus, and negative results in patients with rickettsial disease or Q fever.

A *complement fixation test* employing group-specific rickettsial antigens will differentiate among the most common infections. A rise in titer in a week or two, with a fall in titer later, is specifically diagnostic of rickettsiae.

ACTINOMYCOSIS

The causative organism of this disease is *Actinomyces israelii, A. naeslundii, A. odontolyticus, A. viscosus, A. meyeri*, and *Arachnia propionica*. These organisms exist normally in the mouth and in the female genital tract, with cases of pelvic actinomycosis being reported in users of the intrauterine device. It may manifest following tooth extraction or mandibular fracture as a painful indurated lesion over the jaw. From the original foci the organism may spread to the liver, kidneys, spleen, brain, genitalia, and subcutaneous tissues.

When clumps (called sulfur granules) of the organism have formed, they can be crushed and a *Gram stain* used. If the sulfur granules are not present an anaerobic culture is used. Biopsies are employed when the culture is negative.

Newer methods employ *immunofluorescent techniques* for direct identification of *Actinomyces* and *Arachnia*.

NOCARDIOSIS

Nocardiosis is caused by an aerobic actinomycete found in the soil, which is either inhaled or introduced into the subcutaneous tissue by trauma. The infection is usually chronic and is usually seen in immunosuppressed individuals. Lung abscesses may result and they may spread to the central nervous system. Diagnosis is made by isolation of the gram-positive organism from sputum or abscesses.

MYCOSES (DISEASES CAUSED BY FUNGI)

Cryptococcosis

Cryptococcosis is a pulmonary infection caused by *Cryptococcus neoformans*, an encapsulated yeast. The most virulent strain of this organism is found in pigeon droppings, the dust of which may be inhaled. The organism has an affinity for the central nervous system, with lesions developing in the meninges at the base of the brain. This is one of the causes of aseptic meningitis.

Because the clinical symptoms are often suppressed by corticosteroid therapy, the diagnosis is first made by *culture* or *serological evidence*. The traditional india ink preparation has a low positivity rate and has been replaced by the *cryptococcal latex test for antigen*.

Screening tests for cryptococcosis include *the rapid urease test, levodopa–ferric citrate test (phenol oxidase production)*, and *rapid nitrate reductase test*.

Blastomycosis

The organism *Blastomyces dermatitidis* causes a chronic granulomatous and suppurative infection that gains entrance to the body through the lungs and may eventually involve not only the lungs but also long bones, soft tissue, and skin. Diagnosis is made by *culturing* the organism from sputum, pus, or biopsied material on Sabouraud's dextrose agar. The identification of the organism is conclusive using the *exoantigen test*.

Coccidioidomycosis

This infection is caused by inhalation of the organism *Coccidioides immitis*. After inhalation the organism may be killed or arrested, causing an acute respiratory disease, or in some cases the organism will disseminate and involve meninges, bone, skin, lymph nodes, and subcutaneous tissue. Diagnosis is made by *culturing* the organism on Sabouraud's dextrose agar. The identification of the organism is conclusive using the *exoantigen test*.

Histoplasmosis

This infection is caused by inhalation of the organism *Histoplasma capsulatum*. After being inhaled from the soil, a pulmonary infection ensues very similar clinically to tuberculosis. The infection eventually invades the reticuloendothelial system. Diagnosis is made by *culturing* the organism on Sabouraud's dextrose agar. The identification of the organism is conclusive using the *exoantigen test*.

Candidiasis

This mucocutaneous infection is caused by the *Candida* species. *Candida albicans* is the most frequent causative agent. The *germ tube test* provides a definitive diagnosis.

SEXUALLY TRANSMITTED DISEASES

Syphilis

This is a systemic infection caused by *Treponema pallidum*. It is usually transmitted sexually with the initial manifestation being a chancre. *Microscopic dark-field examination* is essential in evaluating the moist lesions of primary syphilis. This test must be repeated at least once daily for 3 days before the result can be declared to be negative. In the secondary stage, when the lesions are nonpruritic, it is more difficult to obtain the organism from the lesion. However, the diagnosis can be made without the microscopic dark-field examination if the lesions are characteristic and the results of the serological tests are positive.

Serological diagnosis depends on two types of antibodies being produced, the nonspecific reaginic antibody and the specific antitreponemal antibody. The presence of reaginic antibodies is detected by *flocculation tests*, the most common being the VDRL (Venereal Disease Research Laboratories) test. All of these tests are nonspecific, with false-positive results occurring in a significant number of cases.

The *fluorescent treponemal antibody absorption test (FTA-ABS)* is a specific test and detects the presence of antitreponemal antibodies.

Chlamydia *infection*

Chlamydia trachomatis causes a purulent cervicitis in women. The diagnosis is made by direct examination smears prepared from tissues or scrapings. The typical inclusions can be seen in infections of the conjunctiva, urethra, and cervix.

Acquired immune deficiency syndrome (AIDS)

The cause of this serious epidemic is an RNA virus known as human T-cell lymphotrophic virus type III (HTLV-III or HLV). The French have named it the lymphadenopathy virus (LAV). The virus is specific for the type IV T-lymphocytes, which are crucial to immune competence. Once AIDS develops, the patient is markedly immune deficient and develops all the opportunistic infections that are of no clinical consequence to the immunocompetent patient. The two most common complications of immune deficiency include Kaposi's sarcoma and pulmonary infections *(Pneumocystis carinii).*

The diagnosis is made by the *clinical picture* and *serological tests*, which demonstrate antibodies against the viral antigen. Methods used to detect these antibodies are ELISA, the Western blotch method, and immunofluorescence assay. The ELISA method is used for screening and the Western blotch method is more specific. A negative result with the ELISA method indicates absence of AIDS. A positive result in a patient without the clinical syndrome may be false-positive or the individual may be a carrier of the virus; the Western blotch method is used to differentiate. Even a positive result in a high-risk group should be confirmed with the Western blotch method, which is more specific and checks the antibody against the virus.

These tests are also used to diagnose AIDS-related complex (ARC) (a high-risk group with lymphadenopathy and positive serologies for AIDS), and to screen blood donors and high-risk population. There is an extreme urgency to develop a *DNA probe* that may be more specific than the serologic tests and may facilitate the diagnosis of this disease.

In some patients in whom the disease is far advanced and who are unable to produce any immunoglobins against the virus, the virus can be cultured readily. Usually such patients are at the end stage of the disease. In the very early stages of the disease, before antibodies can be formed, the individual may be infectious and the blood infected.

Gonococcal infections

In gonorrhea the organism *Neisseria gonorrhoeae,* transmitted by sexual contact, penetrates the mucous membrane of the urogenital tract. In the male there is a purulent urethritis; in the female, Bartholin's and Skene's glands and the uterine cervical glands are usually infected.

A *Gram stain* of the urethral or endocervical discharge reveals intracellular gram-negative diplococci, which are characteristic and nearly diagnostic.

The *ELISA* system is more rapid than culture and is very sensitive and specific for the gonococcal antigen in the urethral or endocervical discharge.

A *culture* is necessary if ELISA is not available and one cannot find intracellular gram-negative diplococci by Gram stain and the diplococci are extracellular. The culture medium in such a case should have 3% to 10% carbon dioxide to promote growth. In homosexual males, cultures must be taken from the nasopharynx and rectum. In females, the *limulus amebocyte lysate (LAL) assay* has been found to be diagnostic for gonococcal infection.

Chancroid

Chancroid is a sexually transmitted disease caused by *Hemophilus ducreyi*, which penetrates mucous membranes of broken skin. The disease is manifested as a painful ulcer on the genitals. Diagnosis is made by exclusion of other genital lesions with which it can be confused, such as herpes progenitalis.

Other infections

The sexual practices of homosexual men (oral-genital, anal-genital, and oral-anal activities and multiple partners) predispose them to:

Painful lesions of gonorrhea, syphilis (the primary chancre may be hidden in the rectum), and herpes in the usual genital sites, in the oropharynx, and as a cause of proctitis

Neisseria meningitidis (isolated from the oropharynx, anus, and urethra)

"Gay bowel syndrome." Inflammatory bowel disease, ulcerative bowel disease, and diarrhea (caused by *Entamoeba histolytica*, *Giardia lamblia*, *Cryptosporidium*, *Salmonella* species, *Shigella* species, or *Campylobacter jejuni*)

Chlamydia infection (lymphogranuloma venereum [LGV] and non-LGV strains)

Cytomegalovirus

Human T-cell lymphotropic virus (HTLV-III), the causative agent in AIDS
Lymphadenopathy-associated virus (LAV)

HERPESVIRUS GROUP

This is a large group of intranuclear, double-stranded DNA viruses that are able to establish a latent infection many years after a primary infection. The group includes herpes simplex virus type I (fever blisters and keratoconjunctivitis), herpes simplex virus type II (sexually transmitted disease), varicella (chickenpox), herpes zoster (shingles), cytomegalovirus (cytomegalic inclusion disease), Epstein-Barr virus, and a recently described virus that infects the B lymphocytes and is associated with B-cell lymphoma. When the active clinical disease resolves, the virus stays latent in the human body, each type of virus occupying different places in the body, and causes clinical disease when it recurs either because of reinfection or reactivation. In a latent form some of these viruses are associated with significant clinical pathology. New technology is beginning to clarify how such viruses are able to evade or suppress the immune response. In the immunosuppressed patient such infections cause serious disability and clinical manifestations.

Herpes simplex type I

Herpes simplex type I virus causes recurring pharyngitis and blister-type cold sores in the mucous membranes of the mouth. Once the acute infection subsides, the virus lodges in the neurons of ganglions. The latency is associated with clinical remission but the virus is either in a low-level replicating state or inactive, compatible with the normal activities of the cell of the involved neurons. Whenever environmental factors or host resistance and immunodeficiency exist there is reactivation of the dormant virus in the ganglion cells with the clinical appearance of mucous membrane lesions. In a severely immunosuppressed patient (e.g., AIDS), herpes simplex type I causes severe invasive mucous membrane lesions of the mouth and throat, and dissemination may occur with meningitis.

Laboratory diagnosis is made by detecting specific antibodies by the *immunofluorescent technique*. Newer tests with DNA hybridization and DNA probing may become available soon. Because immunosuppressed patients cannot produce antibodies, tests for detecting viral particles rather than antibodies are used. The virus can be cultured and the cytopathological effect of the virus can be observed. This is time consuming and not practical. Isolation of the virus, tissue culture, and cytopathology take 48 to 96 hours. Identifying the serotype is a research tool at the present time.

Herpes simplex type II

Herpes simplex type II virus is similar in pathology to herpes simplex type I, except that it has a tendency to lodge in the ganglions of the pelvic nerves rather than the cervical ganglions. However there is a 20% to 30% cross-over in terms of clinical infection and type II is a sexually transmitted disease, causing recurrent vesicles and small ulcers on the cervix, vagina, and perineum of the female and penis of the male. To distinguish type I from type II herpes simplex, the *indirect hemagglutination inhibition test* or *indirect immunofluorescence* is used.

Herpes zoster

Herpes zoster causes a mononeuritis with an apparent rash along the nerve of the infected nerve root. When the clinical disease resolves, the virus lodges in the nerve root similar to the herpes simplex viruses. Usually the diagnosis is clinical; however, a serological test is available for specific antibody diagnosis.

Cytomegalovirus

Cytomegalovirus causes a disease similar to infectious mononucleosis. It usually occurs in patients who receive large amounts of fresh blood. The diagnosis is made by examining a stained sediment of urine, saliva, or gastric washings, which will demonstrate the cytoplasmic inclusion bodies. Serological tests include *complement fixation*, *neutralization*, and *immunofluorescence*.

Epstein-Barr virus

The Epstein-Barr virus in its acute form causes infectious mononucleosis, which is diagnosed because of marked lymphocytosis and Downey cells (atypical lymphocytes). The virus is associated with Burkitt's lymphoma (widespread in South Africa and increasing in the United States), nasopharyngeal carcinoma (widespread in China and increasing in the United States), and chronic Epstein-Barr virus disease, either neuropsychiatric (causing depression) or chronic musculoskeletal (with symptoms of prolonged fatigue but minimal neuropsychiatric symptoms). The virus attacks B cells and the acute form of the disease is a massive infection of the B-lymphocytes (Downey cells on the blood smear). Kaposi's sarcoma of immunosuppressed patients is associated with either Epstein-Barr virus or cytomegalovirus.

After resolution of the acute disease, which lasts from a few days to a week, the virus stays in the B cells, where the virus invades the DNA and multiplies without causing any apparent acute clinical syndrome. How the clinical syndrome is produced is not known.

The standard tests for chronic Epstein-Barr viral syndrome consists of detection of IgG and IgM antibody against the early antigen, and the detection of Epstein-Barr nuclear antibody. The virus has a protein core around it called the capsid. IgG and IgM antibodies are produced because of the capsid antigen and are directed against the capsid. The presence of antibody against the early capsid antigen indicates relatively recent viremia. The Epstein-Barr nuclear antibody is a neutralizing antibody appearing 2 to 3 months after the acute phase of infectious mononucleosis and seems to be associated with resolution of the acute infectious mononucleosis syndrome. The chronic absence of this antibody seems to be associated with the musculoskeletal and psychiatric forms of the Epstein-Barr viral disease. In low titers, this antibody indicates exposure to and some immunity against the virus. The tissue culture of the acute Epstein-Barr virus is extremely difficult and is a research tool, as is the DNA probe.

VIRAL HEPATITIS

Hepatitis is a general term indicating inflammation of the liver. It may be due to viruses, bacteria, fungi, parasites, drugs, toxins, and physical agents such as heat, hyperthermia, and radiation, among others. We will discuss only the hepatitis virus, which is a double-stranded DNA virus and is fairly complex with a surface antigen, an early antigen, and a core antigen. The diagnostic tests that use antibodies usually are directed against one of these viral antigens.

The term "viral hepatitis" includes at least three virus types: hepatitis A, hepatitis B, and non-A–non-B hepatitis. These conditions are clinically similar but etiologically and epidemiologically different. All are characterized by malaise, low-grade temperature elevation, jaundice, and anorexia, along with elevated liver enzymes (aspartate aminotransferase [formerly SGOT], alanine aminotransferase [formerly SGPT] and elevated *bilirubin* and *alkaline phosphatase* levels. A *liver biopsy* is helpful in demonstrating viral hepatitis in any of the three clinical forms; however, only serology identifies the type of virus.

Hepatitis B

Hepatitis B is the most serious type of viral hepatitis. It may become chronic and end in cirrhosis. It was formerly known as "serum hepatitis" or "posttransfusion hepatitis" and is caused by the hepatitis B virus, which is transmitted through blood and blood components and also may be a sexually transmitted disease. Fig. 13-1 demonstrates the serological pattern for hepatitis B.

During the 6 weeks before the onset of the clinical illness, *hepatitis B surface antigen* appears in the patient's blood; its level peaks just before the onset of jaundice and disappears by the third month. One month before the onset of jaundice the *early antigen* appears in the blood and 1 week later the *core antibodies* appear.

If the patient is immunocompetent, antibodies are produced against the different parts of the virus. The *antibodies against the early antigen* may be detected approximately 2 months after the clinical appearance of the disease. *Antibodies against surface antigen* are seen approximately 3½ months after the onset of the clinical disease. Antibodies against the core antigen are of two types, IgM and IgG. The IgM type increases at the height of the disease and tapers off toward the fourth month. The IgG antibody against the core antigen remains, possibly for life. Immunity developed by active immunization against hepatitis B shows antibodies against surface antigen, indicating that the person is vaccinated. In patients who cannot develop antibodies to fight the infection, liver failure develops and death results; hepatoma (cancer of the liver cells) may also be a complication.

Hepatitis A

Type A hepatitis is much less serious than type B in terms of severity of the disease, duration, and complications. It is usually transmitted through the oral route (ingestion of food or water con-

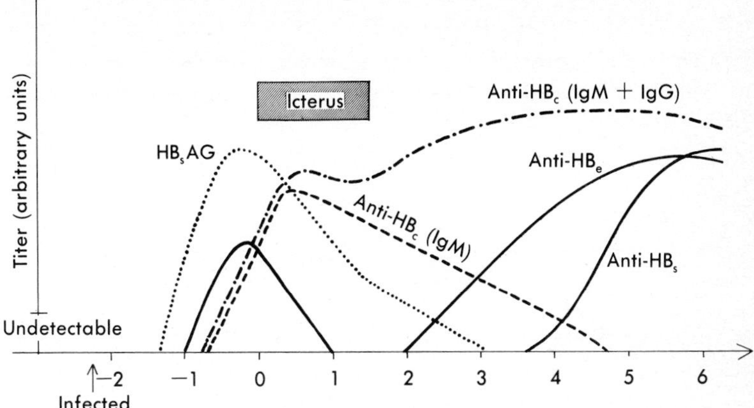

Fig. 13-1. *Serological patterns of hepatitis B infection. The* surface antigen *appears in the blood about 17 days after the patient becomes infected and 5½ weeks before the onset of symptoms (jaundice); however, 5% to 10% of patients with the disease will test negative and 5% to 10% will become carriers of the surface antigen. Levels peak at approximately 7 days before the appearance of jaundice and steadily decline and disappear by the third month following symptoms.*

The early antigen *appears 4 weeks before the onset of symptoms in 80% to 90% of patients, peaks with symptoms, and disappears by the first month of the clinical disease.* Core antibodies *appear shortly after the appearance of the early antigen in all patients. The IgM antibodies steadily decline after peaking with the clinical disease; IgG antibodies remain possibly for life to bestow some immunity.*

By the second month of the clinical illness early antibodies *appear in 70% to 90% of patients, and at 3½ months the* surface antibodies appear *in 80% to 90% of patients. (HB$_s$Ag, hepatitis B surface antigen; HB$_e$Ag, hepatitis B early antigen; anti-HB$_c$, hepatitis B core antibody; anti-HB$_e$, hepatitis B early antibody; anti-HB$_s$, hepatitis B surface antibody.)*

taminated by feces). This virus, also called fecal hepatitis-associated antigen (HAA), is simpler than the hepatitis B virus. Fig. 13-2 demonstrates the serological pattern for hepatitis A. The antigen can be detected in the blood approximately 2 weeks before the onset of the disease. Antibodies against this viral particle are of two types, IgM and IgG. IgM antibodies appear early at the onset of the disease, increase at its height, taper off, and are not detectable 4 months after onset. The IgG antibody remains in the blood, giving some immunity to the patient.

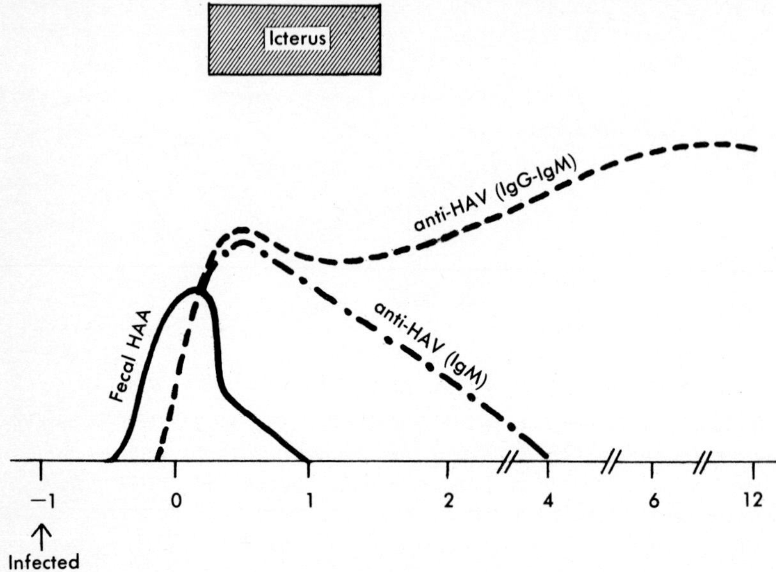

Fig. 13-2. *Serological patterns of hepatitis A infection. The fecal hepatitis-associated antigen (HAA) appears at approximately 2 weeks after infection and 2 weeks before the onset of clinical symptoms in 57% of patients, and then sharply declines. Antibodies appear just before the onset of symptoms, with IgM declining and IgG remaining.*

Hepatitis non-A–non-B

This is a viral hepatitis; the agent is unknown. It is neither type A nor type B by serology, and thus it is called non-A–non-B. Basically diagnosis is by exclusion. The diagnosis of non-A–non-B hepatitis is made when the clinical picture is typical of viral hepatitis and no antigens or antibodies are found to either A or B virus.

LABORATORY TESTS FOR VIRAL HEPATITIS

INITIAL DIAGNOSTIC HEPATITIS PROFILE

- Hepatitis B surface antigen
- Anti-hepatitis A virus antibody (IgM)
- Anti-hepatitis B core antibody (IgG plus IgM)

If the patient has negative values for hepatitis B surface antigen and anti-hepatitis B core antibodies and positive values for anti-hepatitis A virus antibody (IgM), the diagnosis is clear: the patient has hepatitis type A. On the other hand, if the patient has elevated titers for hepatitis B surface antigen and also hepatitis B core antibodies, specifically the IgM type, the patient has acute hepatitis B.

HEPATITIS INFECTIVITY PROFILE

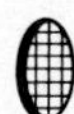

- Hepatitis B early antigen
- Anti-hepatitis B early antibody

The patient's ability to infect other persons with his or her blood may be checked by these tests. If titers are elevated, an ongoing viremia is indicated.

HEPATITIS B IMMUNE PROFILE

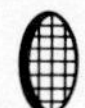

- Anti-hepatitis B core antibody (IgG plus IgM)
- Anti-hepatitis B surface antibody

These tests are performed to determine if the individual should take a vaccine or not. If both hepatitis B core antibodies and hepatitis B surface antibodies are elevated, the patient has had serum hepatitis B in the past, has immunity against the virus, and there is no indication for vaccination. If these levels are not elevated, the patient has never been infected. Usually after vaccination, the anti-hepatitis B surface antibody is elevated, which seems to be protective against hepatitis B.

ACUTE/CHRONIC HEPATITIS PROFILE

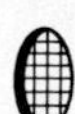

- Anti-hepatitis B surface antibody
- Anti-hepatitis B early antibody

These tests determine if the patient continues to have hepatitis or is going into a chronic hepatitis. The presence of anti-hepatitis B early antibody indicates ongoing production of virus replication (chronic hepatitis).

HEPATITIS B RESOLUTION PROFILE

- Hepatitis B surface antigen
- Hepatitis B early antigen
- Anti-hepatitis B early antibody

These tests are performed to determine complete resolution of the disease, which lasts 2 to 3 months. The disappearance of hepatitis B early antigen and hepatitis B surface antigen within 1 to 3 months, and the appearance of antibodies against early antigen between the third and the fourth month indicates resolution of the hepatitis.

NONTRADITIONAL LABORATORY TECHNIQUES

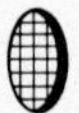

ENZYME-LINKED IMMUNOSORBENT ASSAY (ELISA)

ELISA is a very sensitive technique that detects the presence of either antigens or antibodies. It is valuable because of its speed and broad range. Results are usually stated as positive or negative, but may also be given as end-point titers.

This technique was developed as a substitute for radioimmunoassay. Enzymes are chemically linked to antibodies, which are still able to react with their specific antigen. The enzyme, while attached to the antibody, can catalyze a reaction, yielding an end product that can be seen, and some systems rely on this visual reading, although most rely on automated spectrophotometric reading of end points.

ELISA assay is available for routine diagnostic detection of rotavirus, hepatitis B antigens, *Neisseria gonorrhoeae* antigens, *Chlamydia trachomatis*, Epstein-Barr virus antigens, respiratory syncytial virus, and adenoviruses. Although the sensitivity of the ELISA method has been enhanced by the use of monoclonal antibodies, many organisms (viruses, bacteria, fungi, and *Mycoplasma*) are not detected.

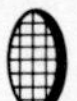

MONOCLONAL ANTIBODIES

Monoclonal antibodies are immunochemically identical antibodies produced from a single cell. These antibodies are highly specific and can be produced in large quantities. This technique eliminates the necessity to immunize animals with the antigen being sought and the subsequent processing of the antibody. Many commercial systems using monoclonal antibodies are being developed.

GENETIC PROBES

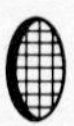

A genetic probe is a small piece of labeled single-stranded nucleic acid (DNA or RNA). It is allowed to react with the culture or material under investigation. For example, a labeled DNA probe is allowed to react with material that has been treated to expose single-stranded DNA. The DNA probe will form strong bonds with complementary DNA present in the material being tested. Such a probe is very stable and can be used on dry material that has been standing for a long time, or it can be used immediately. It can be used among a mixture of other genes and molecules and is able to detect complementary sequences.

LIMULUS AMEBOCYTE LYSATE (LAL) ASSAY

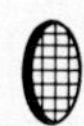

Limulus is a genus of king crab (the horseshoe crab) that has circulating amebocytes in its hemolymph. The lysate of these amebocytes gel in the presence of the endotoxin from gram-negative bacteria. In females, the LAL assay has been found to be diagnostic for gonococcal infection. The specimen is collected on swabs from the endocervical canal and mixed with the lysate fluid from the horseshoe crab. A positive test produces a gel.

LABORATORY TESTS FOR BACTERIAL INFECTION

GRAM STAIN

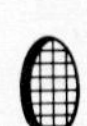

A Gram stain permits the classification of bacteria into four basic groups: gram-positive or gram-negative rods and gram-positive or gram-negative cocci. After staining with gentian violet and Gram's iodine, the morphology can be visualized. A blue stain is gram-positive, a red stain is gram-negative.

Classification of bacteria by Gram stain has important clinical implications. For example, identification of a gram-positive chain of cocci immediately narrows the differential diagnosis to an infectious process, thus guiding therapy 24 to 48 hours before the specific cultural identification and sensitivity testing have been completed. The types of groups in which the bacteria arrange themselves can also be seen on a Gram stain. This is another guide to therapy. For example, the finding of gram-positive diplococci suggests pneumococcus, while the presence of gram-positive organisms in clumps suggests staphylococcus. Of course, eventually the culture and sensitivity tests should be performed for definitive diagnosis and adequate treatment.

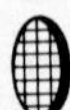

ACID-FAST BACILLI (AFB) STAIN

The acid-fast, or Ziehl-Neelsen, stain is used mainly in the diagnosis of tuberculosis, tuberculous infections, and leprosy. The causative organisms of these diseases appear red against a blue background when stained by this method.

Since it usually takes 2 to 3 weeks to culture the tubercle bacilli, results of the AFB stain can indicate the need for the immediate initiation of therapy. It is diagnostically most helpful if seen in sputum or the cerebrospinal fluid; the AFB stain is used for follow-up evaluation as well.

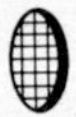

BACTERIAL CULTURE AND SENSITIVITY TESTING

Usually, identification of bacteria and determination of their sensitivity to specific antimicrobial drugs are done after the initial Gram stain analysis. Most frequently, the identification of a specific organism must be accompanied by a sensitivity study. An exception to this generalization is the finding of β-hemolytic streptococci in a throat culture, since the sensitivity of these organisms to antibacterial drugs is well known. However, because of the changing patterns of resistance of other bacteria to antibacterial agents, sensitivity studies are essential.

NURSING ACTION

1. Obtain the specimen before the administration of antimicrobial agents, if at all possible.
2. Avoid external contamination.
3. Be sure to collect a sufficient quantity of the specimen.
4. Ensure that the specimens are delivered to the laboratory promptly.
5. Supply the laboratory with necessary clinical information to ensure the selection of suitable media and techniques.

BILE SOLUBILITY STUDIES

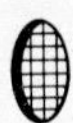

Streptococcus pneumoniae, unlike other streptococci, autolyse under the influence of a bile salt (sodium deoxycholate). This is due to the fact that *S. pneumoniae* possesses a very active autocatalytic enzyme that causes it to dissolve in bile. It differentiates pneumococci from other streptococci and is usually done on sputum or blood cultures after overnight growth. However, if streptococci that resemble pneumococci are found to be insoluble in bile, other tests should be performed since old colonies of pneumococci may lose their active enzyme.

COAGULASE AND THERMONUCLEASE TESTS

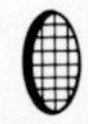

These tests combined together help in the identification of *Staphylococcus aureus*. The slide coagulase test is used to screen quickly for isolates of *S. aureus*. Most strains of *S. aureus* are coagulase-positive; *Staphylococcus epidermidis* and *Micrococcus* are coagulase-negative. The rapid thermonuclease test distinguishes between *Staphylococcus aureus* and coagulase-negative staphylococci.

DELAYED HYPERSENSITIVITY SKIN TEST BATTERY

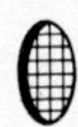

This skin test uses delayed hypersensitivity to detect certain infections, such as tuberculosis or various fungal diseases, detect immunocompetence, and observe an allergy to certain antigens. It is assumed that most adults have been exposed and will react to one of the following antigens within 48 hours after administration: *Candida albicans, Trichophyton,* tetanus toxoid, mumps, and streptokinase-streptodornase. If the patient has intact cell immunity there will be a recall of sensitized T-lymphocytes to the area of the skin that was injected. The reaction is measured by the area of inflammatory induration on the skin. In the absence of cell-mediated immunity, there will be no reaction (negative). The assumption is that if the patient is immune deficient, the reaction will be negative to all of the substances injected, since the patient was surely exposed to one or all of these during his or her lifetime. An immunecompetent individual would have a positive reaction.

SEROLOGICAL TESTS FOR THE DIAGNOSIS OF BACTERIAL DISEASE

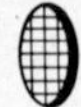

PRECIPITIN TESTS

Precipitates will form when soluble antigens are combined with antiserum containing specific antibodies. These tests are used mainly in the identification of bacterial exotoxins and the antibodies of certain fungi.

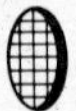

AGGLUTINATION TESTS

Agglutinins are antibodies developed against a specific cell type, and when combined, the clumping of cells results. This method is used instead of culture for the *Brucella* and *Salmonella* bacteria.

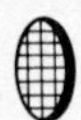

VDRL (VENEREAL DISEASE RESEARCH LABORATORY) TEST

This is a flocculation test for the screening of syphilis. The pathogenic treponemes cause the protein, reagin, to form. Reagin binds to the test antigen, causing flocculation of the particles. Although the VDRL test is negative in very early infection, it detects more than 99% of cases of secondary syphilis. A number of other conditions and infections also cause a positive result.

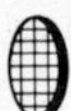

FLUORESCENT TREPONEMAL ANTIBODY ABSORPTION (FTA-ABS) TEST

This is a highly sensitive serological assay that detects antibodies to the causative agent of syphilis *(Treponema pallidum)*. A positive FTA-ABS test remains positive for life.

THE IMMUNE SYSTEM

Reference ranges for the lymphocyte panel

Total WBC count: 3500-11,000/mm^3

Total lymphocyte count: 1200-3900/mm^3

Total T-lymphocytes (T11; PAN T): 74%-86% of lymphocytes

T4 (helper T cells): 38%-52% of lymphocytes

T8 (suppressor T cells): 22%-36% of lymphocytes

T4/T8 ratio: 1.0:2.2
Total B-lymphocytes: 5%-25% of lymphocytes

Human beings are continuously exposed to diseases causing infective particles (bacteria and viruses or parasites) to enter the body. Usually, healthy people with intact immunity either do not contract the disease or they have a brief period of an acute syndrome and recover, indicating the ability to fight and contain disease-causing infective agents.

The immune system comprises *cell-mediated immune responses* (lymphocytes of the T class) and *antibody-mediated immune responses* (lymphocytes of the B class). The cell-mediated immune system is evaluated by skin tests and T-lymphocyte levels and their subpopulations. The humoral system is evaluated by measuring B-lymphocyte and immunoglobulin levels.

Lymphocytes

Lymphocytes are mononuclear leukocytes involved in the production of antibodies, immunological memory, and cell-mediated immunity. There are two main types of lymphocytes, the T-lymphocytes (thymus derived) and the B-lymphocytes (bone marrow derived).

T-lymphocytes

T cells produce cell-mediated immunity. They are generated by stem cells in the bone marrow, mature into thymocytes and multiply rapidly in the thymus gland, and then migrate to the lymph nodes and spleen, where they are known as T cells. They have antigen receptors on their cell membrane. When antigens bind to receptors in the T-cell membranes, the T cells are changed into sensitized T cells. Changes in the number of *total T-lymphocytes (T11; PAN T)* indicate the possibility of aberrations in cell-mediated immunity caused by immunodeficiency, infectious diseases, or T-cell malignancies.

T cells are of three types; T_4 (helper-inducer), T_8 (cytotonic-suppressor), and *null cells* (lymphocytes without T or B characteristics).

Various T lymphocytes travel to the antigen entry point in the body, recognize the particular antigen that originally activated them, bind to it, and destroy it. The cells thus attacked are cells that have been invaded by viruses, are malignant, or have been transplanted (organ rejection).

T_4 cells are stimulated by the antigen to enhance the response of the B cells, which synthesize antibodies. In acquired immune deficiency syndrome (AIDS) a profound decrease in the absolute number of T4 cells is common. Depletion is also seen in numerous other infections.

Suppressor T cells (T_8) are thought to inhibit antibody production either by directly suppressing helper cells or directly inhibiting B-cell differentiation. An absolute or a relative increase of T_8 cells is seen in acute mononucleosis, cytomegaloviral infection, acute and chronic hepatitis B, and possibly also in rheumatoid arthritis and systemic lupus erythymatosus.

Null cells are lymphocytes without T or B characteristics. They are present in systemic lupus erythematosus and can kill tumor cells in vitro.

T4/T8 ratio. In numerous conditions involving altered immunoregulatory function the T4/T8 ratio reverses. Such a reversal is not diagnostic and the clinician should evaluate the absolute number of T4 and T8 cells. A profound decrease in the absolute number of T4 cells results in an inverted T4/T8 ratio. Such is the case in over 95% of AIDS patients who have opportunistic infections and/or Kaposi's sarcoma. Increased numbers of T8+ cells also results in a reversed T_4/T_8 ratio and is often seen in apparently healthy homosexuals.

B-lymphocytes

B cells are generated by the stem cells from bone marrow, where they mature. B cells have antigen receptors on their cell membrane and cause humoral immunity by generating plasma cells that produce antibodies. When antigens bind to antibodies in B-cell membranes (in the lymph nodes and spleen) the B cells are activated and produce plasma cells and more B cells that have a memory for that particular antigen and will undergo repeated mitosis on subsequent exposure.

Antibodies

The plasma cells thus generated secrete large amounts of *antibodies*, proteins of the immunoglobulin family that combine specifically with the antigens that induced their synthesis. *Antigens* are molecules that induce an immune response (the production of antibodies). Antibodies are divided into five different types: immunoglobulin G (IgG), immunoglobulin A (IgA), immunoglobulin M (IgM), immunoglobulin D (IgD), and immunoglobulin E (IgE). Diagnostic serological methods measure only IgM and IgG, and normal individuals produce both in response to most pathogens. IgM is usually produced only during the initial encounter with a particular pathogen, and not in response to a second infection with the same pathogen. Fig. 13-3 traces the relative humoral response to antigen stimulation over time. Usually a second-encounter response is that of IgG with the *anamnestic response*, in which antibodies are produced quicker and more abundantly. IgM differs from IgG in that it cannot cross the placental barrier and cannot bind complement.

As the infectious process continues, the cells that were producing IgM switch to IgG, which is often more specific for the antigen. Thus the presence of IgM is indicative of acute infection. Since IgG persists after the initial infection or is produced because of reinfection, the presence of IgG without IgM indicates the recuperative phase or reinfection with the same pathogen.

Antibodies produce *humoral immunity* by rendering the pathogens more vulnerable to phagocytosis or by exposing *complement*-binding sites on their molecule and thus causing them to be lysed. Antigens are "recognized" by the immunoglobulin, which binds to them (antigen-antibody complex), causing the antibody to expose its complement-binding site. Antigens may also be agglutinated, making it easier for the phagocytes to digest the clumped antigens.

Laboratory tests to evaluate for humoral deficiencies include determination of the number of *B-lymphocytes* (reference range: 5% to 25%) in the peripheral blood and by assay of serum concentrations

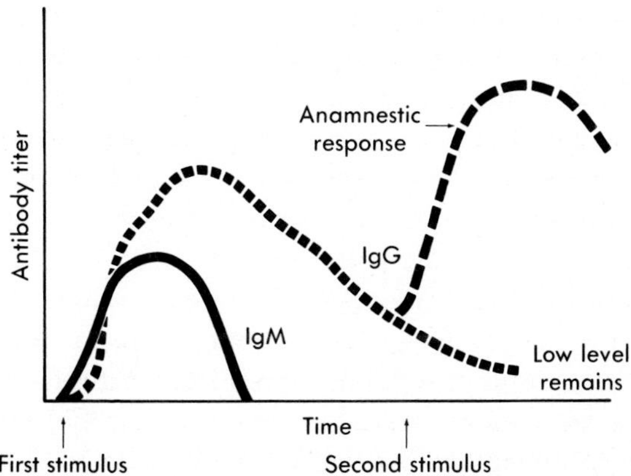

Fig. 13-3. *Relative humoral response to antigen stimulation over time. (From Finegold, S.M., and Baron, E.J.: Bailey and Scott's diagnostic microbiology, ed. 7, St. Louis, 1986, The C.V. Mosby Co.)*

of the *immunoglobulins* that are produced by the B-lymphocytes (IgG, IgA, and IgM). Absence or markedly reduced numbers suggests congenital or acquired immunodeficiency states. Marked increase suggests malignancy states and is helpful in the diagnosis of chronic lymphocytic leukemia. Predominance of B cells with monoclonal phenotype marker is of prognostic value in leukemias and lymphomas.

The complement system

Complements are inactive enzymes that normally exist in the blood serum and kill foreign cells directly by cytolysis, and indirectly by enhancement of phagocytosis and causing vasodilation. There are sites on the antibody molecule that are capable of binding with the complement (complement-binding sites). These sites are exposed during the formation of the antigen-antibody complex. When the binding site becomes available, complement protein C1 is activated and catalyzes the action of the next complement protein and so on down the line in rapid succession. Molecules that result from this complement activity surround the surface of the foreign cell, causing a hole to appear in its membrane. The foreign cell then swells and lyses (cytolysis).

Complements consist of 20 or more protein compounds, which have three components, the classic pathway, the alternate (properdin) pathway, and the final common pathway. The classic pathway is activated by IgG or IgM immunoglobulins, DNA, C-reactive protein, and staphylococcal protein A. The classic pathway and the IgG and IgM complexes are most frequently associated with autoimmune phenomena. The alternate pathway is activated by bacteria, certain fungal infections, and IgA and IgG antibodies induced by viruses. The common terminal pathway is formed by complements C5 to C9 ("membrane attack complex") and is reached either through the classic pathway or the alternate pathway.

Deficiencies of complements C1 and C2 are associated with autoimmune diseases. Deficiencies of other components of the complement system result in systemic lupus erythematosus (C1, C4, C2, C5, C8) and recurrent neisserial infections (C5 to C8).

Evaluation of defects in the complement system

When there is a deficiency of selected components of the complement cascade, a particular disease results. For example, if C3 is deficient, pyogenic infections may result; if one of the components from C5 to C8 are deficient the patient is predisposed to recurrent neisserial infections; reduced levels of any component may indicate systemic lupus erythematosus.

Laboratory tests for the evaluation of complement integrity include CH_{50} and C3 and C4 levels.

CH_{50} (COMPLEMENT HEMOLYTIC 50%)

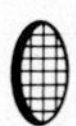

Reference range

100-200 units/ml

This value reflects the amount of serum needed to lyse 50% of a suspension of sheep red cells coated with anti–red cell antibody. Although a normal value rules out complement deficiency, a low value is not specific, since it may indicate selective deficiency of a single factor or an overall activation of the complement system followed by consumption of all components.

C3 AND C4

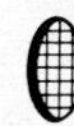

Reference ranges

C4: 10-20 mg/dl   C3: 100-200 mg/dl

C4 levels may reflect activity in the early components of the classic pathway. C3 levels may reflect activity in the alternate pathway.

Evaluation of phagocyte function abnormalities

Abnormalities of phagocyte function usually are associated with congenital immunodeficiency diseases, diabetes, and certain drugs that cause immunosuppression (e.g., corticosteroids). Such patients often develop recurrent infections that should alert the clinician to the possibility of defective phagocytic cell activity. The infections that are particularly noted are sinus and pulmonary infections and/or skin infections, specifically *Staphylococcus aureus*, *Serratia* species, *Aspergillus*, or *Candida*.

Laboratory tests for phagocyte function include

1. Polymorphonuclear leukocytes and monocytes. Determination of the relative and absolute numbers rules out bone marrow dysfunction or peripheral destruction.
2. Peripheral blood film (Wright's stain) for the evaluation of cellular

morphology. One looks for Döhle bodies, toxic granulations, intracellular organisms, or granule deficiency.
3. Peroxidase strains may also be evaluated and may reveal myeloperoxidase deficiency.
4. Chemotaxis may be evaluated in vivo and in vitro.
5. Phagocytosis itself may be evaluated in vitro by exposing the cells to bacteria, fungi, and so forth and determining how many of the bacteria or foreign substances have been engulfed.
6. Examination of the composition and concentration of the granules.

LABORATORY TESTS FOR VIRAL INFECTIONS

When a viral illness is encountered the physician and virologist may determine that a specimen should be collected so that the viral agent can be isolated, the antigen detected by labeled antibody, the antibody response measured, and the standard serological viral tests performed (heterophil antibody test, tests of agglutination, hemagglutination inhibition test, complement fixation test, and the neutralization test). The virus-specific antibodies may also be measured to identify the virus (immunofluorescent technique, immunoradioisotope technique, immunoenzyme technique). There are kits available for the antibody response to specific viral antigens. The clinician should be aware of the different sensitivities among the kits and be in communication with the laboratory for the proper interpretation and management of the patient.

Collection, storage, and transport of specimens

1. Instruct the patient regarding the nature of the test and tell him or her that there are no dietary restrictions before the test.
2. Determine the specimen container to be used. Virology laboratories may supply special containers with transport media.
3. You may be asked to obtain swabs for culture from the nasal passages, posterior wall of the pharynx, conjunctiva, open lesions, or the rectal mucosa or the stool.
4. The physician may wish to obtain deep pharyngeal aspirates. Use a narrow-gauge gavage tube attached to the end of a 5 ml syringe. Aspirate the mucus, cut off the distal 3 to 5 cm of the tube, and drop it into the culture medium.
5. If cerebrospinal fluid is the specimen, collect it in a sterile screw-capped tube; it should not be contaminated with blood.

6. If urine is the specimen, collect 10 ml in a sterile screw-capped tube.
7. Pack the specimen on ice and transport it as soon as possible to the virology laboratory by courier or delivery service. If there must be a delay before transport refrigerate the specimen at 4° C (39.2° F) or place it on wet ice until shipment.
8. If the specimen is tissue, collect approximately 2 cm^2 by sterile instrument in a sterile screw-capped tube without preservatives and place it on wet ice. If the specimen cannot be transported to the laboratory within 48 hours it should be frozen at −70° C (−94° F) and transported on dry ice.
9. Obtain serum from whole blood and refrigerate it or freeze it until testing.
10. As an aid to the laboratory in determining the diagnostic test indicated, include the following information with the specimen: patient's name, address, sex, age, brief clinical summary, date of onset of illness, date of specimen collection, disease suspected, and major clinical and laboratory findings. Also include data regarding recent patient travel, occupational or geographical exposure to infectious diseases, recent vaccination, and contact with animals.

Note: An extra word of caution is in order here, even though the procedure is very routine. Be extremely attentive when drawing blood from patients suspected of having a viral infection so as not to accidentally prick yourself with the needle that has been used to withdraw the specimen.

Isolation of the virus

Viruses cannot be isolated in a culture medium such as is possible with bacteria. A virus multiplies in a living cell; thus viral culture methods involve the use of tissue (tissue culture cell monolayer). The diagnosis is also aided by observations regarding the tissue culture in which the virus grows, cytological changes, and the time required for these effects. Once the virus begins to grow in the culture, a specific diagnosis can be made by hemagglutination tests, immunofluorescence, immunoenzyme and immunoradioisotope detection, and electron microscopy can be performed. More antibodies can be produced for use in identifying virus isolates by injecting a viral suspension from the culture into an animal host.

Detection of antigen by labeled antibody

Measurement of virus-specific IgM and IgG antibodies can be useful in identifying current or past infection, since in response to acute infection, IgM levels are the first to rise and remain elevated into convalescence before declining. Serum levels of IgG usually rise several days after those of IgM and persist for months or years. The techniques employed are *immunofluorescence, radioimmunoassay (RIA),* and *ELISA* (p. 520).

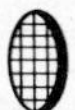

IMMUNOFLUORESCENT TECHNIQUE

The immunofluorescent technique detects the antigen using the specific antiviral antibody that has been tagged with a fluorochrome label (direct method) or uses a known virus-specific antibody to bind to the antigen from the clinical specimen (indirect method). Results are based on the presence or absence of fluorescence and are either positive or negative.

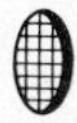

RADIOIMMUNOASSAY (RIA)

Radioimmunoassay (RIA) uses antibodies labeled with a radioisotope to detect the specific antigen or antibody. This method requires an instrument for counting radioactive emissions. Results are stated as positive or negative.

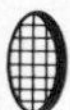

ELECTRON MICROSCOPY

After preparation with negative staining techniques, feces, serum, urine, CSF, and biopsy material can be examined by the electron microscope for the identification of viral agents. The sensitivity of the method is increased with immune electron microscopy in that viral particles are aggregated by adding specific antibodies, allowing them to be differentiated from morphologically similar nonviral particles.

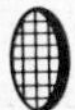

MEASUREMENT OF ANTIBODY RESPONSE

The diagnosis of viral infection may be based on the titer of antibodies in the patient's serum in the acute phase of the illness as compared with the convalescent phase. This test requires that both specimens (acute and convalescent) be processed at the same time in the laboratory so that the antibody titers can be compared. A rise in the antibody titer of the convalescent serum can be of diagnostic value. Serum and cerebrospinal fluid (CSF) titers should also be compared because their ratios may be diagnostically significant.

Measurement of antibody response provides evidence of infection with a specific viral agent, is useful in screening for evidence of prior infection and presence of protective immunity (e.g., rubella titers), detects viral encephalitis (cerebrospinal fluid), and aids in the diagnosis of congenital infections by testing the antibody titers in maternal and neonatal serum. For example, in herpes encephalitis the ratio of serum to CSF antibody titers is less than 20:1; and with intrauterine infection IgM is present in cord or neonatal serum. IgM antibodies, unlike IgG, do not cross the placental barrier and represent fetal response to infection. IgG can cross the placental barrier and, therefore, if it is found in neonatal serum it may indicate that the fetus has passively acquired the maternal antibodies.

HETEROPHIL ANTIBODY TEST

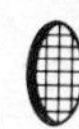

This is a test for acute infectious mononucleosis, which is caused by the Epstein-Barr virus. The antibody usually is not detected in the chronic Epstein-Barr viral syndrome. There are several rapid slide tests available to screen for the heterophil antibody–positive infectious mononucleosis. If this rapid test is equivocal the specimen should be sent to an experienced laboratory for a quantitative test. Even with a positive serological test, the diagnosis is only made when it is also indicated by the clinical setting and the presence of 50% or more lymphocytes with 10% or more atypical cells in the differential white blood cell count.

TESTS OF AGGLUTINATION

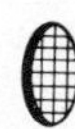

Tests of agglutination are screening tests that rapidly measure antibody response. They are especially useful in screening for antibody levels to rubella virus. The *hemagglutination inhibition test* is based on the ability of certain viruses to agglutinate the erythrocytes of such animals as geese and chickens, monkeys, or sheep. This test is ordered if infection with arboviruses, influenza, rubella, mumps, or measles virus is suspected.

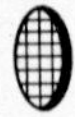

COMPLEMENT FIXATION TEST

The complement fixation test is gradually being replaced by more sensitive tests with quicker results. Complement is a complex system of proteins and glycoproteins and the chief humoral mediator of antigen-antibody reactions. The complement components C1 to C9 cause lysis of antibody-coated bacteria by causing a hole in the cell membrane through which water and ions may enter and produce cell bursting. The complement fixation test is performed in two stages and measures a variety of antigens and antibodies. Results are expressed as the highest serum (antibody) dilution showing complete first-stage fixation (consumption) of complement and prevention of hemolysis.

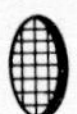

NEUTRALIZATION TEST

The neutralization test is the principal method used to identify virus isolates. The test is based on the ability of a specific antibody in the patient's serum to render neutral a known virus that is added to the serum. The end-point titer is the highest dilution of serum showing no hemolysis (no cell infection). Sometimes an end point of 50% hemolysis is used, but it is not widely accepted.

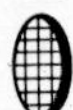

HISTOCYTOPATHOLOGICAL EXAMINATION

Several well-known viral diseases may be diagnosed by histological examination of tissues. Conventional staining and immunofluorescent techniques are used. The Papanicolaou smear and the Tzanck smear can be prepared in the office and sent to the laboratory for interpretation.

Herpes simplex and varicella-zoster show intranuclear inclusions and/or multinucleated giant cells in infected cells (Papanicolaou smear of the uterine cervix or Tzanck smear on vesicular skin lesions).

Vaccinia and variola show intracytoplasmic inclusions (Guarnieri bodies).

Rabies shows intracytoplasmic inclusions in brain tissue (Negri bodies).

LABORATORY TESTS FOR MYCOSES

GERM TUBE TEST

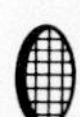

This test is an economical method of identifying yeasts. It diagnoses the *Candida albicans* species within 3 hours. The test gets its name from the filamentous outgrowths ("germ tubes") produced by *C. albicans* cells after incubation. For the definitive diagnosis of *C. albicans* the organism is cultured on Sabouraud's dextrose agar which takes 3 days to complete.

RAPID UREASE TEST

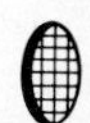

Several bacteria and fungi produce the enzyme urease. These include *Proteus* species, *Klebsiella* species, some *Citrobacter* species, some *Hemophilus* species, and the yeast *Cryptococcus neoformans*. Urease hydrolyzes urea into ammonia, water, and carbon dioxide and the alkaline end products change the indicator, phenol red, from yellow to pink.

LEVODOPA–FERRIC CITRATE TEST

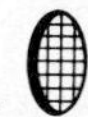

This test is based on the fact that *Cryptococcus neoformans* can be identified because it is the only member of this genus that produces phenol oxidase. The C/N Screen (Flow Laboratories) provides a product that uses levodopa for the detection of phenol oxidase. This test takes 48 to 72 hours for a positive reaction to be visible.

EXOANTIGEN TEST

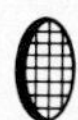

This new method is now available commercially to all laboratories. It provides a conclusive identification of *Blastomyces dermatitidis*, *Coccidioides immitis*, *Histoplasma capsulatum*, and *Paracoccidioides brasiliensis*. The test requires a mature fungous culture on Sabouraud's dextrose agar and is based on the fact that soluble antigens from the organism can be added to serum known to contain antibodies against the specific antigen. Instructions are included by the manufacturer with the package.

Michael M. Stevenson, Ph.D.

14

Diagnostic tests for sleep disorders

PHYSIOLOGY

Sleep is a complex and active process, the control of which, along with wakefulness, resides in diffuse brain areas that generate three relatively distinct states of consciousness. These states are waking or arousal, dreaming or rapid eye movement sleep (REM), and non–rapid eye movement sleep (NREM).

Sleep and wakefulness alternate in a periodic way during every 24 hours. During the sleep phase, REM sleep occurs in a cyclic fashion, alternating with periods of NREM sleep. Each REM-NREM cycle lasts 70 to 120 minutes. A single night of normal sleep consists of four to six cycles, each of which includes both NREM sleep and REM sleep, as shown in Fig. 14-1.

NREM sleep normally begins as a person falls asleep and becomes decreasingly conscious of the external environment. It is divided into stages 1, 2, 3, and 4, with stage 1 representing the lightest sleep and stages 3 to 4 the deepest sleep. A normal young adult would be expected to spend 5% of the night in stage 1, 45% in stage 2, 25% in stages 3 to 4, and 25% in REM sleep.

NREM sleep is quiet, passive, and restful. Breathing, heart rate, and blood pressure become lower and more regular in NREM sleep, but as the brain enters REM sleep, profound physiological changes occur.

REM sleep is characterized by an intensely active brain within a paralyzed body (relatively low voltage, mixed frequency EEG, episodic rapid eye movements, and a low amplitude EMG). Active inhibition of spinal reflexes prevents all reflex and voluntary movements. Transient release of inhibition results in occasional twitches of the face and limbs, with rapid eye movements occurring in phasic bursts. Respiration, heart rate, and blood pressure become more variable. Cerebral blood flow increases and a loss of thermoregulatory response occurs in the hypothalamus. Reports of highly visual, storylike dreams are associated with waking from REM sleep. Penile erections are associated with REM and are independent of dream content. Fig. 14-2 distinguishes REM sleep from NREM sleep on the basis of polysomnographic differences.

Sleep duration and patterns in normal individuals vary extensively and change with age. Most normal adults sleep 7 to 8 hours, although normal sleep can be as short as 4 hours and as long as 10 to 12 hours. Infants sleep up to 18 hours a day, and they spend more time in stage 4 sleep and in REM sleep than children or adults. With increasing age, stage 4 sleep diminishes, sleep latency (the time required to fall asleep) increases, and sleep disturbances become more frequent. Some of these changes are considered to be part of the normal aging process, while others are potentially correctable.

PATHOPHYSIOLOGY AND CLINICAL APPLICATION OF LABORATORY TESTS

The scientific study of sleep and sleep disorders is a relatively new development in clinical medicine. During the past decade, var-

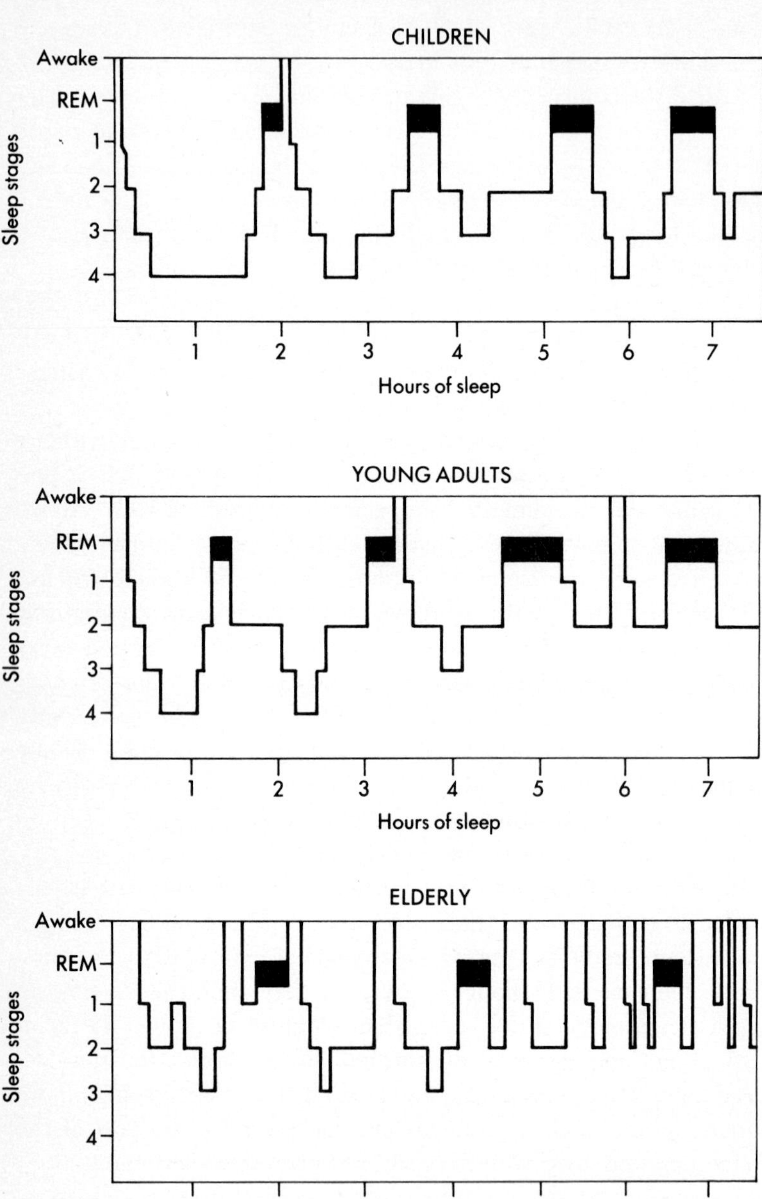

Fig. 14-1. *An idealized night's sleep in children, normal young adults, and the elderly.*

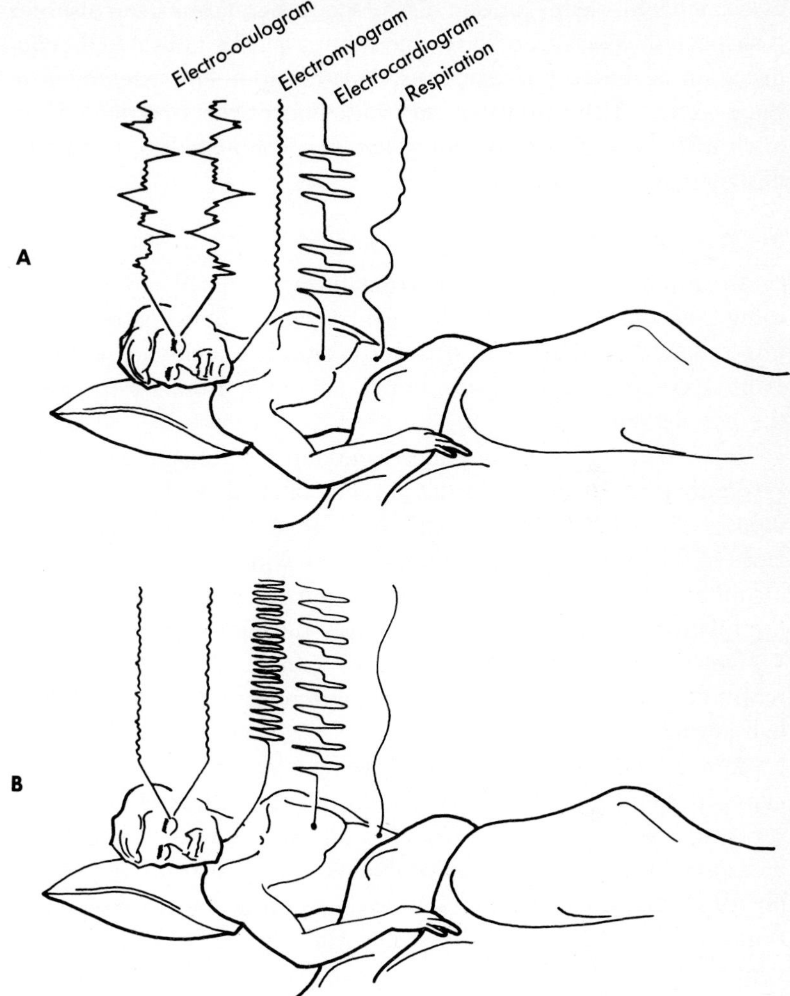

Fig. 14-2. *Polysomnographic records during REM (**A**) and NREM (**B**) sleep.*

ious sleep-related medical disorders have been described and treatment methods have been proposed. The medical history and the patient's presentation and complaints remain the most important diagnostic clues. These complaints tend to fall into three broad categories: (1) difficulty falling asleep and/or staying asleep (insomnia), (2) excessive daytime sleepiness (EDS), and (3) abnormal behaviors associated with sleep (parasomnias). Once a significant sleep disorder is suspected, specialized diagnostic studies may be indicated for confirmation of the clinical diagnosis, quantification and assessment of the severity of the disorder, and initiation of the treatment plan. Such a study, called *polysomnography,* is conducted in a specially designed sleep laboratory.

Sleep apnea syndrome

Breathing abnormalities occurring during sleep fall into two broad categories, obstructive apnea and central apnea. Some patients have mixed apnea in which both patterns occur. The incidence of significant sleep apnea is unknown, but it may range from 1% to 15% of the population.

In *obstructive apnea,* the most common type of apnea in adults, respiratory efforts persist in the absence of air flow at the nose and mouth. The mechanism of obstruction seems to be related to a collapse of the structures of the upper airway while the individual is in a supine position, combined with the normal reduction of tone in the dilating muscles of the upper airway during sleep.

During obstructions, typically lasting from 10 to 60 seconds or more, arterial oxygen saturation can plummet to levels of less than half normal.

Apnea incidences exceeding 6 per hour of sleep are considered clinically significant. However, the level and duration of *oxygen desaturation* and the extent of *sleep fragmentation* are more important measures of potential clinical problems. Patients exhibiting severe obstructive episodes should always be referred for ear, nose, and throat (ENT) evaluation for possible surgical or mechanical intervention.

Central apnea, the less common form in adults, occurs when both air flow and respiratory efforts are absent as a result of defects in central (brain) respiratory control during sleep. Reflexive responses to airway irritation during sleep may also contribute. In normal healthy individuals, short central apneas may occur at sleep onset or in REM sleep without arousal, sleep state changes, or major oxygen desaturation. In more severe cases, a key symptom of central sleep apnea is insomnia with few or any complaints concerning the disordered breathing itself.

Narcolepsy

Narcolepsy is a genetically transmissible disease, characterized by excessive daytime sleepiness (EDS), which may be exacerbated by monotonous activity or reduced stimulation (e.g., reading or driving). It is considered to be an organic neurological disorder rather than a psychogenic one. However, emotional factors are still thought to be important, particularly in the precipitation of cataplectic episodes.

The majority of narcoleptics also suffer from one or more associated symptoms including cataplexy, hypnagogic hallucinations, and sleep paralysis. *Cataplexy* is the partial to complete loss of tone in the skeletal muscles, usually in association with a strong emotional stimulus such as laughter or anger. Normal consciousness is maintained, although the patient may experience difficulty breathing and speaking. Hypnagogic hallucinations are vivid dreamlike experiences that may be difficult to distinguish from reality. These usually occur at sleep onset or transition to waking and may be associated with sleep paralysis or a feeling of being unable to move. Hypnagogic hallucinations and sleep paralysis may also occur on occasion in the normal population. The narcoleptic patient commonly experiences the onset of symptoms in late puberty to the early twenties, and once present it is a lifelong illness.

The *multiple sleep latency test (MSLT)* helps to diagnose the narcoleptic, since abnormal manifestations of REM sleep account for much of the pathology of the disorder. The narcoleptic patient will typically exhibit REM sleep within a few minutes following sleep onset. In contrast, the normal patient will first exhibit REM sleep at approximately 90 minutes after sleep onset.

Insomnia

Insomnia is a transient or chronic sleep disorder characterized by the inability to fall asleep or the inability to maintain sleep. Insomnia is a symptom activated by a number of causes including psychiatric disturbances, the abuse of drugs or alcohol, sleep apnea, nocturnal myoclonus, restless legs, psychophysiological causes (such as an acute emotional arousal, chronic tension, or negative conditioning to sleep), various medical and environmental conditions, and biological rhythm disturbances. The incidence of insomnia in the general population ranges between 15% and 30%.

The differential diagnosis of insomnia can usually be made in the office by thoroughly evaluating the patient's sleep/wake history. If the patient or bed partner reports nocturnal choking, gagging, loud snoring, or apnea, *nocturnal polysomnography* is indicated to exclude sleep-related respiratory impairment. If the bed partner has noticed repetitive jerking motions of the limbs, the possibility of nocturnal myoclonus should be ruled out through polysomnography. The management of insomnia requires a complete understanding of the conditions causing it before an effective treatment plan can be initiated.

Parasomnias

Parasomnias are dysfunctions associated with sleep or made worse by sleep, not disorders of the process of sleep itself. Disorders such as sleepwalking, sleep terrors, bed-wetting, and bruxism always occur in NREM sleep. Dream anxiety attacks (nightmares) and sleep paralysis are associated with REM sleep.

The differential diagnosis of parasomnias can sometimes be made through evaluation of the sleep/wake history but can require *polysomnography* to differentiate sleep apnea, sleep-related epileptic seizures, and sleep terrors.

THE SLEEP LABORATORY

Sleep disorder centers are primarily diagnostic units where patients are seen on a consultation basis. Here a specialized investigation of a suspected sleep disorder is undertaken. Sleep studies are performed in a specially designed laboratory, which provides an optimal environment for sleep. These laboratories are equipped with television cameras and microphones to observe patient movements and noises while sleeping. Cables lead from the patient's bed to a recording laboratory to permit continuous recording of various data on a polygraph with minimal interference with the patient's sleep.

Standard sleep laboratory equipment also includes ear oximeters to measure oxygen saturation, thermistors to monitor air flow, and strain gauges that sense respiratory effort. Some laboratories may also use equipment to monitor nocturnal penile tumescence.

LABORATORY TESTS FOR SLEEP DISORDERS

THE STANDARD POLYSOMNOGRAM

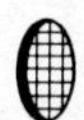

EXPLANATION OF THE TEST

The polysomnograph (Fig. 14-3) is the basic diagnostic tool in the sleep laboratory. It consists of a multichannel (8, 12, or 16) recording that continuously monitors sleep state (electroencephalo-

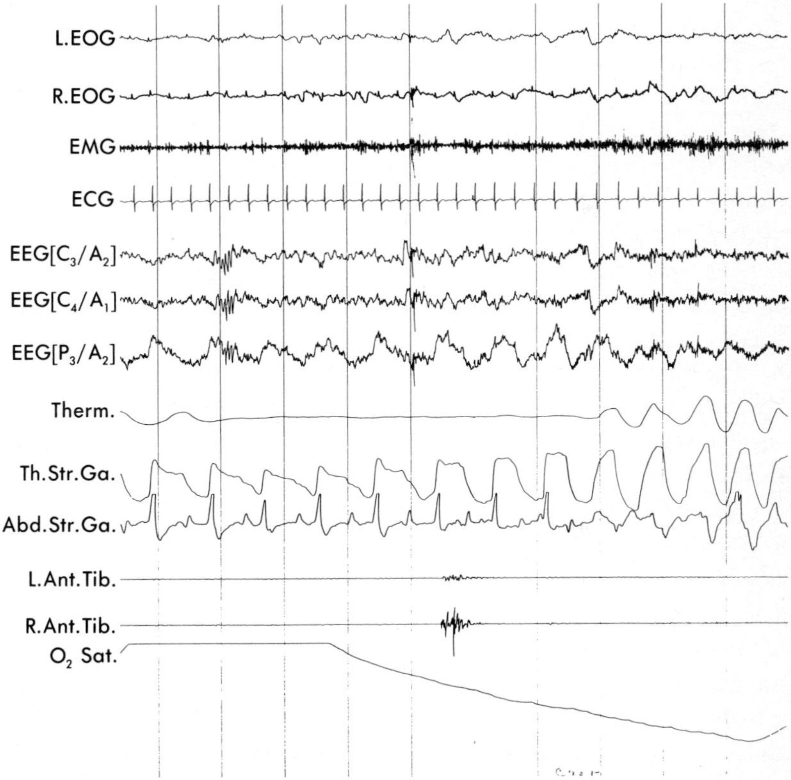

Fig. 14-3. *Polygraphic recording during sleep in a patient with obstructive sleep apnea. The patient's airway occludes at sleep onset and remains obstructed for 19 seconds. The event is terminated following arousal. (EOG, electrooculogram; EMG, electromyogram; ECG, electrocardiogram; EEG, electroencephalogram; Therm, thermister; Th. Str. Ga., thoracic strain gauge; Abd. Str. Ga., abdominal strain gauge; L. Ant. Tib., left anterior tibialis; R. Ant. Tib., right anterior tibialis;* O_2 *Sat., oxygen saturation)*

gram, electrooculogram, electromyogram), heart (electrocardiogram), and respiratory functions. These recordings indicate the presence or absence of sleep, the type of sleep, and cardiac and respiratory problems.

The *electroencephalogram (EEG)* records a portion of the brain's electrical activity. Sleep state scoring relies exclusively on electrode placements in the central region of the scalp (C_3 and C_4), with occipital (O_1 or O_2) or parietal (P_3 or P_4) leads used as an aid in determining sleep onset. Electrode placements on the scalp are referred to A_1 or A_2, which are located on the mastoid bone behind each ear.

The *electrooculogram (EOG)* is a recording of eye movement essential in determining the onset of sleep and in scoring REM sleep. Standard EOG placements are the left outer corner of the left eye and right outer corner of the right eye. By offsetting one electrode above and the other slightly below horizontal, both horizontal and vertical eye movements can be detected.

The *chin electromyogram (EMG)* aids in the scoring of REM sleep. During REM sleep, a profound reduction in muscle tone occurs.

The *electrocardiogram (ECG)* monitors heart rate variations and rhythm changes. Increased cardiac arrhythmias and periods of bradycardia and tachycardia may occur because of breathing difficulties during sleep.

Respirations are measured by evaluating the air flow at the nose and mouth and the respiratory effort at the abdomen and chest. Air flow is monitored by measuring changes in temperature of inspired versus expired air by placing a thermistor at the nose and mouth. The respiratory effort at the abdomen and chest is measured by encircling the rib cage and abdominal cavity with mercury strain gauges or coils of wire. The expansion and contraction of these coils during breathing are monitored by an electronic system producing signals that may be recorded.

Oxygen saturation is measured with an ear oximeter that computes oxygen saturation by analyzing the absorption of certain wavelengths of light passing through the pinna of the ear. This method is reliable at oxygen saturations greater than 50%; however, anemia or darkly pigmented skin may give spurious readings.

A *peripheral electromyogram (EMG)* from the anterior tibialis muscle is important in evaluating patients who have stereotyped, repetitive movements of the lower extremities during sleep called nocturnal myoclonus.

CLINICAL IMPLICATIONS

Aids in the diagnosis of sleep apnea, nocturnal myoclonus, some forms of insomnia, and abnormal behavior associated with sleep. Fig. 14-3 is a polygraphic recording during sleep in a patient with obstructive sleep apnea.

NURSING ACTION

1. Instruct the patient that medications which may interfere with sleep (stimulants or sedatives) should not be taken for at least 1 week before the test. This does not include medications for chronic medical conditions.
2. The patient should be instructed in every aspect of the test.
3. Carefully secure the electrodes, using electrode paste and surgical tape. Collodion-soaked gauze patches are used to maintain EEG electrodes for up to 24 hours if needed.

SPECIAL STUDIES

In addition to the standard nocturnal polysomnogram, the following tests can also be performed.

NOCTURNAL PENILE TUMESCENCE

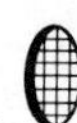

EXPLANATION OF THE TEST

Erection of the penis normally occurs during REM sleep. Penile-circumference changes are monitored by a mercury-filled strain gauge placed on the base as far down the penile shaft as possible and near the tip of the penis, just behind the corona in circumcized men. Evaluation of penile rigidity requires a device to measure the force that causes the penis to buckle. Photographs of erection episodes may provide important diagnostic clues. Obtaining both the patient's and technician's subjective evaluation of the degree and adequacy of the patient's erection on awakening is also useful.

The standard evaluation protocol usually includes 2 to 3 nights of polygraphic and penile-circumference monitoring.

CLINICAL IMPLICATIONS

Determines whether the patient's impotence is primarily organic (vascular or neural) as evidenced by the absence of any adequate penile changes, or whether the condition is psychogenic, in which case normal tumescence of the penis occurs during sleep

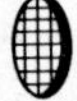

MULTIPLE SLEEP LATENCY TEST (MSLT)

EXPLANATION OF THE TEST

The technique of polygraphically monitoring sleep at various times during the normal waking period through multiple naps, is used to measure excessive daytime sleepiness (EDS). This technique can precisely detect the onset of sleep and evaluate sleep architecture to diagnose such abnormalities as sleep-onset REM periods often present in narcolepsy. Normally, 4 to 6 20-minute nap periods are used separated by 2-hour intervals.

CLINICAL IMPLICATIONS

Highly effective in identifying those patients with pathological sleepiness

Differentiates narcoleptics from other patients who manifest EDS

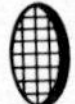

INTRAESOPHAGEAL pH MONITORING

EXPLANATION OF THE TEST

Gastroesophageal reflux and resultant esophagitis are often associated with recumbent reflux occurring during sleep. This may result from an increased number of reflux episodes, as well as from delayed esophageal acid clearing.

Esophageal pH is monitored with standard stomach pH probes. Techniques to measure the phenomenon of acid clearing may also be used.

CLINICAL IMPLICATIONS

Determines the frequency and duration of gastroesophageal reflux

CONTINUOUS POSITIVE AIRWAY PRESSURE (CPAP)

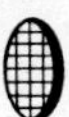

EXPLANATION OF THE TEST

Obstructive apnea can be prevented in many patients by applying a low level (2.5 to 15 cm H_2O) of positive air pressure continuously through the nose. Patients who have already been diagnosed as having obstructive apnea are adapted to wearing a snug surgical mask applying 2.5 to 5 cm H_2O pressure while awake. During sleep, pressures are increased until a patent airway is consistently maintained during REM sleep. Most patients require pressures between 5 to 10 cm H_2O to eliminate airway occlusion.

CLINICAL IMPLICATIONS

Determination of the pressures required for a patent airway so that patients may be given a prescription for a CPAP home unit using a pressure suited to their condition

15

Diagnostic tests in nutritional disorders

An adequate nutritional state is important to protein synthesis, resistance to infection, and wound healing. Protein and calorie requirements are increased by surgery, stress, sepsis, trauma, or hypermetabolic disease processes, and dramatically increased by burns. Thus, attendance to the caloric needs of a patient is often a critical factor in the prognosis.

Tests for nutritional assessment are employed for the following purposes:

1. Pretreatment evaluation of a nutritionally deficient patient
2. Evaluation of the progress of a patient while he or she is being treated

3. Differentiation between nutritional deficiencies—for example, kwashiorkor (protein-calorie malnourishment) versus marasmus (generalized malnourishment)
4. Diagnosis of individual nutritional deficiencies, such as iron deficiency or folic acid deficiency
5. Evaluation of subclinical nutritional deficiency, as yet an ill-defined area in clinical medicine

The quickest and easiest way to determine the presence or absence of malnutrition is to evaluate the body height/weight index and the anthropometric measurements (body measurements). The anthropometric measurements include the *triceps skinfold* and the *arm muscle circumference*, which is calculated from the *mid—upper arm circumference* and the triceps skinfold. Visceral protein status is determined from the serum albumin and/or transferrin levels; it is a guide to the level of immune competence. The status of metabolically active tissue is evaluated by creatinine height index analysis.

THE ANTHROPOMETRIC MEASUREMENTS

Anthropometric measurements are converted to percentages of standard. Anything less than 60% is classified as severe malnutrition. Moderate malnutrition is indicated when a measurement falls in the 60% to 80% range.

TRICEPS SKINFOLD

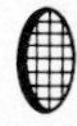

Measurement of the triceps skinfold provides an indication of available fat stores, which are a reflection of the body's caloric reserve. Fat stores are significantly diminished in marasmus (Table 15-1).

The midpoint of the upper portion of the patient's nondominant arm is identified. The skinfold at this point is measured over the

Table 15-1 Triceps skinfold measurements (mm), adults

		Percent of standard			
	Standard	**90**	**80**	**70**	**60**
Male	12.5	11.3	10.0	8.8	7.5
Female	16.5	11.9	13.2	11.6	9.9

triceps muscle with a skinfold caliper. Three separate measurements are made, and the two closest results are averaged.

It should be remembered that body fat stores may remain normal, or may even be excessive, in the face of moderate to severe malnutrition. Therefore, the triceps skinfold measurement lacks sensitivity in the detection of malnutrition.

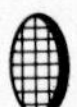

MID–UPPER ARM CIRCUMFERENCE (MUAC)

The mid–upper arm circumference provides an indication of the available fat and protein stores and facilitates an assessment of current nutritional status in either kwashiorkor, a syndrome produced by severe protein deficiency, or marasmus, a condition characterized by generalized wasting and emaciation (Table 15-2).

The circumference at the midpoint of the upper portion of the nondominant arm is measured with the arm hanging freely.

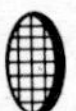

ARM MUSCLE CIRCUMFERENCE (AMC)

The arm muscle circumference provides an indication of the amount of muscle protein, which is usually diminished in kwashiorkor as opposed to pure marasmus (Table 15-3). The measurement is

Table 15-2 Mid–upper arm circumferences (mm), adults

		Percent of standard			
	Standard	**90**	**80**	**70**	**60**
Male	29.3	26.3	23.4	20.5	17.6
Female	28.5	25.7	22.8	20.0	17.1

Table 15-3 Arm muscle circumferences (mm), adults

		Percent of standard			
	Standard	**90**	**80**	**70**	**60**
Male	25.3	22.8	20.2	17.7	15.2
Female	23.2	20.9	18.6	16.2	13.9

obtained by using the following formula:

Arm muscle circumference =
arm circumference (cm) − (0.314 × triceps skinfold [mm])

A significant decrease in this measurement reflects a decrease in total muscle protein, and usually indicates kwashiorkor. If both total body fat and muscle protein are diminished, both kwashiorkor and marasmus should be suspected.

BIOCHEMICAL MEASUREMENTS

SERUM ALBUMIN LEVEL

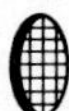

Reference range

Mild decrease: 3.0-3.5 g/dl
Moderate decrease: 2.1-3.0 g/dl
Severe decrease: <2.1 g/dl

The serum albumin level provides an indication of visceral protein reserve; the albumin level is usually reduced when protein stores are lost. A serum albumin concentration of less than 3.4 g/dl, in the absence of liver disease, indicates protein malnutrition.

VALUE AND LIMITATIONS OF THE TEST

The serum albumin level correlates with changes in arm muscle circumference, and it is a reliable indicator of visceral protein activity.

Because the half-life of albumin synthesis is long (16 to 18 days), serious protein and calorie depletion is already present by the time it is reflected in the serum albumin level, and early response to treatment is somewhat unpredictable. The half-life for albumin may be decreased in patients with infection, burns, severe injuries, and protein-losing enteropathies.

SERUM TRANSFERRIN LEVEL

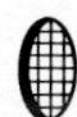

Reference range

Mild decrease: 150-175 mg/dl
Moderate decrease: 100-150 mg/dl
Severe decrease: <100 mg/dl

Transferrin is a serum β-globulin that binds and transports iron. Therefore the transferrin level can be measured directly, or it can be estimated by multiplying the total iron-binding capacity by 0.8 and subtracting 43.

VALUE AND LIMITATIONS OF THE TEST

Since transferrin has a shorter half-life than albumin, its level is reduced earlier, making it a more sensitive indicator of visceral secretory protein status.

The transferrin level and the iron-binding capacity may be influenced by iron metabolism and low iron stores. Thus iron deficiency anemia can produce falsely elevated transferrin levels.

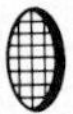

THYROXINE-BINDING PREALBUMIN AND RETINOL-BINDING PROTEIN

These levels are probably better indicators of subclinical nutritional deficiency than of a substantial deficiency. Thyroxine-binding prealbumin has a half-life of only 2 days, and that of retinol-binding protein is only 12 hours. Both substances are sensitive to changes in protein and calories and respond rapidly to refeeding.

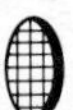

CREATININE HEIGHT INDEX

Creatinine is a product of muscle metabolism; the 24-hour urinary excretion of creatinine is roughly proportional to the lean body mass or metabolically active tissue. A decrease in the 24-hour urinary output of creatinine reflects muscle protein depletion and a decrease in muscle mass.

The creatinine height index is obtained by multiplying the actual 24-hour urinary creatinine output by 100 and dividing by the ideal urinary creatinine output of a normal male or female of the same height as the person being tested. Table 15-4 lists the ideal 24-hour urinary creatinine outputs according to sex and height. To convert height in inches to height in centimeters, multiply the height in inches by 2.54. This index is a fairly accurate indicator of muscle protein depletion and decreases in muscle mass.

Table 15-4 Ideal urinary creatinine values

Male		Female	
Height (cm)	**Value (mg/24 hr)**	**Height (cm)**	**Value (mg/24 hr)**
157.5	1288	147.3	830
160.0	1325	149.9	851
162.6	1359	152.4	875
165.1	1386	154.9	900
167.6	1426	157.5	925
170.2	1467	160.0	949
172.7	1513	162.6	977
175.3	1555	165.1	1006
177.8	1596	167.6	1044
180.3	1642	170.2	1076
182.9	1691	172.7	1109
185.4	1739	175.3	1141
188.0	1785	177.8	1174
190.5	1831	180.3	1206
193.0	1891	182.9	1240

IMMUNOLOGIC TESTS

In malnutrition (both marasmus and kwashiorkor) there are apparently immunologic deficiencies, which disappear after malnutrition has been corrected. The following tests are usually performed.

TOTAL LYMPHOCYTE COUNT

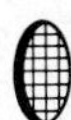

Reference range

Moderate decrease: 800-1200/mm^3

Severe decrease: <800/mm^3

Lymphocytes are sensitive to deficiencies in calories and precursor amino acids. Thus when protein malnutrition exists, the synthesis of lymphocytes is depressed, which in turn contributes to the impaired ability of the white cells to fight infection.

The total lymphocyte count is equal to the percentage of lymphocytes multiplied by the white blood cell (WBC) count. This figure is then converted to a percentage of the standard, which is considered to be 1500/mm^3.

$$\text{Percentage of standard} = \frac{\text{total lymphocyte count} \times 100}{1500/\text{mm}^3}$$

SKIN TESTING

An impaired ability of the white cells to fight infection, a situation that is linked to a decreased total lymphocyte count, can be recognized by means of skin testing. The usual antigens for skin testing are used, including streptokinase-streptodornase (SK-SD), mumps virus, *Candida* organisms, and purified protein derivative of tuberculin (PPD). The results are read in 24 to 48 hours. A normal response is positive, indicated by the appearance of a wheal 5 mm or more in diameter within 24 to 48 hours. An abnormal response is negative (anergy). Some clinicians try to quantitate the response, arguing that a wheal between 10 and 15 mm indicates mild deficiency, a wheal between 5 and 10 mm indicates moderate deficiency, and a wheal of less than 5 mm indicates severe immune deficiency and anergy. However, such a classification is not very accurate, and it is probably better simply to characterize the reaction as positive (indicating cellular immunity) or negative (indicating depressed cellular immunity).

LIMITATIONS OF THE TEST

Anergy also occurs as a result of acute fevers, sepsis, steroid treatment, certain tumors, shock, and circulating inhibitors of lymphocyte function, making the results of skin testing less than completely reliable.

TESTS FOR DEFICIENCIES OF VITAMINS OR NUTRIENTS

Deficiencies of specific vitamins or nutrients can be identified by means of laboratory tests, as follows:

Vitamin A: Deficiency evaluated by serum assay. A low serum vitamin A level plus a low serum carotene level strongly suggests a vitamin A deficiency, although serum carotene levels themselves reflect only the recent dietary intake.

Vitamin B_1 (thiamine): Deficiency best identified by recognition of diminished erythrocyte transketolase activity, the test for which is not readily available

Vitamin B_2 (riboflavin): Deficiency best assessed through the use of the glutathione reductase assay, not readily available

Vitamin B_6: Deficiency detected by an enzymatic assay, not readily available

Vitamin B_{12}: Assays readily available clinically

Vitamin D: Serum 25-OH-D_3 assay, not routinely employed; serum alkaline phosphatase level, easily determinable but indirect measure; serum calcium and phosphorous levels, also easily available but indirect measures

Vitamin E: Serum tocopherol measurement, not readily available. (Tocopherols are substances possessing vitamin E activity.)

Vitamin K: Level indirectly measured by prothrombin time

Folic acid: Serum levels readily available. The red cell folate level is more accurate in the diagnosis of chronic deficiency and depletion of tissue stores, and correlates well with the clinical syndromes associated with folic acid deficiency.

Iron and iron-binding capacity: Serum assay readily available. However, the results can be variable, inaccurate, and sometimes misleading.

Ferritin: Determination of serum ferritin level. Such a determination is fairly accurate, and the ferritin level is a good index of iron stores, correlating very well with a bone marrow iron stain level for the diagnosis of iron deficiency. One pitfall is that the ferritin level is elevated in acute inflammatory diseases, infections, and lymphomas; such an elevation thus does not reflect iron stores.

DIAGNOSIS OF SUBCLINICAL NUTRITIONAL DEFICIENCIES

Subclinical nutritional deficiency is not an established clinical entity. In the future it may or may not be considered clinically significant. However, we would like to alert you to the possibility that it may. For example, although clinical beriberi is very rare in the United States, the majority of alcoholics have red cell transketolase levels that are significantly diminished, indicating subclinical deficiencies of vitamin B_1, which respond to the administration of thiamine. It is difficult to establish the significance of such a decreased transketolase level in the clinical setting. However, one can say that in alcoholics, in view of the decreased transketolase level, there is subclinical B_1 deficiency.

The serum ferritin level is another example. A ferritin level of 10 mg/dl or less with microcytic anemia is diagnostic of iron deficiency anemia. However, in the absence of anemia and in the presence of apparent microcytosis, a ferritin level of 10 to 40 mg/dl is definitely associated with decreased bone marrow iron levels, as shown by bone marrow stains, and with decreased bone marrow stores. Before iron deficiency anemia sets in or before there is a decrease in hemoglobin level, or hematocrit, the levels of certain iron-dependent enzymes decrease. There is strong clinical evidence that these decreases contribute significantly to the symptoms of iron deficiency anemia, suggesting that a ferritin level between 10 and 40 mg/dl indicates a subclinical deficiency of iron. For example, in a patient who is complaining of fatigue and who has a ferritin level of 20 mg/dl without anemia, there is evidence to suggest that before frank anemia develops there is a definite decrease in the iron-dependent enzyme levels, and that this decrease is the cause of the symptoms.

These are just two examples to alert you to future developments in the area of subclinical nutritional deficiency.

16

Prenatal diagnostic tests

CLINICAL APPLICATION OF LABORATORY TESTS

Prenatology is a relatively new and rapidly advancing field. First trimester diagnosis has been made possible because of advances in *ultrasonographic technique* for diagnosis and guidance of needles and aspiration catheters; advances in *tissue culture,* which makes it feasible to grow chorionic tissue or amniocytes; and because of *recombinant DNA* technology.

First trimester

This technology in the first trimester involves *sampling of chorionic villi* for culture and cytogenetic studies. With the added help of recombinant DNA technology, this information may be attainable within 4 to 5 hours of sample acquisition.

Second and third trimesters

In the second and third trimesters, *amniocentesis* and *ultrasonography* are the diagnostic tests used. However, there is a 2- to 3-week delay for tissue culture and chromosome studies.

Diabetic mothers

In the monitoring of high-risk pregnancy in diabetic mothers the level of *unconjugated estriol* is measured. For the more specific detection of fetal distress syndrome in diabetes, the *lecithin/sphingomyelin (L/S) ratio* is measured. In addition, the simultaneous determination of *phosphatidylglycerol* (PG) is measured.

Maternal hypertension

In high-risk pregnancy when the mother has hypertension, the serum level of *human placental lactogen (HPL)* is measured.

Chromosome abnormalities

Normally there are 46 chromosomes in the human cells—44 somatic chromosomes and 2 sex chromosomes. The somatic chromosomes are numbered and the sex chromosomes are designated either X (female) or Y (male). A normal female is designated 46XX (44 normal somatic chromosomes and 2 female sex chromosomes); a normal male is designated 46XY (44 somatic chromosomes, 1 male sex chromosome, and 1 female sex chromosome).

The three categories of chromosome abnormalities are the trisomies (an additional chromosome), the deletion syndromes (too few chromosomes), and sex chromosome abnormalities. It is possible to make the definitive diagnosis by *chromosome analysis* of amniotic fluid in the second trimester.

Trisomy 21 (Down's syndrome) causes mental retardation, musculoskeletal malformation, and cardiac anomalies.

Trisomy D_1 is rarer than Down's syndrome and involves additional chromosomes in positions 13 through 15. When the additional chromosomes are in the 16 to 18 group (E group), the disorder is designated trisomy E. The definitive diagnosis is made by cytological chromosomal analysis (karyotyping) of smears of either buccal mucosa or amniotic fluid.

Polysomy X (super female) syndrome is relatively rare and is usually characterized by mental retardation and ovarian dysfunction.

The diagnosis is made by chromosomal analysis, in which 1 or more extra X chromosomes are found (e.g., 47XXX, 48XXXX, 49XXXXX). As the number of extra chromosomes increases, so does the severity of the clinical picture.

XYY (super male) syndrome is a relatively common abnormality of males, with an estimated frequency of 1 in 1000 male births. This abnormality has been associated with mental illness and criminal tendencies. Affected persons are often male pseudohermaphrodites with female phenotypes, individuals with intersexual genitalia (true hermaphrodites), or tall males with normal genitalia and behavioral abnormalities. Infertility is not associated with this syndrome and offspring have been normal. Laboratory diagnosis is made by chromosome analysis, which shows an additional Y chromosome (47XYY).

The deletion syndromes cause mental retardation, congenital cardiac abnormalities, and musculoskeletal and genitourinary tract abnormalities and are designated 4 P/P syndrome (deletion of the short arm of chromosome 4), cri du chat syndrome (deletion of chromosome 5), 13Q syndrome (deletion of the long arm of chromosome 13), and 18Q syndrome (deletion of the long arm of chromosome 18).

Turner's syndrome affects females and is usually characterized by primary amenorrhea, sexual infantilism, short stature, absence or agenesis of ovaries, musculoskeletal and cardiac abnormalities, and mental deficiency. In the classic form the second X chromosome is absent, resulting in the syndrome being designated 45XO.

Klinefelter's syndrome (XXY syndrome) affects only males and is characterized by testicular hypoplasia, underdevelopment of secondary sex characteristics, gynecomastia, azoospermia, and a high incidence of mental retardation. The pubic hair may have the distribution characteristic of females.

PRENATAL DIAGNOSTIC LABORATORY TESTS

AMNIOCENTESIS

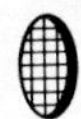

EXPLANATION OF THE TEST

Amniocentesis is the transabdominal needle aspiration of amniotic fluid for laboratory analysis of color, bilirubin, meconium, creatinine, L/S ratio, phosphatidylglycerol, glucose, α-fetoprotein, bacteria, chromosome analysis, and acetycholinesterase.

Value of the test in the second trimester

Helpful in the detection of neural tube defects
Diagnostic of chromosome abnormalities

Value of the test in the third trimester

Aids in the diagnosis of respiratory distress syndrome
Aids in the management of isoimmunization and hemolytic disease
Monitors high-risk pregnancies, including hypertension and diabetes

NURSING ACTION

1. Inform the patient that there are no dietary restrictions before this test.
2. Explain the procedure to the patient and inform her that the test evaluates fetal health and maturity. Explain that some fetal abnormalities are undetected by this test.
3. Obtain informed consent.
4. Ask the patient to void just before the procedure.
5. Provide an amber or foil-covered collection tube. Exposure to light may cause abnormally low bilirubin levels.
6. Provide a glass syringe for aspiration; a plastic disposable syringe can be toxic to amniotic fluid cells.
7. Following the procedure, monitor fetal heart rate and maternal vital signs at least twice in the first half-hour.
8. Position the patient on her left side to avoid uterine pressure on the vena cava.
9. Instruct the patient to call her physician immediately if she notices vaginal bleeding or secretions or has abdominal pain, chills, or fever. She should also be aware of fetal hyperactivity or lethargy and notify her physician in these events.

INTERFERING FACTORS

Maternal blood in the amniotic fluid may lower creatinine levels, and blood or meconium affect the L/S ratio.

Improper collection of specimen (i.e., use of plastic syringes and failure to use amber or foil-covered collection tube) can affect test results.

The α-fetoprotein test is invalidated if there is fetal blood in the specimen, and levels are increased as a result of infectious mononucleosis, cirrhosis, hepatic cancer, teratoma, endodermal sinus tumor, gastric carcinoma, pancreatic carcinoma, and subacute hereditary tyrosinemia.

CLINICAL IMPLICATIONS OF SECOND TRIMESTER AMNIOCENTESIS

α-Fetoprotein. High amniotic fluid levels indicate neural tube defects. Elevated levels may also occur in multiple pregnancy, omphalocele, congenital nephrosis, esophageal or duodenal atresia, cystic fibrosis, exomphalos, Turner's syndrome, fetal bladder neck obstruction with hydronephrosis, and impending fetal death.

Acetylcholinesterase (AChE). Levels increase with neural tube defects, exomphalos (hernia of the abdominal viscera into the umbilical cord), and other serious malformations.

Chromosome analysis. Karyotyping of amniotic fluid is done to observe for too many or too few chromosomes, and for abnormalities in the sex chromosomes.

L/S ratio. The lecithin/sphingomyelin measurement evaluates fetal pulmonary maturity. An L/S ratio greater than 2 confirms fetal pulmonary maturity; an L/S ratio less than 2 suggests a risk of respiratory distress, especially in a diabetic pregnancy.

CLINICAL IMPLICATIONS OF THIRD TRIMESTER AMNIOCENTESIS

Surfactant is decreased in respiratory distress syndrome.

Bilirubin (tested at the twenty-sixth week) in large amounts may indicate hemolytic disease of the newborn.

Phosphatidylglycerol levels appear with pulmonary maturity.

Phosphatidylinositol levels decrease with pulmonary maturity.

PELVIC ULTRASONOGRAPHY

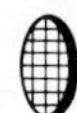

EXPLANATION OF THE TEST

High frequency sound waves are reflected to a transducer, which converts them into electrical energy and forms images on an oscilloscope; selected views are photographed for a permanent record. With the combination of ultrasonography and amniotic fluid analysis of α-fetoprotein and acetylcholinesterase, a fairly precise diagnosis of fetal abnormalities can be made.

VALUE OF THE TEST

Evaluates symptoms that suggest pelvic disease
Determines fetal growth and multiple pregnancy
Evaluates fetal viability, position, and length of gestation
Confirms fetal abnormalities. Among the fetal abnormalities that can be detected are hydrocephalus, microcephaly, renal abnormalities, obstructive lesions of the genitourinary tract, and urinary tract masses.
Guides the amniocentesis needle

NURSING ACTION

1. Inform patient that there are no dietary restrictions before test.
2. Explain the procedure to the patient and tell her that it is entirely painless and completely safe.
3. Explain that the procedure requires a full bladder as a landmark to define pelvic organs, so that she should drink and not void before the procedure.
4. A water enema may be necessary to produce a better outline of the large intestine.
5. Explain to the patient that her pelvic area will be coated with water-soluble jelly to increase sound wave conduction.

INTERFERING FACTORS

The image may be impossible to interpret if the patient is obese, the bladder is empty, or the fetal head is positioned deep in the pelvis.

SERUM UNCONJUGATED ESTRIOL (E_3)

EXPLANATION OF THE TEST

This is a hormone assay that estimates whether placental function is normal and predicts impending fetal death. Estriol is produced by the placenta and is unconjugated when it reaches the maternal blood and has a half-life of about 20 minutes. It is conjugated in the maternal liver and excreted in the urine. Estriol levels in the serum slowly increase from the ninth week of gestation until the last trimester, when they increase more dramatically.

VALUE OF THE TEST

Evaluates placental function and fetal well-being

CLINICAL IMPLICATIONS

Failure of the estriol level to increase steadily or an abrupt decrease of 40% from the previous mean level of the same patient indicates fetal distress or placental malfunction. It is recommended that the assay then be done twice a week during the first 32 to 34 weeks and daily after that. For a more specific detection of fetal distress syndrome in diabetic mothers the L/S ratio and the level of phosphatidylglycerol in the amniotic fluid are measured. An L/S ratio of less than 2:1 is very likely an indicator of fetal distress, especially in diabetic pregnancy.

SERUM HUMAN PLACENTAL LACTOGEN (HPL)

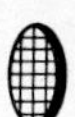

Reference ranges

Weeks of gestation	*Reference range*
5-27	<4.6 μg/ml
28-31	2.4-6.1μg/ml
32-35	3.7-7.7 μg/ml
36-term	5.0-8.6 μg/ml

EXPLANATION OF THE TEST

Human placental lactogen (HPL) is a polypeptide hormone secreted by placental syncytial trophoblasts. During pregnancy, in combination with prolactin, HPL prepares the breasts for lactation. It also has a role in maternal metabolism, fetal nutrition, and protein synthesis.

Plasma levels of HPL are measured by radioimmunoassay and are roughly proportional to placental mass. For example, the levels are higher in multiple pregnancy. Levels rise during the first and second trimesters and reach a plateau during the last 2 to 3 months of pregnancy.

VALUE OF THE TEST

Monitors the hypertensive patient
Assesses placental function

Aids in the diagnosis of hydatidiform mole and choriocarcinoma (although human chorionic gonadotropin levels are more diagnostic)
Aids in the diagnosis and monitors the treatment of nontrophoblastic tumors that secrete HPL ectopically

NURSING ACTION

1. Inform the patient that there are no dietary restrictions before this test.
2. Explain the purpose of the test to the patient and tell her that a blood sample is required.
3. Withdraw venous blood in a 7-ml red-top tube. Handle the sample gently to prevent hemolysis and transport it to the laboratory immediately.

CLINICAL IMPLICATIONS

Hypertension. In high-risk pregnancies when the mother has hypertension, the reduction of HPL in the serum is related to the severity and duration of the hypertension.

Neoplasm is suggested when the levels of HPL decrease in the second trimester along with increased HCG.

17

Miscellaneous diseases and laboratory tests

ALLERGY

Allergy in the true sense of the word means an adverse reaction to an antigen-antibody interaction, or, in some cases, an abnormal effect induced by an antigen in certain primed cells called T-lymphocytes. However, in general use the term has taken on a wider meaning. For example, patients with histories of rashes caused by ampicillin or sulfa drugs are told that they are "allergic" to those substances and never take them again. Such rashes, however, do not truly represent allergic reactions, because they have no immunologic basis. These rashes appear idiosyncratic in origin and absolutely unrelated to any antigen-antibody interaction. Several studies have shown that if a patient is rechallenged with a drug to which he or she is "allergic," there is no "allergy."

Allergic reactions may be divided into four types, only the first of which is discussed here:

1. Processes caused by interactions of antigens with IgE antibodies
2. Reactions resulting from antibodies that are directed toward membranes, as in an autoimmune hemolytic anemia
3. Pathologic damage caused by deposition of immune complexes, as in serum sickness
4. Adverse reactions resulting from cellular immunity, as in graft rejection

A type I (immediate hypersensitivity) allergic reaction occurs as follows: Immunoglobulin E, or IgE, is a circulating and tissue-fixed antibody that is present in extremely small amounts (10 to 200 ng/ml) in normal, nonatopic people but in excessive amounts in atopic individuals. This circulating antibody attaches itself to IgE receptors that are located mainly on circulating basophils and tissue-fixed mast cells. When all of the receptors on a cell are saturated with IgE, the cell becomes surrounded by molecules of excess IgE, all of which are extending their arms into the spaces between cells. When an antigen comes along, such as a drug, pollen, or grain, it can latch on to the free-floating arms of IgE, which is now attached to the cell. If two different IgE molecules are thereby brought together, a reaction in the cell is triggered through an extremely complex set of biochemical and biophysical interactions to ultimately allow calcium to enter the cell, which in turn triggers the release of endogenous substances. All of these substances, when released, can lead to an extremely noxious reaction that is manifested as allergic rhinitis (hay fever), allergic asthma, hives (urticaria), angioedema, or even frank anaphylaxis.

PORPHYRIAS

Porphyrias are hereditary metabolic disorders of heme synthesis, the biochemical hallmark of which is overproduction of porphyrins and their precursors. Similar biochemical abnormalities are found in lead poisoning (both acute and chronic), which is a differential diagnosis. Several syndromes of porphyria have been described, two of which are mentioned here.

Erythropoietic porphyria is mainly characterized by skin lesions, photosensitivity, burning, and pruritus. Laboratory diagnosis is made on the basis of elevated uroporphyrin and coproporphyrin levels in the urine and in the red blood cells. In erythropoietic protoporphyria the erythrocyte protoporphyrin level is elevated.

Hepatic porphyria is characterized by acute intermittent abdominal pain and by neurologic abnormalities, neuropathies, and psychiatric disturbances. Laboratory diagnosis is made during an acute attack, on the basis of elevated urine levels of porphobilinogen (PBG) and δ-aminolevulinic acid (ALA). The RBC porphyrin level is normal.

Lead poisoning is also characterized by elevated urine levels of ALA and coproporphyrins and by high RBC levels of protoporphyrins. The elevated serum lead level, however, is diagnostic.

VAGINAL DISCHARGE

The usual cause of vaginal discharge is infection with *Candida* organisms, *Trichomonas vaginalis,* or *Hemophilus vaginalis*.

For candidiasis, a wet potassium hydroxide smear is the method of laboratory diagnosis. One can see the spores and filaments characteristic of this fungal infection.

For a *Trichomonas vaginalis* infection, a wet saline smear is the mode of diagnosis. The active motile organism is seen in most cases, and one seldom has to grow a culture.

Hemophilus vaginalis is the cause of nonspecific vaginitis; the presence of this organism is usually suspected because of the character of the discharge and the odor. After ruling out a *Trichomonas* infection and candidiasis, a clinician should use a wet saline smear to test for a *Hemophilus vaginalis* infection. The appearance of the epithelial granular-looking cells called Clue cells suggests this diagnosis. The diagnosis can be confirmed by culturing the organism.

AMYLOIDOSIS

Amyloidosis is a disorder of protein metabolism in which fibrillar protein is deposited in the extracellular spaces. Clinically this manifests as hepatomegaly, congestive heart failure, neuropathies, and malabsorption syndrome. The diagnosis is made by *rectal mucosal biopsy* with staining for amyloid with Congo red.

WILSON'S DISEASE (HEPATOLENTICULAR DEGENERATION)

Wilson's disease is an inherited abnormality in the hepatic excretion of copper; the disorder results in toxic levels of copper accumulating in various organs. Clinically, the disorder may manifest as a neurologic disease (athetoid chorea) and liver cirrhosis. Pathologically, there is abnormal deposition of copper in the brain, kidneys, cornea, and liver.

The diagnosis is suspected when the serum level of *ceruloplasmin* (a copper protein) is low, the *urinary excretion of copper* is greater than 150 μg/day, and *biopsies* of the kidney and the liver show increased deposition of copper.

Reference ranges

Serum ceruloplasmin: 27-37 mg/dl (SI units: 1.8-2.5 μmol/L)
Serum copper (total): 100-106 mEq/L (SI units: 16-31 μmol/L)
Urine copper: 0-100 μg/24 hr (SI units: 0–1.6 μmol/24 hr)
Liver copper: 10-35 μg/g dry weight

IRON STORAGE DISEASE (HEMOCHROMATOSIS)

Iron storage disease is characterized by increased deposition of iron in the liver, heart, and pancreas. Clinically the disorder presents as diabetes, liver cirrhosis, congestive heart failure, and arrhythmias. The diagnosis is made because the *serum iron* level is elevated (usually greater than 200 μg/dl) and the serum *iron-binding capacity* is nearly at its maximum. The serum ferritin level is also elevated. The final diagnosis is made by liver and bone marrow *biopsies*, which show abnormal deposition of iron.

Reference ranges

Serum iron: 50-150 μg/dl (higher in males) (SI units: 9.0-26.9 μmol/L)
Iron-binding capacity: 250-410 μg/dl (44.8-73.4 μmol/L)
Liver iron: 530-900 μg/g dry weight

MISCELLANEOUS LABORATORY TESTS

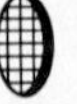

INTRADERMAL SKIN TESTS FOR ALLERGIES

EXPLANATION OF THE TEST

For intradermal skin testing, small amounts of allergens are injected into the superficial dermis, where there are large numbers of mast cells. The reaction of these mast cells to the injected antigens occurs within 15 to 20 minutes and triggers a release of histamine, causing a wheal at the site of injection.

VALUE OF THE TESTS

The intradermal skin tests are the most convenient, sensitive, highly reproducible, rapid, and economical means of determining if a patient has specific IgE antibodies against common environmental antigens.

NURSING ACTION

1. Inform the patient that there are no dietary restrictions before this test.
2. Explain to the patient that this test will help to determine the particular substance to which he or she is allergic.
3. Choose a space several fingerwidths away from the antecubital space. Avoid hairy or blemished areas.
4. Prepare the skin with an alcohol swab. Do not use an agent that discolors the skin and do not rub so hard that the skin becomes reddened.
5. Hold the patient's forearm with your nondominant hand and stretch the skin with your thumb.
6. The needle should be almost flat against the skin with the bevel of the needle up.
7. Insert the needle through the skin until it is resting ⅛ inch (3 mm) below the surface.
8. Inject the allergen slowly and gently; you should feel some resistance if the needle is properly located. A small wheal should form. Withdraw the needle and apply gentle pressure; do not massage the puncture site.

CLINICAL IMPLICATIONS

If a skin test profile correlates well with a patient's history, it is fairly certain that there is an allergic phenomenon present, and desensitizing shots can be initiated.

BREAST BIOPSY

EXPLANATION OF THE TEST

Biopsy and histological examination of breast tissue is the only definitive means of making a cytological diagnosis in a case of breast tumor. The biopsy specimen may be obtained by needle biopsy, fine needle (22-gauge) biopsy, or open biopsy.

VALUE OF THE TEST

Differentiates between benign and malignant breast tumors

Needle biopsy is restricted to fluid-filled cysts and advanced malignant lesions and has limited diagnostic value.

Interpretation requires special training.

NURSING ACTION

1. If the patient is to receive a local anesthetic, inform her that there are no dietary restrictions before the test.
2. Obtain a signed consent. Explain that this test permits microscopic examination of breast tissue.

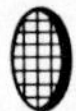

MAMMOGRAPHY

EXPLANATION OF THE TEST

Mammography is a radiographic technique by which breast tumors or cysts may be detected. Xeromammography is the making of photographs or photocopies of the x-ray images by means of an electrostatically charged plate.

VALUE AND LIMITATIONS OF THE TEST

Detection of breast cancer (biopsy is still essential for all breast lesions)

The test has a 75% false-positive result rate.

It involves exposure to ionizing radiation and requires special training and proper technique to avoid overexposure.

Useful in indicating the biopsy site when there is more than one breast mass

Detects tumors in the opposite breast
Demonstrates foci elsewhere in the breast

NURSING ACTION

1. Explain the test to the patient and let her know that there is a high incidence of false-positive results.
2. Ask the patient to remove all jewelry.

CYTOLOGICAL EXAMINATION OF NIPPLE DISCHARGE

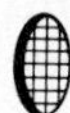

EXPLANATION OF THE TEST

This test is ordered when there is unexplained discharge from the nipple.

VALUE AND LIMITATIONS OF THE TEST

Differentiates between malignant and benign conditions
A negative result does not rule out carcinoma.

NURSING ACTION

1. Explain the procedure to the patient.
2. Before obtaining the specimen, wash the patient's nipple and dry it.
3. Ask the patient to express the fluid from her nipple. Discard the first drop and place a glass slide across the nipple to collect the next drop. Immediately spray the specimen with a cytological spray or place it in 95% ethanol solution. Send the specimen to the laboratory immediately after these steps are taken.
4. Note on laboratory slip which breast specimen is from and any pertinent history (medications, pregnant, perimenopausal).

ESTROGEN RECEPTOR ASSAY; PROGESTERONE RECEPTOR ASSAY

Normal results (femtomoles/mg)

The degree of positivity correlates with prognosis and the potential responsiveness of the tumor to hormonal manipulation.

Estrogen receptor	*Progesterone receptor*
Positive: >10	>5
Intermediate: 3-10	
Negative: <3	<5

EXPLANATION OF THE TEST

The presence or absence of estrogen receptor protein and progesterone receptor protein is an important prognostic factor in breast cancer in addition to the size of tumor and axillary nodes involved. These assays require tissue slices or cytoplasm extracts from the tumor.

VALUE OF THE TEST

Positive results indicate that the tumor will respond to hormonal manipulation.

NURSING ACTION

The tissue specimen (at least 1 g) should be frozen by dry ice within 15 minutes of being secured and sent to the laboratory packed in dry ice. Failure to quick-freeze the specimen results in false-negative results.

PAPANICOLAOU SMEAR

EXPLANATION OF THE TEST

This is a cytological test that is noted as a screening test for uterine carcinoma. It requires scrapings directly from the cervix. A positive or suspicious smear should be followed with a biopsy.

VALUE AND LIMITATIONS OF THE TEST

Detects cervical carcinoma
A single-scrape smear has a false-negative probability of about 30%.

NURSING ACTION

1. Schedule the test for midmenstrual cycle if possible.
2. Instruct the patient not to douche or insert vaginal medications for 24 hours before the test.

3. Inform the patient that there is no pain associated with the procedure, although there may be slight discomfort from the speculum.
4. The specimen is spread on a slide and immediately fixed according to laboratory instructions.

PREGNANCY TEST (URINE HUMAN CHORIONIC GONADOTROPIN)

EXPLANATION OF THE TEST

The laboratory diagnosis of pregnancy is based on the detection of human chorionic gonadotropin (HCG), a placental hormone, in the urine. A test may be positive as early as 4 days after the expected date of menstruation. It is more than 95% reliable by the tenth to the fourteenth day.

The placental trophoblastic cells begin to produce HCG, a glycoprotein that prevents degeneration of the corpus luteum at the end of the normal menstrual cycle. The HCG levels rise rapidly until the tenth week of gestation, after which they fall off to less than 10% of peak levels.

VALUE OF THE TEST

Detects pregnancy as early as 10 days after a missed menstrual period
Evaluates suspected hydatidiform mole or HCG-secreting tumors

NURSING ACTION

1. Explain the test to the patient. A qualitative test requires a first-voided morning specimen; a quantitative test requires a 24-hour specimen.
2. Refrigerate the 24-hour specimen or keep it on ice during the collection period.

CLINICAL IMPLICATIONS

Positive

For a one-time urine specimen, agglutination fails to occur and the individual is assumed to be pregnant.

In quantitative analysis HCG levels are:
First trimester: Up to 500,000 IU/24 hr
Second trimester: 5,000 to 15,000 IU/24 hr
Postpartum: Undetectable within a few days

Negative

For a one-time urine specimen, agglutination occurs and the individual is assumed not to be pregnant.

In quantitative analysis HCG is not found in the urine of the male or nonpregnant female.

Bibliography

Andiman, W.A., and others: Opportunistic lymphoproliferations associated with Epstein-Barr viral DNA in infants and children with AIDS, Lancet, Dec. 21, 1985, p. 1390.

Berlin, N.I., and others: Recommended methods for the measurement of vitamin B_{12} absorption, J. Nucl. Med. **22**:1091, 1981.

Bessman, J.D., Gilmer, P.R., and Gardner, F.H.: Improved classification of anemias by MCV and RDW, Am. J. Clin. Pathol. **80**(3):322, 1983.

Boyd, J., and others: Value of laboratory tests in the differential diagnosis of hypercalcemia, Am. J. Med. **77**:863, 1984.

Bravo, E., and others: The changing clinical spectrum of primary aldosteronism, Am. J. Med. **74**:641, 1983.

Chopra, I., and others: Thyroid function in nonthyroidal illnesses, Ann. Intern. Med. **98**:946, 1983.

Comerci, G.D.: Diagnosis: inhibited growth and delayed puberty, Hosp. Med. **14**:138, 1983.

Cooper, B.A.: Megaloblastic anemia, when to suspect it, how to treat it, Drug Ther., April 1984, p. 65.

Corey, L., and Spear, P.G.: Infections with herpes simplex viruses (first of two parts), N. Engl. J. Med. **314**(11):686, 1986.

Corey, L., and Spear, P.G.: Infections with herpes simplex viruses (second of two parts), N. Engl. J. Med. **314**(12):749, 1986.

Das, K.C., and others: Unmasking covert folate deficiency in iron-deficient subjects with neutrophil hypersegmentation: dU suppression tests on lymphocytes and bone marrow, Br. J. Haematol. **39**:357, 1978.

De Pablo, F., and others: Plasma prolactin in acromegaly before and after treatment, J. Clin. Endocrinol. **53**:344, 1981.

Dembert, M.L., and Kaiser, C.: Laboratory diagnosis of viral infections, Am. Fam. Physician **28**(4):125, 1983.

Edelstein, P.H.: Legionnaires' disease laboratory manual. Legionnaires' disease laboratory, Los Angeles, Calif., 1985, Wadsworth V.A. Medical Center.

Edelstein, P.H., Meyer, R.D., and Finegold, S.M.: Laboratory diagnosis of Legionnaires' disease, Am. Rev. Respir. Dis. **121**:317, 1980.

English, E.C., and Finch, C.A.: Iron deficiency: a systematic approach, Drug Ther., April 1984, p. 45.

Fairbanks, V.F., and Elveback, L.R.: Tests for pernicious anemia: serum vitamin B_{13} assay, Mayo Clin. Proc. **58**:135, 1983.

Fajaus, S., and Floyd, J.C.: Fasting hypoglycemia in adults, N. Engl. J. Med. **294**(14):766, 1976.

Fajaus, S., and Floyd, J.: Diagnosis and medical management of insulinomas, Annu. Rev. Med. **30**:313, 1979.

Felig, P., and others, editors: Endocrinology and metabolism, San Francisco, Calif., 1981, McGraw-Hill Book Co.

Finch, C.A., and Huebers, H.: Perspectives in iron metabolism, N. Engl. J. Med. **306**:1520, 1982.

Finegold, S.M., and Baron, E.J.: Bailey and Scott's diagnostic microbiology, ed. 7, St. Louis, 1986, The C.V. Mosby Co.

Fitzsimons, E.J., and Kaplan, K.: Rapid drop in serum iron concentration in myocardial infarction, Am. J. Clin. Pathol. **73**:552, 1980.

Gold, E.: The Cushing syndromes: changing views of diagnosis and treatment, Ann. Intern. Med. **90**:829, 1979.

Gondos, B.: Diagnosis of abnormalities in gonadal development, Ann. Clin. Lab. Sci. **12**:276, 1982.

Halliday, J.W., and Powell, L.W.: Iron overload, Semin. Hematol. **19**:6, 1982.

Herbert, V.: Hematology and the anemias. In Schneider, H.A., Anderson, C.E., and Coursin, D.B,. editors: Nutritional support of medical practice, ed. 2, New York, 1983, Harper & Row.

Herbert, V.: Megaloblastic anemia with two nutrient deficiencies: two cases, Med. Grand Rounds **1**:320, 1983.

Herbert, V.: Inroads in diagnosing and treating anemias, Drug Ther., April 1984, p. 38.

Hines, J.D.: The normochromic-normocytic anemias, Drug Ther., April 1984, p. 77.

Kaplan, L.A., and Pexce, A.J.: Clinical chemistry, theory, analysis, and correlation, St. Louis, 1984, The C.V. Mosby Co.

Koppelman, M., and others: Hyperprolactinemia, amenorrhea, and galactorrhea, Ann. Intern. Med. **100**:115, 1984.

Lafferty, F.W.: Primary hyperparathyroidism, Arch. Intern. Med. **141**:1761, 1981.

Marwick, C.: 'Molecular level' view gives immune system clues, JAMA **253**(23):3371, 1985.

Matsen, J.M., editor: Symposium on bacterial identification systems, Clin. Lab. Med. **5**(1), 1985.

Mazzaferri, E.L.: Thyrotoxicosis, Postgrad. Med. **73**:85, 1983.

Morley, J.E., and Shafer, R.B.: Thyroid function screening in new psychiatric admissions, Arch. Intern. Med. **142**:591, 1982.

Nakamura, R.M., and Rowlands, D.T., Jr., editors: Advances in immunopathology, Clin. Lab. Med. **6**(1):3, 1986.

Ney, R., editor: Investigations of endocrine disorders, Clin. Endocrinol. Metab. **14**(1):150, 1985.

Nyhan, W.L.: Cytogenetic diseases, Clin. Symp. **35**(1):1, 1983.

Petersdorf, R.G., and others, editors: Harrison's principles of internal medicine, ed. 10, New York, 1983, McGraw-Hill Book Co.

Ravel, R.: Conditions which affect interpretation of thyroid function tests, Ill. Med. J. **160**:155, 1981.

Ravel, R.: Clinical laboratory medicine, ed. 4, Chicago, 1984, Year Book Medical Publishers.

Reeves, W.B., and Haurani, F.I.: Clinical applicability and usefulness of ferritin measurements, Ann. Clin. Lab. Sci. **10**:529, 1980.

Rude, R.K., and others: Urinary and nephrogenous adenosine 3,5-monophosphate in the hypercalcemia of malignancy, J. Clin. Endocrinol. **52**:765, 1981.

Salahuddin, S.Z., and others: Isolation of a new virus HBLV in patients with lymphoproliferative disorder, Science **234**:596, 1986.

Sauberlich, H.E.: Implications of nutritional status on human biochemistry, physiology, and health, Clin. Biochem. **17**:132, April 1984.

Schilling, R.F.: Vitamin B_{12}: assay and absorption testing, Lab. Management **20**:31, 1982.

Schumann, G.B., editor: Symposium on body fluid analysis, Clin. Lab. Med. **5**(2):195 June 1985.

Scully, R.E., McNeely, B.U., and Mark, E.J., editors: Case records of the Massachusetts General Hospital: normal reference laboratory values, N. Engl. J. Med. **314**(1):39, 1986.

Siegel, R.S., and Lessin, L.S.: The hemolytic anemias, guidelines for rational management, Drug Ther., April 1984, p. 87.

Southern, P., and Oldstone, M.B.A.: Medical consequences of persistent viral infection, New Engl. J. Med. **314**(6):359, 1986.

Spivak, J.L.: Masked megaloblastic anemia, Arch. Intern. Med. **142**:2111, 1982.

Tolis, G.: Prolactin: physiology and pathology, Hosp. Pract. **15**:85, 1980.

Watson, L., and others: Hydrocortisone suppression test and discrimant analysis in differential diagnosis of hypercalcemia, Lancet **1**:1320, 1980.

Weibe, R.H.: Endocrine evaluation of hyperprolactinemia, Clin. Obstet. Gynecol. **23**:349, 1980.

Weinberger, M., and others: Primary aldosteronism, Ann. Intern. Med. **90**:386, 1979.

Wenk, R.E., editor: Symposium on Perinatal Diagnosis. In Clin. Lab. Med. **1**(2):151, June 1981.

Wilson, J., and Foster, D., editors: Textbook of endocrinology, ed. 7, Philadelphia, 1985, W.B. Saunders Co.

Young, L.S., and others: Epstein-Barr virus receptors on human pharyngeal epithelia, Lancet, Feb. 1, 1986, p. 240.

Appendices

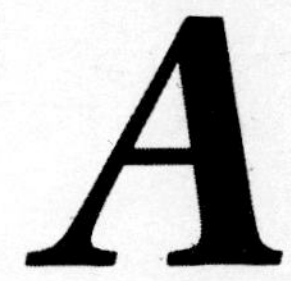

Normal reference laboratory values*†

Abbreviations used in tables

<	= less than
>	= greater than
dl	= deciliter (100 ml)
g	= gram
IU	= international unit
kg	= kilogram
L	= liter
mEq	= milliequivalent
mg	= milligram
ml	= milliliter
mM	= millimole
mm Hg	= millimeters of mercury
ImU	= international milliunit
mOsm	= milliosmole
mμ	= millimicron
mU	= milliunit
ng	= nanogram
pg	= picogram
μEq	= microequivalent
μg	= microgram
IμU	= international microunit
μl	= microliter
μU	= microunit
U	= unit

Scully, R.E., editor: Case records of the Massachusetts General Hospital, N. Engl. J. Med. 314:39-49, January 2, 1986. Reprinted by permission of The New England Journal of Medicine.

*Both conventional and SI units are listed. The SI for the Health Professions. World Health Organization, Office of Publications, Geneva, Switzerland, 1977.

†Abbreviations used: SI, Système International d'Unités; P, plasma; S, serum; B, blood; and U, urine.

Blood, plasma or serum values

Determination	Reference range	
	Conventional	SI
Acetoacetate plus acetone	Negative	
Aldolase	1.3–8.2 U/liter	22-137 nmol·sec^{-1}/liter
Ammonia	12-55 μmol/liter	12-55 μmol/liter
Amylase	4-25 units/ml	4-25 arb. unit
Ascorbic acid	0.4-1.5 mg/100 ml	23-85 μmol/liter
Bilirubin	Direct: up to 0.4 mg/100 ml. Total: up to 1.0 mg/100 ml	Up to 7 μmol/liter Up to 17 μmol/liter
Blood volume	8.5-9.0% of body weight in kg	80-85 ml/kg
Calcium	8.5-10.5 mg/100 ml (slightly higher in children)	2.1-2.6 mmol/liter
Carbamazepine	4.0-12.0 μg/ml	17-51 μmol/liter
Carbon dioxide content	24-30 meq/liter	24-30 mmol/liter
Carbon monoxide	Less than 5% of total hemoglobin	
Carotenoids	0.8-4.0 μg/ml	1.5-7.4 μmol/liter
Ceruloplasmin	27-37 mg/100 ml	1.8-2.5 μmol/liter
Chloramphenicol	10-20 μg/ml	31-62 μmol/liter
Chloride	100-106 meq/liter	100-106 mmol/liter
CK isoenzymes	5% MB or less	
Copper	Total: 100-200 μg/100 ml	16-31 μmol/liter
Creatine kinase (CK)	Female: 10-79 U/liter Male: 17-148 U/liter	167-1317 nmol·sec^{-1}/liter 283-2467 nmol·sec^{-1}/liter
Creatinine	0.6-1.5 mg/100 ml	53-133 μmol/liter
Ethanol	0 mg/100 ml	0 mmol/liter

Minimal ml required	Note	Method
1-B		Behre: J Lab Clin Med 13:770, 1928 (modified)
2-S	Use unhemolyzed serum	Beisenherz et al.: Z Naturforsch 86:555, 1963
2-B	Collect in heparinized tube; deliver *immediately* packed in ice	Da Fonseca-Wolheim: J Clin Chem Clin Biochem 11:421, 1973
1-S		Zinterhofer et al.: Clin Chim Acta 43:5, 1973
7-B	Collect in heparinized tube before any food is given	Roe, Kuether: J Biol Chem 147:399, 1943
1-S		Gambino: Standard Methods Clin Chem 5:55, 1965
		Isotope dilution technique with ^{131}I albumin
1-S		Spectrophotometry using cresolphthalein complexone
1-S	Fill tube to top	By CO_2 electrode
		Liquid chromatography
3-B	Fill tube to top	Multi-wavelength spectrophotometry
3-S	Vitamin A may be done on same specimen	Natelson: Microtechniques of Clinical Chemistry, 2nd ed., 1961, p. 454
2-S		Ravin: J Lab Clin Med 58:161, 1961
0.2-S		Liquid chromatography
1-S		Cotlove: Standard Methods Clin Chem 3:81, 1961
0.2-S		Electrophoresis
1-S		Atomic-absorption spectrophotometry
1-S		Szasz: Clin Chem 22:650, 1976
1-S		Fabiny, Ertingshausen: Clin Chem 17:696, 1971
2-B	Collect in oxalate and refrigerate	Gas-liquid chromatography

Continued.

Blood, plasma or serum values—cont'd

Determination	Reference range	
	Conventional	**SI**
Glucose	Fasting: 70-110 mg/100 ml	3.9-5.6 mmol/liter
Iron	50-150 μg/100 ml (higher in males)	9.0-26.9 μmol/liter
Iron-binding capacity	250-410 μg/100 ml	44.8-73.4 μmol/liter
Lactic acid	0.6-1.8 meq/liter	0.6-1.8 mmol/liter
Lactic dehydrogenase	45-90 U/liter	750-1500 nmol·sec^{-1}/liter
Lead	50 μg/100 ml or less	Up to 2.4 μmol/liter
Lipase	2 units/ml or less	Up to 2 arb. unit
Lipids		
Cholesterol	120-220 mg/100 ml	3.10-5.69 mmol/liter
Triglycerides	40-150 mg/100 ml	0.4-1.5 g/liter
Lipoprotein electrophoresis (LEP)		
Lithium	0.5-1.5 meq/liter	0.5-1.5 mmol/liter
Magnesium	1.5-2.0 meq/liter	0.8-1.3 mmol/liter
5′ Nucleotidase	1-11 U/liter	17-183 nmol·sec^{-1}/liter
Osmolality	280-296 mOsm/kg water	280-296 mmol/kg
Oxygen saturation (arterial)	96-100%	0.96-1.00
PCO_2	35-45 mm Hg	4.7-6.0 kPa
pH	7.35-7.45	Same

Minimal ml required	Note	Method
1-P	Collect with oxalate-fluoride mixture	Bergmeyer: Methods of Enzymatic Analysis, 1965, p. 117
1-S		Spectrophotometry using Ferrozine
1-S		Spectrophotometry using Ferrozine
2-B	Collect with oxalate-fluoride; deliver immediately packed in ice	Hadjivassiliou, Rieder: Clin Chim Acta 19:357, 1968
1-S	Unsuitable if hemolyzed	Gay, McComb, Bowers: Clin Chem 14:740, 1968
2-B	Collect with oxalate-fluoride mixture	Berman: Atom Absorp Newslett 3:9, 1964 (modified)
1-S		Zinterhofer: Clin Chim Acta 44:173, 1973
1-S	Fasting	Siedel: J Clin Chem Clin Biochem 19:838, 1981
1-S	Fasting	Ziegenhorn: Clin Chem 21:1627, 1975
2-S	Fasting, do not freeze serum	Lees, Hatch: J Lab Clin Med 61:518, 1963
1-S		Pybus, Bowers: Clin Chem 16:139, 1970
1-S		Willis: Clin Chem 11:251, 1965 (modified)
1-S		Arkesteijn: J Clin Chem Clin Biochem 14:155, 1976
1-S		Osmometry using freezing-point depression
3-B	Deliver in sealed heparinized syringe packed in ice	Gordy, Drabkin: J Biol Chem 227:285, 1957
2-B	Collect and deliver in sealed heparinized syringe	By CO_2 electrode
2-B	Collect without stasis in sealed heparinized syringe; deliver packed in ice	Glass electrode

Continued.

Blood, plasma or serum values—cont'd

Determination	Reference range: Conventional	Reference range: SI
PO_2	75-100 mm Hg (dependent on age) while breathing room air Above 500 mm Hg while on 100% O_2	10.0-13.3 kPa
Phenobarbital	15-50 μg/ml	65-215 μmol/liter
Phenytoin (Dilantin)	5-20 μg/ml	20-80 μmol/liter
Phosphatase (acid)	Male—Total: 0.13-0.63 sigma U/ml	36-175 nmol·sec^{-1}/liter
	Female—Total: 0.01-0.56 sigma U/ml	2.8-156 nmol·sec^{-1}/liter
	Prostatic: 0-0.5 Fishman-Lerner U/100 ml	
Phosphatase (alkaline)	13-39 U/liter; infants and adolescents up to 104 U/liter	217-650 nmol·sec^{-1}/liter; up to 1.26 μmol·sec^{-1}/liter
Phosphorus (inorganic)	3.0-4.5 mg/100 ml (infants in first year up to 6.0 mg/100 ml)	1.0-1.5 mmol/liter
Potassium	3.5-5.0 meq/liter	3.5-5.0 mmol/liter
Primidone (Mysoline)	4-12 μg/ml	18-55 μmol/liter
Procainamide	4-10 μg/ml	17-42 μmol/liter
Protein: Total	6.0-8.4 g/100 ml	60-84 g/liter
Albumin	3.5-5.0 g/100 ml	35-50 g/liter
Globulin	2.3-3.5 g/100 ml	23-35 g/liter
Electrophoresis	(% of total protein)	
Albumin	52-68	
Globulin:		
$Alpha_1$	4.2-7.2	
$Alpha_2$	6.8-12	
Beta	9.3-15	
Gamma	13-23	
Pyruvic acid	0-0.11 meq/liter	0-0.11 mmol/liter

Minimal ml required	Note	Method
2-B		Oxygen electrode
1-S		Liquid chromatography
1-S		Liquid chromatography
1-S	Must always be drawn just before analysis or stored as frozen serum; avoid hemolysis	Bessey et al.: J Biol Chem 164:321, 1946
		Babson et al.: Clin Chim Acta 13:264, 1966
1-S		Stevens, Thomas: Clin Chim Acta 37:541, 1972
1-S		Daly, Ertingshausen: Clin Chem 18:263, 1972
1-S	Serum must be separated promptly from cells	Ion-selective electrode
1-S		Enzyme immunoassay
1-S		Liquid chromatography
1-S		Weichselbaum: Am J Clin Pathol 16:40, 1946
1-S		Doumas et al.: Clin Chim Acta 31:87, 1971
	Globulin equals total protein minus albumin	
1-S	Quantitation by densitometry	Kunkel, Tiselius: J Gen Physiol 35:89, 1951
		Durrum: J Am Chem Soc 72:2943, 1950
2-B	Collect with oxalate fluoride. Deliver immediately packed in ice	Hadjivassiliou, Rieder: Clin Chim Acta 19:357, 1968

Continued.

Blood, plasma or serum values—cont'd

Determination	Reference range	
	Conventional	**SI**
Quinidine	1.2-4.0 μg/ml	3.7-12.3 μmol/liter
Salicylate:	0	
Therapeutic	20-25 mg/100 ml; 25-30 mg/100 ml to age 10 yr 3 hr post dose	1.4-1.8 mmol/liter 1.8-2.2 mmol/liter
Sodium	135-145 meq/liter	135-145 mmol/liter
Sulfonamide	5-15 mg/100 ml	
Transaminase, SGOT (aspartate aminotransferase)	7-27 U/liter	117-450 nmol·sec^{-1}/liter
Transaminase, SGPT (alanine aminotransferase)	1-21 U/liter	17-350 nmol·sec^{-1}/liter
Urea nitrogen (BUN)	8-25 mg/100 ml	2.9-8.9 mmol/liter
Uric acid	3.0-7.0 mg/100 ml	0.18-0.42 mmol/liter
Vitamin A	0.15-0.6 μg/ml	0.5-2.1 μmol/liter

Minimal ml required	Note	Method
1-S		Liquid chromatography
2-P		Keller: Am J Clin Pathol 17:415, 1947
1-S		Ion-selective electrode
2-P		Bratton, Marshall: J Biol Chem 128:537, 1939
1-S		Karmen et al.: J Clin Invest 34:126, 1955
1-S		Henry et al.: Am J Clin Pathol 34:381, 1960
1-S		Paulson et al.: Clin Chem 17:644, 1971
1-S		Spectrophotometry using uricase
3-S		Natelson: Microtechniques of Clinical Chemistry, 2nd ed. 1961, p. 451

Urine values

Determination	Reference range	
	Conventional	SI
Acetone plus aceto-acetate (quantitative)	0	0 mg/liter
Amylase	24-76 units/ml	24-76 arb. unit
Calcium	300 mg/day or less	7.5 mmol/day or less
Catecholamines	Epinephrine: under 20 μg/day	<109 nmol/day
	Norepinephrine: under 100 μg/day	<590 nmol/day
Chorionic gonadotropin	0	0 arb. unit
Copper	0-100 μg/day	0-1.6 μmol/day
Coproporphyrin	50-250 μg/day	80-380 nmol/day
	Children under 80 lb (36 kg): 0-75 μg/day	0-115 nmol/day
Creatine	Under 100 mg/day or less than 6% of creatinine. In pregnancy: up to 12%. In children under 1 yr: may equal creatinine. In older children: up to 30% of creatinine.	<0.75 mmol/day
Creatinine	15-25 mg/kg of body weight/day	0.13-0.22 mmol·kg^{-1}/day
Cystine or cysteine	0	0
Hemoglobin and myoglobin	0	
5-Hydroxyindoleacetic acid	2-9 mg/day (women lower than men)	10-45 μmol/day
Lead	0.08 μg/ml or 120 μg/day or less	0.39 μmol/liter or less

Minimal quantity required	Note	Method
2 ml		Behre: J Lab Clin Med 13:770, 1928
		Zinterhofer et al.: Clin Chim Acta 43:5, 1973
24-hr specimen	Collect in special bottle with 10 ml of concentrated HCl	Atomic-absorption spectrophotometry
24-hr specimen	Should be collected with 10 ml of concentrated HCl (pH should be between 2.0 and 3.0)	Fluorometry
1st morning void		Immunologic technique
24-hr specimen		Atomic-absorption spectrophotometry
24-hr specimen	Collect with 5 g of sodium carbonate	Schwartz: J Lab Clin Med 37:843, 1951 With: Scand J Clin Lab Invest 7:193, 1955
24-hr specimen	Also order creatinine	Folin: Laboratory Manual of Biological Chemistry, 5th ed., 1933, p. 163
24-hr specimen		Fabiny, Ertingshausen: Clin Chem 17:696, 1971
10 ml	Qualitative	Hawk et al.: Practical Physiological Chemistry, 13th ed., 1954, p. 141
Freshly voided sample	Chemical examination with benzidine	Spectroscopy
24-hr specimen	Collect with 10 ml of concentrated HCl	Sjoerdsma et al.: JAMA 159:397, 1955
24-hr specimen		Willis: Anal Chem 34:614, 1962 (modified)

Continued.

Urine values—cont'd

Determination	Reference range	
	Conventional	**SI**
Phosphorus (inorganic)	Varies with intake; average, 1 g/day	32 mmol/day
Porphobilinogen	0	0
Protein:		
Quantitative	<150 mg/24 hr	<0.15 g/day
Steroids:		
17-Ketosteroids (per day)	Age / Male / Female 10 / 1-4 mg / 1-4 mg 20 / 6-21 / 4-16 30 / 8-26 / 4-14 50 / 5-18 / 3-9 70 / 2-10 / 1-7	μmol/day / μmol/day 3-14 / 3-14 21-73 / 14-56 28-90 / 14-49 17-62 / 10-31 7-35 / 3-24
17-Hydroxysteroids	3-8 mg/day (women lower than men)	8-22 μmol/day as tetrahydrocortisol
Sugar:		
Quantitative glucose	0	0 mmol/liter
Urobilinogen	Up to 1.0 Ehrlich U	To 1.0 arb. unit
Uroporphyrin	0-30 μg/day	<36 nmol/day
Vanilmandelic acid (VMA)	Up to 9 mg/24 hr	Up to 45 μmol/day

Minimal quantity required	Note	Method
24-hr specimen	Collect with 10 ml of concentrated HCl	Daly, Ertingshausen: Clin Chem 18:263, 1972
10 ml	Use freshly voided urine	Watson, Schwartz: Proc Soc Exp Biol Med 47:393, 1941
24-hr specimen		Meulmans: Clin Chim Acta 5:757, 1951
24-hr specimen	Not valid if patient is receiving meprobamate	Vestergaard: Acta Endocrinol 8:193, 1951. Normal values taken from Hamburger: Acta Endocrinol 1:19, 1948
24-hr specimen	Keep cold: chlorpromazine and related drugs interfere with assay	Epstein: Clin Chim Acta 7:735, 1962
24-hr or other timed specimen		Stein. In: Bergmeyer: Methods of Enzymatic Analysis, 1965, p. 117
2-hr sample (1-3 p.m.)		Watson et al.: Am J Clin Pathol 15:605, 1944
See Coproporphyrin		Schwartz et al.: Proc Soc Exp Biol Med 79:463, 1952
24-hr specimen	Collect as for catecholamines	Pisano et al.: Clin Chim Acta 7:285, 1962

Special endocrine tests: Steroid hormones

Determination	Reference range	
	Conventional	SI
Aldosterone	Excretion: 5-19 μg/24 hr	14-53 nmol/day
	Supine: 48 ± 29 pg/ml	133 ± 80 pmol/liter
	Upright (2 hr): 65 ± 23 pg/ml	180 ± 64 pmol/liter
	Supine: 107 ± 45 pg/ml	279 ± 125 pmol/liter
	Upright (2 hr): 239 ± 123 pg/ml	663 ± 341 pmol/liter
	Supine: 175 ± 75 pg/ml	485 ± 208 pmol/liter
	Upright (2 hr): 532 ± 228 pg/ml	1476 ± 632 pmol/liter
Cortisol	8 a.m.: 5-25 μg/100 ml	0.14-0.69 μmol/liter
	8 p.m.: Below 10 μg/100 ml	0-0.28 μmol/liter
	4-hr ACTH test: 30-45 μg/100 ml	0.83-1.24 μmol/liter
	Overnight suppression test: Below 5 μg/100 ml	0.14 nmol/liter
	Excretion: 20-70 μg/24 hr	55-193 nmol/day
Dehydroepiandrosterone (DHEA)	Male: 0.5-5.5 ng/ml	1.7-19 nmol/liter
	Female: 1.4-8.0 ng/ml	4.9-28 nmol/liter
	0.3-4.5 ng/ml	1.0-15.6 nmol/liter

Minimal ml required	Note	Method
5/day	Keep specimen cold	Bayard et al.: J Clin Endocrinol Metab 31:507, 1970
3-S, P	Fasting, at rest, 210-meq sodium diet	Poulson et al.: Clin Immunol Immunopathol 2:373, 1974
	Upright, 2 hr, 210-meq sodium diet	
	Fasting, at rest, 110-meq sodium diet	
	Upright, 2 hr, 110-meq sodium diet	
	Fasting, at rest, 10-meq sodium diet	
	Upright, 2 hr, 10-meq sodium diet	
1-P	Fasting	Catt, Tregear: Science 158:1670, 1967
1-P	At rest	
1-P	20 U ACTH, IV per 4 hr	
1-P	8 a.m. sample after 0.5 mg dexamethasone by mouth at midnight	
2/day	Keep specimen cold	
2-S, P		Sekihara, Ohsawa: Steroids 24:317, 1974
	Adult	
	Post-menopausal	

Continued.

Special endocrine tests: Polypeptide hormones—cont'd

Determination	Reference range: Conventional	Reference range: SI
Dehydroepiandrosterone sulfate (DHEA-S)	Male:	
	151-446 μg/100 ml	3.9-11.4 μmol/liter
	Female:	
	84-433 μg/100 ml	2.2-11.1 μmol/liter
	1.7-177 μg/100 ml	0.04-4.5 μmol/liter
11-Deoxycortisol	Responsive:	
	Over 7.5 μg/100 ml	>0.22 μmol/liter
Estradiol	Male: <50 pg/ml	<184 pmol/liter
	Female: 23-361 pg/ml	84-1325 pmol/liter
	<30 pg/ml	<110 pmol/liter
	<20 pg/ml	<73 pmol/liter
Progesterone	Male: <1.0 ng/ml	<3.2 nmol/liter
	Female:	
	0.2-0.6 ng/ml	0.6-1.9 nmol/liter
	0.3-3.5 ng/ml	0.95-11 nmol/liter
	6.5-32.2 ng/ml	21-102 nmol/liter
Testosterone	Adult male:	
	300-1100 ng/100 ml	10.4-38.1 nmol/liter
	Adolescent male:	
	Over 100 ng/100 ml	>3.5 nmol/liter
	Female:	
	25-90 ng/100 ml	0.87-3.12 nmol/liter
Unbound testosterone	Adult male:	
	3.06-24.0 ng/100 ml	106-832 pmol/liter
	Adult female:	
	0.09-1.28 ng/100 ml	3.1-44.4 pmol/liter

Minimal ml required	Note	Method
2-S, P		Buster, Abraham: Anal Lett 5:543, 1972
	Adult	
	Post-menopausal	
1-P	8 a.m. sample, preceded by 4.5 g of metyrapone by mouth per 24 hr or by single dose of 2.5 g by mouth at midnight	Mahajan et al.: Steroids 20:609, 1972
5-S, P		Mikhail et al.: Steroids 15:333, 1970
	Adult	
	Post-menopausal	
	Pre-pubertal	
5-S, P		Furuyama, Nugent: Steroids 17:663, 1971
	Follicular phase	
	Midcycle peak	
	Post-ovulatory	
1-P	a.m. sample	Catt, Tregear: Science 158:1670, 1967
2-P	a.m. sample	Forest et al.: Steroids 12:323, 1968

Special endocrine tests: Polypeptide hormones

	Reference range	
Determination	**Conventional**	**SI**
Adrenocortico-tropin (ACTH)	15-70 pg/ml	3.3-15.4 pmol/liter
Alpha subunit	<0.5-2.5 ng/ml	<0.4-2.0 nmol/liter
	<0.5-5.0 ng/ml	<0.4-4.0 nmol/liter
Calcitonin	Male: 0-14 pg/ml	0-4.1 pmol/liter
	Female: 0-28 pg/ml	0-8.2 pmol/liter
	>100 pg/ml in medullary carcinoma	>29.3 pmol/liter
Follicle-stimulating hormone (FSH)	Male: 3-18 mU/ml	3-18 arb. unit
	Female: 4.6-22.4 mU/ml	4.6-22.4 arb. unit
	13-41 mU/ml	13-41 arb. unit
	30-170 mU/ml	30-170 arb. unit
Growth hormone	Below 5 ng/ml	<233 pmol/liter
	Children: Over 10 ng/ml	>465 pmol/liter
	Male: Below 5 ng/ml	<233 pmol/liter
	Female: Up to 30 ng/ml	0-1395 pmol/liter
	Male: Below 5 ng/ml	<233 pmol/liter
	Female: Below 5 ng/ml	<233 pmol/liter
Insulin	6-26 μU/ml	43-187 pmol/liter
	Below 20 μU/ml	<144 pmol/liter
	Up to 150 μU/ml	0-1078 pmol/liter
Luteinizing hormone (LH)	Male: 3-18 mU/ml	3-18 arb. unit
	Female: 2.4-34.5 mU/ml	2.4-34.5 arb. unit
	43-187 mU/ml	43-187 arb. unit
	30-150 mU/ml	30-150 arb. unit
Parathyroid hormone	<25 pg/ml	<2.94 pmol/liter
Prolactin	2-15 ng/ml	0.08-6.0 nmol/liter

Minimal ml required	Note	Method
5-P	Place specimen on ice and send promptly to laboratory. Use EDTA tube only.	Gonzales: Clin Chem 26:1228, 1980
2-S	Adult male or female Postmenopausal female	Kourides et al.: Endocrinology 94:1411, 1974
5-S	Test done only on known or suspected cases of medullary carcinoma of the thyroid	Deftos et al.: Metabolism 20:1129, 1971 Deftos et al.: Metabolism 20:428, 1971
5-S, P	Same sample may be used for LH Pre- or post-ovulatory Mid-cycle peak Post-menopausal	Midgley: J Clin Endocrinol Metab 27:295, 1967
1-S	Fasting, at rest After exercise	Glick et al.: Nature 199:784, 1963
	After glucose load	
1-S	Fasting During hypoglycemia After glucose load	Morgan, Lazarow: Proc Soc Exp Biol Med 110:29, 1962
5-S, P	Same sample may be used for FSH	Odell et al.: J Clin Invest 46:248, 1967
	Pre- or post-ovulatory	
	Mid-cycle peak Post-menopausal	
5-P	Keep blood on ice, or plasma must be frozen if it is to be sent any distance; a.m. sample	Stewart et al.: N Engl J Med 306:1136, 1982
2-S		Sinha et al.: J Clin Endocrinol Metab 36:509, 1973

Continued.

Special endocrine tests: Polypeptide hormones—cont'd

Determination	Reference range	
	Conventional	**SI**
Renin activity	Supine:	
	1.1 ± 0.8 ng/ml/hr	0.9 ± 0.6 nmol/liter/hr
	Upright:	
	1.9 ± 1.7 ng/ml/hr	1.5 ± 1.3 nmol/liter/hr
	Supine:	
	2.7 ± 1.8 ng/ml/hr	2.1 ± 1.4 nmol/liter/hr
	Upright:	
	6.6 ± 2.5 ng/ml/hr	5.1 ± 1.9 nmol/liter/hr
	Diuretics:	
	10.0 ± 3.7 ng/ml/hr	7.7 ± 2.9 nmol/liter/hr
Somatomedin C (Sm-C, IGF-1)	0.08-2.8 U/ml	0.08-2.8 arb. unit
	0.9-5.9 U/ml	0.9-5.9 arb. unit
	0.34-1.9 U/ml	0.34-1.9 arb. unit
	0.45-2.2 U/ml	0.45-2.2 arb. unit

Special endocrine tests: Thyroid hormones

Determination	Reference range	
	Conventional	**SI**
Thyroid-stimulating hormone (TSH)	0.5-5.0 μU/ml	0.5-5.0 arb. unit
Thyroxine-binding globulin capacity	15-25 μg T_4/100 ml	193-322 nmol/liter
Total triiodothyronine (T_3)	75-195 ng/100 ml	1.16-3.00 nmol/liter
Reverse triiodothyronine (rT3)	13-53 ng/ml	0.2-0.8 nmol/liter
Total thyroxine by RIA (T_4)	4-12 μg/100 ml	52-154 nmol/liter
T_3 resin uptake	25-35%	0.25-0.35
Free thyroxine index (FT_4I)	1-4	

Minimal ml required	Note	Method
4-P	EDTA tubes, on ice, normal diet	Haber et al.: J Clin Endocrinol Metab 29:1349, 1969
	Low-sodium diet	
	Low-sodium diet	
2-P	EDTA plasma Prepubertal During puberty Adult males Adult females	Furlanetto et al.: J Clin Invest 60:648, 1977

Minimal ml required	Note	Method
2-S		Ridgway et al.: J Clin Invest 52:2785, 1973
2-S		Levy et al.: J Clin Endocrinol Metab 32:372, 1971
2-S		Larsen et al.: J Clin Invest 51:1939, 1972
2-S		Cooper et al.: J Clin Endocrinol Metab 54:101, 1982
1-S		Chopra: J Clin Endocrinol Metab 34:938, 1972
2-S		Taybearn et al.: J Nucl Med 8:739, 1967
2-S		Sarin, Anderson: Arch Intern Med 126:631, 1970

Vitamin D derivatives

Determination	Reference range	
	Conventional	SI
1,25-Dihydroxy-vitamin D	26-65 pg/ml	62-155 pmol/liter
25-Hydroxy-vitamin D	8-55 ng/ml	19.4-137 nmol/liter

Hematologic values

Determination	Reference range	
	Conventional	SI
Coagulation factors:		
Factor I (fibrinogen)	0.15-0.35 g/100 ml	4.0-10.0 μmol/liter
Factor II (prothrombin)	60-140%	0.60-1.40
Factor V (accelerator globulin)	60-140%	0.60-1.40
Factor VII-X (proconvertin-Stuart)	70-130%	0.70-1.30
Factor X (Stuart factor)	70-130%	0.70-1.30
Factor VIII (antihemophilic globulin)	50-200%	0.50-2.0
Factor IX (plasma thromboplastic cofactor)	60-140%	0.60-1.40
Factor XI (plasma thromboplastic antecedent)	60-140%	0.60-1.40
Factor XII (Hageman factor)	60-140%	0.60-1.40
Coagulation		
Screening tests:		
Bleeding time (Simplate)	3-9.5 min	180-570 sec

Minimal ml required	Note	Method
1-S		Reinhardt et al.: J Clin Endocrinol Metab 58:91, 1984
1-S		Preece et al.: Clin Chim Acta 54:235, 1974

Minimal ml required	Note	Method
4.5-P	Collect in Vacutainer containing sodium citrate	Ratnoff, Menzies: J Lab Clin Med 37:316, 1951
4.5-P	Collect in plastic tubes with 3.8% sodium citrate	Owren, Aas: Scand J Clin Lab Invest 3:201, 1951
4.5-P	Collect as in factor II determination	Lewis, Ware: Proc Soc Exp Biol Med 84:640, 1953
4.5-P	Collect as in factor II determination	Same as factor II
4.5-P	Collect as in factor II determination	Bachman et al.: Thromb Diath Haemorrh 2:29, 1958
4.5-P	Collect as in factor II determination	Tocantins, Kazal: Blood Coagulation, Hemorrhage and Thrombosis, 2nd ed., 1964
4.5-P	Collect as in factor II determination	*Idem*
4.5-P	Collect as in factor II determination	*Idem*
4.5-P	Collect as in factor II determination	*Idem*
		Simplate Bleeding Time Device (General Diagnostics)

Continued.

Hematologic values—cont'd

Determination	Reference range: Conventional	Reference range: SI
Prothrombin time	Less than 2-sec deviation from control	Less than 2-sec deviation from control
Partial thromboplastin time (activated)	25-38 sec	25-38 sec
Whole-blood clot lysis	No clot lysis in 24 hr	0/day
Fibrinolytic studies:		
Euglobin lysis	No lysis in 2 hr	0/2 hr
Fibrinogen split products	Negative reaction at >1:4 dilution	0 (at 1:4 dilution)
Thrombin time	Control ±5 sec	Control ±5 sec
"Complete" blood count:		
Hematocrit	Male: 45-52% Female: 37-48%	Male: 0.45-0.52 Female: 0.37-0.48
Hemoglobin	Male: 13-18 g/100 ml Female: 12-16 g/100 ml	Male: 8.1-11.2 mmol/liter Female: 7.4-9.9 mmol/liter
Leukocyte count	4300-10,800/mm^3	4.3-10.8 × 10^9/liter
Erythrocyte count	4.2-5.9 million/mm^3	4.2-5.9 × 10^{12}/liter
Mean corpuscular volume (MCV)	86-98 μm^3/cell	86-98 fl
Mean corpuscular hemoglobin (MCH)	27-32 pg/RBC	1.7-2.0 pg/cell
Mean corpuscular hemoglobin concentration (MCHC)	32-36%	0.32-0.36
Erythrocyte sedimentation rate	Male: 1-13 mm/hr Female: 1-20 mm/hr	Male: 1-13 mm/hr Female: 1-20 mm/hr

Minimal ml required	Note	Method
4.5-P	Collect in Vacutainer containing 3.8% sodium citrate	Colman et al.: Am J Clin Pathol 64:108, 1975
4.5-P	Collect in Vacutainer containing 3.8% sodium citrate	Babson, Babson: Am J Clin Pathol 62:856, 1974
2.0-whole blood	Collect in sterile tube and incubate at 37° C	Page, Culver: Syllabus, Laboratory Examination and Clinical Diagnosis, 1960, p. 207
4.5-P	Collect as in factor II determination	Sherry et al.: J Clin Invest 38:810, 1959
4.5-S	Collect in special tube containing thrombin and epsilon aminocaproic acid	Carvalho: Am J Clin Pathol 62:107, 1974
4.5-P	Collect as in factor II determination	Stefanini, Dameshek: Hemorrhagic Disorders, 1962, p. 492
1-B	Use EDTA as anticoagulant; the seven listed tests are performed automatically on the Ortho ELT 800, which directly determines cell counts, hemoglobin (as the cyanmethemoglobin derivative), and MCV and computes hematocrit, MCH, and MCHC	
5-B	Use EDTA as anticoagulant	Modified Westergren method. Gambino et al.: Am J Clin Pathol 35:173, 1965

Continued.

Hematologic values—cont'd

Determination	Reference range: Conventional	SI
Erythrocyte enzymes:		
Glucose-6-phosphate dehydrogenase	5-15 U/g Hb	5-15 U/g
Pyruvate kinase	13-17 U/g Hb	13-17 U/g
Ferritin (serum)		
Iron deficiency	0-12 ng/ml	0-4.8 nmol/liter
Borderline	13-20	5.2-8 nmol/liter
Iron excess	>400 ng/liter	>160 nmol/liter
Folic acid		
Normal	>3.3 ng/ml	>7.3 nmol/liter
Borderline	2.5-3.2 ng/ml	5.75-7.39 nmol/liter
Haptoglobin	40-336 mg/100 ml	0.4-3.36 g/liter
Hemoglobin studies:		
Electrophoresis for abnormal hemoglobin		
Electrophoresis for A_2 hemoglobin	3.0%	0.015-0.035
Borderline	0.3-3.5%	0.03-0.035
Hemoglobin F (fetal hemoglobin)	Less than 2%	<0.02
Hemoglobin, met- and sulf-	0	0
Serum hemoglobin	2-3 mg/100 ml	1.2-1.9 μmol/liter
Thermolabile hemoglobin	0	0
Lupus anticoagulant	0	0
LE (lupus erythematosus) preparation:		
Method I	0	0
Method II	0	0

Minimal ml required	Note	Method
9-B	Use special anticoagulant (ACD solution)	Beck: J Biol Chem 232:251, 1958
8-B	Use special anticoagulant (ACD solution)	Beutler: Red Cell Metabolism, 2nd ed., 1975, p. 60
		Addison et al.: J Clin Pathol 25:326, 1972
1-S		Waxman, Schreiber: Blood 42:281, 1973
1-S		
1-S		Behring Diagnostic Reagent Kit
5-B	Collect with anticoagulant	Singer: Am J Med 18:633, 1955
5-B	Use oxalate as anticoagulant	Abraham: Hemoglobin 1: 27, 1976
5-B	Collect with anticoagulant	Maile: Laboratory Medicine—Hematology, 2nd ed., 1962, p. 845
5-B	Use heparin as anticoagulant	Michel, Harris: J Lab Clin Med 29:445, 1940
2-S		Hunter et al.: Am J Clin Pathol 20:429, 1950
1-B	Any anticoagulant	Dacie et al.: Br J Haematol 10:388, 1964
4.5-P	Collect as in factor II determination	Boxer et al.: Arthritis Rheum 19:1244, 1976
5-B	Use heparin as anticoagulant	Hargraves et al.: Proc Staff Meet Mayo Clin 24:234, 1949
5-B	Use defibrinated blood	Barnes et al.: J Invest Dermatol 14:397, 1950

Continued.

Hematologic values—cont'd

Determination	Reference range	
	Conventional	**SI**
Leukocyte alkaline phosphatase:		
Qualitative method	Males: 33-188 U	33-188 U
	Females (off contraceptive pill): 30-160 U	30-160 U
Muramidase	Serum, 3-7 μg/ml	3-7 mg/liter
	Urine, 0-2 μg/ml	0-2 mg/liter
Osmotic fragility of erythrocytes	Increased if hemolysis occurs in over 0.5% NaCl; decreased if hemolysis is incomplete in 0.3% NaCl	
Peroxide hemolysis	Less than 10%	0.10
Platelet count	150,000-350,000/mm^3	150-350 × 10^9/liter
Platelet function tests:		
Clot retraction	50-100%/2 hr	0.50-1.00/2 hr
Platelet aggregation	Full response to ADP, epinephrine, and collagen	1.0
Platelet factor 3	33-57 sec	33-57 sec
Reticulocyte count	0.5-2.5% red cells	0.005-0.025
Vitamin B_{12}	205-876 pg/ml	150-674 pmol/liter
Borderline	140-204 pg/ml	102.6-149 pmol/liter

Minimal ml required	Note	Method
20-Isolated blood leuko-cytes	Special handling of blood necessary	Valentine, Beck: J Lab Clin Med 38:39, 1951
Smear-B		Kaplow: Am J Clin Pathol 39:439, 1963
1-S 1-U		Osserman, Lawlor: J Exp Med 124:921, 1966
5-B	Use heparin as anticoagulant	Beutler. In: Williams et al., eds. Hematology, McGraw-Hill, 1972, p. 1375
6-B	Use EDTA as anticoagulant	Gordon et al.: Am J Dis Child 90:669, 1955
0.5-B	Use EDTA as anticoagulant; counts are performed on Clay Adams Ultraflow; when counts are low, results are confirmed by hand counting	(Hand count): Brecher et al.: Am J Clin Pathol 23:15, 1955
4.5-P	Collect as in factor II determination	Benthaus: Thromb Diath Haemorrh 3:311, 1959
18-P	Collect as in factor II determination	Born: Nature 194:927, 1962
4.5-P	Collect as in factor II determination	Rabiner, Hrodek: J Clin Invest 47:901, 1968
0.1-B		Brecher: Am J Clin Pathol 19:895, 1949
12-S		Difco Manual, 9th ed., 1953, p. 221 (modified)

Cerebrospinal fluid values

Determination	Reference range	
	Conventional	**SI**
Bilirubin	0	0
Cell count	0-5 mononuclear cells	
Chloride	120-130 meq/liter	120-130 mmol/liter
Colloidal gold	0000000000-0001222111	Same
Albumin	Mean: 29.5 mg/100 ml ±2 SD: 11-48 mg/100 ml	0.295 g/liter ±2 SD: 0.11-0.48
IgG	Mean: 4.3 mg/100 ml ±2 SD: 0-8.6 mg/100 ml	0.043 g/liter ±2 SD: 0-0.086
Glucose	50-75 mg/100 ml	2.8-4.2 mmol/liter
Pressure (initial)	70-180 mm of water	70-180 arb. unit
Protein:		
Lumbar	15-45 mg/100 ml	0.15-0.45 g/liter
Cisternal	15-25 mg/100 ml	0.15-0.25 g/liter
Ventricular	5-15 mg/100 ml	0.05-0.15 g/liter

Miscellaneous values

Determination	Reference range	
	Conventional	**SI**
Carcinoembryonic antigen (CEA)	0-2.5 ng/ml	0-2.5 μg/liter
Chylous fluid		
Digitoxin	17 ± 6 ng/ml	22 ± 7.8 nmol/liter
Digoxin	1.2 ± 0.4 ng/ml	1.54 ± 0.5 nmol/liter
	1.5 ± 0.4 ng/ml	1.92 ± 0.5 nmol/liter

Minimal ml required	Note	Method
2		See Blood Bilirubin (adapted)
0.5		
0.5		See Blood Chloride
0.1		Wuth, Faupel: Bull Johns Hopkins Hosp 40:297, 1927
2.5		Mancini et al.: Immunochemistry 2:235, 1965
0.5		See Blood Glucose
1		Meulmans: Clin Chim Acta 5:757, 1960
1		
1		

Minimal ml required	Note	Method
20-P	Must be sent on ice	Hansen et al.: J Clin Res 19:143, 1971
	Use fresh specimen	Todd et al.: Clinical Diagnosis, 12th ed., 1953, p. 624
1-S	Medication with digitoxin or digitalis	Smith, Butler, Haber: N Engl J Med 281:1212, 1969
1-S	Medication with digoxin 0.25 mg per day	Smith, Haber: J Clin Invest 49:2377, 1970
1-S	Medication with digoxin 0.5 mg per day	

Continued.

Miscellaneous values—cont'd

Determination	Reference range: Conventional	Reference range: SI
Duodenal drainage		
pH (urine)	5-7	5-7
Gastric analysis	Basal:	
	Females: 2.0 ± 1.8 mEq/hr	0.6 ± 0.5 μmol/sec
	Males: 3.0 ± 2.0 mEq/hr	0.8 ± 0.6 μmol/sec
	Maximal (after histalog or gastrin):	
	Females: 16 ± 5 mEq/hr	4.4 ± 1.4 μmol/sec
	Males: 23 ± 5 mEq/hr	6.4 ± 1.4 μmol/sec
Gastrin-I	0-200 pg/ml	0-95 pmol/liter
Immunologic tests:		
Alpha fetoprotein	Undetectable in normal adults	
Alpha-1-antitrypsin	85-213 mg/100 ml	0.85-2.13 g/liter
Rheumatoid factor	<60 IU/ml	
Antinuclear antibodies	Negative at a 1:8 dilution of serum	
Anti-DNA antibodies	Negative at a 1:10 dilution of serum	
Antibodies to Sm and RNP (ENA)	None detected	
Antibodies to SS-A (Ro) and SS-B (La)	None detected	
Autoantibodies to:		
Thyroid colloid and microsomal antigens	Negative at a 1:10 dilution of serum	

Minimal ml required	Note	Method
	pH should be in proper range with minimal amount of gastric juice	
		Marks: Gastroenterology 41:599, 1961
4-P	Heparinized sample	Dent et al.: Ann Surg 176:360, 1972
2-S		
10-B		Nephelometric assay
10 ml clotted blood	Fasting sample preferred	Nephelometric assay
2-S	Send to laboratory promptly	Immunofluorescence assay
2-S		*Crithidia lucilliae* assay
10 ml clotted blood		Double diffusion
10 ml clotted blood		Double diffusion
2-S	Low titers in some elderly normal women	Doniach, Bottazzo, Drexhage: The autoimmune endocrinopathies. In: Lachmann, Peters, eds. Clinical Aspects of Immunology. Vol. 2. Oxford: Blackwell Scientific, 1982, p. 903

Continued.

Miscellaneous values—cont'd

Determination	Reference range: Conventional	Reference range: SI
Gastric parietal cells	Negative at a 1:20 dilution of serum	
Smooth muscle	Negative at a 1:20 dilution of serum	
Mitochondria	Negative at a 1:20 dilution of serum	
Interstitial cells of the testes	Negative at a 1:10 dilution of serum	
Skeletal muscle	Negative at a 1:60 dilution of serum	
Adrenal gland	Negative at a 1:10 dilution of serum	
Bence Jones protein	No Bence Jones protein detected in a 50-fold concentrate of urine	
Complement, total hemolytic	150-250 U/ml	
Cryoprecipitable proteins	None detected	0 arb. unit
C3	Range, 83-177 mg/100 ml	0.83-1.77 g/liter
C4	Range, 15-45 mg/100 ml	0.15-0.45 g/liter
Factor B	12-30 mg/100 ml	
C1 esterase inhibitor	13.2-24 mg/100 ml	
Hemoglobin A_{1c}	3.8-6.4%	0.038-0.064
Hypersensitivity pneumonitis screen	No antibodies to those antigens assayed	
Immunoglobulins:		
IgG	639-1349 mg/100 ml	6.39-13.49 g/liter
IgA	70-312 mg/100 ml	0.7-3.12 g/liter
IgM	86-352 mg/100 ml	0.86-3.52 g/liter
Viscosity	1.4-1.8 relative viscosity units	

Minimal ml required	Note	Method
2-S		
2-S		
2-S		
2-S		
2-S		
2-S		Doniach et al.: Protocol of Autoimmunity Laboratories. London: Middlesex Medical School
50-U		
10-B	Must be sent on ice	Hook, Muschel: Proc Soc Exp Biol Med 117:292, 1964
10-S	Collect and transport at 37° C	Barr et al.: Ann Intern Med 32:6, 1950 (modified)
2-S		Nephelometric assay
2-S		Nephelometric assay
5 ml clotted blood		Nephelometric assay
5 ml clotted blood		Nephelometric assay
5-P	Send EDTA tube on ice promptly to laboratory	Nathan et al.: Clin Chem 28:512, 1982
5 ml clotted blood		Double diffusion
2-S		
2-S		
2-S		
10-B	Expressed as the relative viscosity of serum compared with water	Barth: Viscosimetry of serum in relation to the serum globulins. In: Sunderman, Sunderman, eds. Serum Proteins and the Dysproteinemias, 1964, p. 102

Continued

Miscellaneous values—cont'd

Determination	Reference range: Conventional	Reference range: SI
Iontophoresis	Children: 0-40 meq sodium/liter	0-40 mmol/liter
	Adults: 0-60 meq sodium/liter	0-60 mmol/liter
Propranolol (includes bioactive 4-OH metabolite)	100-300 ng/ml	386-1158 nmol/liter
Stool fat	Less than 5 g in 24 hr or less than 4% of measured fat intake in 3-day period	<5 g/day
Stool nitrogen	Less than 2 g/day or 10% of urinary nitrogen	<2 g/day
Synovial fluid:		
Glucose	Not less than 20 mg/100 ml lower than simultaneously drawn blood sugar	See Blood Glucose
D-Xylose absorption	5-8 g/5 hr in urine; 40 mg per 100 ml in blood 2 hr after ingestion of 25 g of D-xylose	33-53 mmol/day 2.7 mmol/liter

Minimal ml required	Note	Method
	Value given in terms of sodium	Gibson, Cooke: Pediatrics 23:545, 1959
1-S	Obtain blood sample 4 hr after last dose of beta-blocking agent	M.G.H. method of Rockson, Homcy, Haber: by radioimmunoassay
24-hr or 3-day specimen		Jover et al.: J Lab Clin Med 59:878, 1962
24-hr or 3-day specimen		Peters, Van Slyke: Quantitative Clinical Chemistry, Vol. 2 (Methods), 1932, p. 353
1 ml of fresh fluid	Collect with oxalate-fluoride mixture	See Blood Glucose
5-U 5-B	For directions see Benson et al.: N Engl J Med 256:335, 1957	Roe, Rice: J Biol Chem 173:507, 1948

B

Gastric fluid

Test	Normal value
Fasting residual volume	20-100 ml
pH	<2.0
Basal acid output (BAO)	0-6 mEq/hr
Maximal acid output (MAO) after histamine stimulation	5-40 mEq/hr
BAO/MAO ratio	<0.4

C

Oxygen saturation, oxygen content, and left-to-right shunt

Table I. Normal blood oxygen saturation at various sites in cardiac chambers and great vessels

Site	Oxygen saturation (%)
IVC	80 ± 5
SVC	70 ± 5
RA	70 ± 5
RV	70 ± 5
PA	70 ± 5
LA	96 ± 2
LV	96 ± 2
AO	96 ± 2

Table II. Minimal percentage of oxygen saturation changes between cardiac chambers indicative of left-to-right shunts

	Minimal saturation increase (%)		
	Sets of samples		
Position	1	2	3
SVC-RA	10	7	5
RA-RV	7	5	3
RV-PA	5	3	3

Table III. Normal blood oxygen content at various sites in cardiac chambers and great vessels

Site	Oxygen content (vol%)
IVC	16 ± 1
SVC	14 ± 1
RA	15 ± 1
RV	15.2 ± 1
PA	15.2 ± 1
Arterial	19.1 ± 0.2

Table IV. Maximal normal variation in oxygen content between right heart chambers and the pulmonary artery

Site	Maximal step-up in oxygen content over proximal chamber (vol%)
PA	0.5
RV	0.9
RA	1.9

Table V. Typical blood oxygen contents at various sites with specific left-to-right shunts

	Oxygen content (vol%)		
Site	ASD	VSD	PDA
IVC	16	16	16
SVC	14	14	14
RA	17	14	14
RV	17	17	14
PA	17	17	17
Arterial	19	19	19

IVC, inferior vena cava; *SVC*, superior vena cava; *RA*, right atrium; *RV*, right ventricle; *PA*, pulmonary artery.

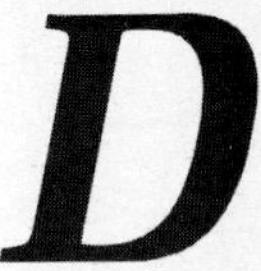

Normal intracardiac and intravascular pressures in adults

Pressures (mm Hg)		
Right atrium (RA)	Mean	0-8
	a Wave	2-10
	v Wave	2-10
Right ventricle (RV)	Systolic	15-30
	End diastolic	0-8
Pulmonary artery (PA)	Systolic	15-30
	Diastolic	5-14
	Mean	10-22
Pulmonary artery wedge (PAW)	Mean	4-12
Left atrium (LA)	Mean	4-12
	a Wave	5-15
	v Wave	5-15
Left ventricle (LV)	Systolic	90-150
	End diastolic	4-12
Aortic (AO)	Systolic	90-150
	Diastolic	60-90
	Mean	70-105

E

Cardiovascular function: derived data

Cardiovascular function tests—formulas

Oxygen (O_2) capacity = Hemoglobin (Hgb) (g/dl) × 1.39 (ml O_2/g Hgb)
O_2 content = O_2 capacity × % saturation

O_2 consumption (basal state estimate)
Arteriovenous oxygen difference (aVO_2 difference) = arterial O_2 content − venous O_2 content
Cardiac output (Fick principle) = O_2 consumption (ml/min)/AVo_2 difference (vol%) × 10
O_2 delivery = Cardiac output × arterial O_2 content × 10
Cardiac index = Cardiac output/body surface area
Stroke volume = End-diastolic volume − end-systolic volume or Cardiac output (ml/min)/heart rate
Stroke index (SI) = Cardiac index (ml/min)/heart rate
LV stroke work index = [SI × (mean arterial pressure − mean PA wedge pressure) × 1.36]/100
Systemic vascular resistance (SVR) = (mean arterial pressure − mean central venous pressure)/cardiac output

Pulmonary vascular resistance (PVR) = (Mean PA pressure − mean PAW or LA pressure)/cardiac output
Total pulmonary resistance (TPR) = mean PA pressure/cardiac output

$$\text{Mitral valve area} = \frac{\text{Mitral valve flow (ml/sec)}}{37.7\sqrt{\text{Diastolic gradient across the mitral valve}}}$$

$$\text{where: Mitral valve flow} = \frac{\text{Cardiac output (ml/min)}}{\text{Diastolic filling period (sec/min)}}$$

Diastolic filling period (sec/min) = diastolic period per beat (sec/beat) × heart rate (beats/min)

From Tilkian, A.G. and Daily, E.K.: Cardiovascular procedures: Diagnostic techniques and therapeutic procedures, St. Louis, 1986, C.V. Mosby Co.

Units	Normal values
vol%	17-23.5 (Hgb 12-17)
vol%	19 ± 1 (arterial) 15.2 ± 1 (mixed venous)
ml/min/m^2	130 ± 10
vol%	4.1 ± 0.6
L/min	6.0 ± 2.0 (varies with body size)
ml/min	1000
L/min/m^2	2.5-4.2
ml/beat	60-130
ml/beat/m^2	30-65
gram − m/m^2	30-100
Hybrid resistance units (HRU) (mm Hg/L/min)	9-20
HRU	0.2-1.5
HRU	1.2-3.5
cm^2	4.0-6.0

Continued.

Cardiovascular function: derived data—cont'd

Cardiovascular function tests—formulas
Diastolic gradient across the mitral valve (mm Hg) = left atrial mean pressure (mm Hg) − left ventricular mean diastolic pressure (mm Hg)
37.7 = Empirical constant
Aortic valve area = $\frac{\text{Aortic valve flow (ml/sec)}}{44.3\sqrt{\text{Systolic pressure gradient across the aortic valve}}}$
where: Aortic valve flow (ml/sec) = $\frac{\text{Cardiac output (ml/min)}}{\text{Systolic ejection period (sec/min)}}$
Systolic ejection period (sec/min) = systolic ejection period per beat (sec/beat) × heart rate (beats/min)
Systolic pressure gradient across the aortic valve (mm Hg) = left ventricular mean systolic pressure (mm Hg) − aortic mean systolic pressure (mm Hg)
44.3 = Empirical constant
Coronary perfusion pressure = arterial diastolic pressure − LVEDP (or mean PAW pressure)
Left ventricular volumes
End systolic volume (ESV)
End diastolic volume (EDV)
Ejection fraction (ESV/EDV × 100)

Units	Normal values
cm^2	2.6-3.5
mm Hg	60-80
ml/m^2	24-36
	70-100
%	58-75

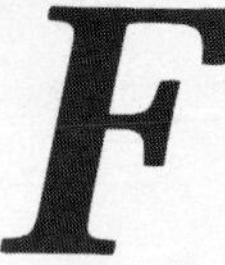

Echocardiographic measurements: normal values

Table F-1 Adult normal values

	Range (cm)	Mean (cm)	Number of subjects
Age (years)	13-54	26	134
Body surface area (m^2)	1.45-2.22	1.8	130
RVD-flat	0.7-2.3	1.5	84
RVD-left lateral	0.9-2.6	1.7	83
LVID-flat	3.7-5.6	4.7	82
LVID-left lateral	3.5-5.7	4.7	81
Posterior LV wall thickness	0.6-1.1	0.9	137
Posterior LV wall amplitude	0.9-1.4	1.2	48
IVS wall thickness	0.6-1.1	0.9	137
Mid IVS amplitude	0.3-0.8	0.5	10
Apical IVS amplitude	0.5-1.2	0.7	38
Left atrial dimension	1.9-4.0	2.9	133
Aortic root dimension	2.0-3.7	2.7	121
Aortic cusps' separation	1.5-2.6	1.9	93
Mean rate of circumferential shortening (Vcf)	1.02-1.94 circ/sec	1.3 circ/sec	38

From Feigenbaum, H.: Echocardiography, ed. 4, Philadelphia, 1985, Lea and Febiger.

Table F-2 Adult normal values, corrected for body surface area

	Range (cm)	Mean (cm)	Number of subjects
RVD/m²—flat	0.4-1.4	0.9	76
RVD/m²—left lateral	0.4-1.4	0.9	79
LVID/m²—flat	2.1-3.2	2.6	77
LVID/m²—left lateral	1.9-3.2	2.6	81
LAD/m²	1.2-2.2	1.6	127
Aortic root/m²	1.2-2.2	1.5	115

Table F-3 Normal values for children, arranged by body surface area

	BSA (m²)	Mean (cm)	Range (cm)	Number of subjects
RVD	0.5 or less	0.8	0.3-1.3	24
	0.6 to 1.0	1.0	0.4-1.8	39
	1.1 to 1.5	1.2	0.7-1.7	29
	over 1.5	1.3	0.8-1.7	11
LVID	0.5 or less	2.4	1.3-3.2	24
	0.6 to 1.0	3.4	2.4-4.2	39
	1.1 to 1.5	4.0	3.3-4.7	29
	over 1.5	4.7	4.2-5.2	11
LV and IV septal wall thickness	0.5 or less	0.5	0.4-0.6	24
	0.6 to 1.0	0.6	0.5-0.7	39
	1.1 to 1.5	0.7	0.6-0.8	29
	over 1.5	0.8	0.7-0.8	11
LA dimension	0.5 or less	1.7	0.7-2.4	24
	0.6 to 1.0	2.1	1.8-2.8	39
	1.1 to 1.5	2.4	2.0-3.0	29
	over 1.5	2.8	2.1-3.7	11
Aortic root	0.5 or less	1.2	0.7-1.5	24
	0.6 to 1.0	1.8	1.4-2.2	39
	1.1 to 1.5	2.2	1.7-2.7	29
	over 1.5	2.4	2.0-2.8	11
Aortic valve opening	0.5 or less	0.8	0.5-1.0	24
	0.6 to 1.0	1.3	0.9-1.6	39
	1.1 to 1.5	1.6	1.3-1.9	29
	over 1.5	1.8	1.5-2.0	11

Table F-4 Normal values for children, arranged by weight

	Weight (lbs)	Mean (cm)	Range (cm)	Number of subjects
RVD	0-25	0.9	0.3-1.5	26
	26-50	1.0	0.4-1.5	26
	51-75	1.1	0.7-1.8	20
	76-100	1.2	0.7-1.6	15
	101-125	1.3	0.8-1.7	11
	126-200	1.3	1.2-1.7	5
LVID	0-25	2.4	1.3-3.2	26
	26-50	3.4	2.4-3.8	26
	51-75	3.8	3.3-4.5	20
	76-100	4.1	3.5-4.7	15
	101-125	4.3	3.7-4.9	11
	126-200	4.9	4.4-5.2	5
LV and IV septal wall thickness	0-25	0.5	0.4-0.6	26
	26-50	0.6	0.5-0.7	26
	51-75	0.7	0.6-0.7	20
	76-100	0.7	0.7-0.8	15
	101-125	0.7	0.7-0.8	11
	126-200	0.8	0.7-0.8	5
LA dimension	0-25	1.7	0.7-2.3	26
	26-50	2.2	1.7-2.7	26
	51-75	2.3	1.9-2.8	20
	76-100	2.4	2.0-3.0	15
	101-125	2.7	2.1-3.0	11
	126-200	2.8	2.1-3.7	5
Aortic root	0-25	1.3	0.7-1.7	26
	26-50	1.7	1.3-2.2	26
	51-75	2.0	1.7-2.3	20
	76-100	2.2	1.9-2.7	15
	101-125	2.3	1.7-2.7	11
	126-200	2.4	2.2-2.8	5
Aortic valve opening	0-25	0.9	0.5-1.2	26
	26-50	1.2	0.9-1.6	26
	51-75	1.4	1.2-1.7	20
	76-100	1.6	1.3-1.9	15
	101-125	1.7	1.4-2.0	11
	126-200	1.8	1.6-2.0	5

Index

Boldface indicates main discussion of test.

B

D

F

Q